PSYCHIATRIC DISORDERS
IN AMERICA

PSYCHIATRIC DISORDERS IN AMERICA

The Epidemiologic Catchment Area Study

EDITED BY

Lee N. Robins, Ph.D., and Darrel A. Regier, M.D., M.P.H.

With Foreword by DANIEL X. FREEDMAN, M.D.

GERALD. A. GROVES, M.D.
654 STATE RD
PRINCETON, NJ 08540
TEL. 609-924-1486

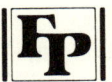

THE FREE PRESS
A Division of Macmillan, Inc.
NEW YORK

Collier Macmillan Canada
TORONTO

Maxwell Macmillan International
NEW YORK   OXFORD   SINGAPORE   SYDNEY

The Free Press
A Division of Macmillan, Inc.
866 Third Avenue, New York, N.Y. 10022

Collier Macmillan Canada, Inc.
1200 Eglinton Avenue East
Suite 200
Don Mills, Ontario M3C 3N1

Printed in the United States of America

printing number
1 2 3 4 5 6 7 8 9 10

Library of Congress Cataloging-in-Publication Data

Psychiatric disorders in America : the epidemiologic
    catchment area study / edited by Lee N. Robins
    and Darrel A. Regier.
        p.   cm.
      ISBN 0-02-926571-1
      1. Psychiatric epidemiology—United States.
    2. Health service areas—United States. [1. Includes
    bibliographical references.] I. Robins, Lee N. II. Regier,
    Darrel A.
      [DNLM: 1. Catchment Area (Health)—
    United States. 2. Mental Disorders—epidemiology—United States.
    WM 100 P9735]
    RC455.2.E64P78   1990
    362.2′ 0422′ 0973—dc20
    DNLM/DLC
    for Library of Congress   90–3168
                                                            CIP

Contents

List of Figures

FIGURE

List of Tables

ix

TABLE

TABLE

TABLE

TABLE

TABLE

TABLE

TABLE

TABLE

TABLE

TABLE

TABLE

TABLE

Foreword

DANIEL X. FREEDMAN, M.D.

Less than a month after President Carter's 1977 inauguration, Rosalynn Carter was authorized to assemble a commission to examine the nation's needs for mental health services and new knowledge about disorders. Sitting with her in a basement office of the White House East Wing as the initial plans were made, one could not mistake Mrs. Carter's clear respect for and interest in sound information. Her questions were unerringly straightforward. How many are suffering from these illnesses, who are they, and how are they treated? Embarrassingly, equally straightforward answers could not be provided. The base of information about the scope and boundaries of mental illnesses was simply inadequate. Fifteen months later her commission had sparked a remarkable decade-long journey to this singular volume.

Psychiatric Disorders in America is an unprecedented atlas that clearly maps a near dozen different mental illnesses, both treated and untreated, with their varying symptoms, severity, and impairments, as they occur across rural and urban America. Individual symptoms and their aggregations that define disorders are described precisely. We can now accurately chart the relative peaks and valleys of disease prevalences against which illnesses studied in any particular hospital or clinic or in any targeted genetic, psychosocial, familial, or therapeutic research can be matched to gain necessary perspective. In brief, to answer the questions of how much and what kinds of illness are "out there" we no longer must blindly grope and guess. Everyone has problems. But not everyone has symptoms, and fewer have a disorder. As a group the various psychiatric disorders appear to have about the same prevalence as hypertension. Significant numbers are at risk for mild to severe impairments, and the studies have already pointed to hitherto undetected or unappreciated risks and dysfunctions.

The appearance and course of any disease entail variations that are difficult to quantify and track. The scope of the natural history of disease, so essential for identifying genetic and cultural factors that determine risk and resistance, is rarely within our grasp. The journey, presaged by the

tentative epidemiological probes of the 1950s and 1960s and enabled by the
objective diagnostic methods pioneered in the early 1970s, has now
brought us a rich lode of new information on the natural history of psychiatric disorders.

In their modern-day voyage of the Beagle, the crew encountered many
obstacles and conflicts and steered around them with the aid of the sophisticated tools and research designs of contemporary epidemiology. With
respect to the entire span of medical diseases, no data base can rival this one
for psychiatric disorders. The sheer size of the study is important; it was
intentionally large enough to permit the detection and tracking of rare as
well as common disorders. The sophisticated research design permits
follow-ups of this data base, and evaluation of change and factors associated
with it and of the effects of health services on frequencies as well. The
design permits "instant replication" of a hypothesis generated in one region, permitting its test across the country. Here then is the soundest
fundamental information about the range and extent and variety of psychiatric disorders ever assembled. In psychiatry, no single volume of the twen-
tieth century has such importance and utility not only for the present but
for the decades ahead.

Preface

The completion of a book containing results from a major collaborative, multisite research project is a time for reflection on the contributions made by literally hundreds of people. From the time of inception and refinement of the concept at the National Institute of Mental Health (NIMH) in 1977, through the completion of data collection from 20,000 people in five sites, data analysis, and finally data presentation, every imaginable scientific, administrative, and political problem has arisen and been addressed. An effort of this magnitude may come along only once in many scientists' lifetime—which, given the amount of energy required, may be a source of solace.

This study has raised the level of epidemiologic and services research in the mental health field far beyond the point to which the efforts of any single individual or research group could have brought it. In the process of carrying out the project, major contributions have been made to the development of assessment instruments for mental and substance abuse disorders that are critical for all clinical research in this field. We now have a data base to define the prevalence of mental disorders, syndromes, and symptoms in this country—matched by a parallel description of how our mental health, general medical, and other human services systems respond to individuals with these disorders. The utility of this data base is enhanced by its placement in the public domain to be used by any interested research investigator. One such application is its current use as an empirical data source to develop refinements in the next generation of offical diagnostic criteria, including the fourth edition of the *Diagnostic and Statistical Manual* (DSM-IV) and the tenth edition of the *International Classification of Diseases* (ICD-10).

As a summary of the research, this book provides our best current estimates and descriptions of psychiatric disorders in America. It includes tabular breakdowns on each disorder by age, sex, and ethnic backgrounds—to facilitate comparison with samples in many other national and international studies that have adopted the instruments and methods developed for this study. We hope that in the following multi-authored chapters you will be able to sense the collegial stimulation and excitement that have characterized this effort to reduce the ignorance surrounding these much stigmatized mental and substance abuse disorders. For despite the often cumbersome nature of so large a project, it has been a privilege for its participants to work together, and it is a joy now to see the fruits of their sustained and well-executed research labors on behalf of the mentally ill.

Special recognition should be given to Rosalynn Carter and the President's Commission on Mental Health, who saw the need for such a study and facilitated its early financial and administrative support. Four NIMH directors and many higher-level U.S. Public Health Service administrators have provided sustained support for this program of research. Many members appointed to NIMH scientific Initial Review Groups reviewed the initial NIMH staff concept and the proposals from the academic community for carrying it out; many journal editors and referees have also provided useful critiques of its publications. All of them have thus made significant contributions to its character and success. Their contributions have "justified" our procedural goal, which has been to ensure transparency of methods and symptom criteria, of their operationalization, and of their assembly into diagnoses. The openness with which each stage of this project has been conducted has enabled it to benefit from the critiques of gifted colleagues along the way.

In a special category are the principal investigators, collaborators, and project officers who guided the implementation of the project for over a decade. Their institutions and names, as contained in the "boilerplate" acknowledgment reproduced below,* are inscribed on each of the over 100 scientific publications that have emanated from this effort. Although these publications and their contributors cannot all be mentioned in this space—and would be instantly out of date in any case because new ones are being added rapidly—a continuously updated listing may be obtained from the Epidemiology and Psychopathology Research Branch, Division of Clinical Research, NIMH, Rm 10C-05, 5600 Fishers Lane, Rockville, MD 20857.

Finally, it is appropriate that we use this occasion to recognize the contribution of Carl A. Taube, who was intimately involved in the conceptualization of the project and served as its project officer from 1978 to 1985. His untimely death this year deprived the nation of an outstanding research scientist, renowned for his work on behalf of the mentally ill in developing the field of mental health services research, and it deprived his colleagues of a highly esteemed friend.

Darrel A. Regier
Lee N. Robins
December 12, 1989

*The ECA is a series of five epidemiological research studies performed by independent research teams in collaboration with staff of the Division of Biometry and Epidemiology—reorganized in 1985 with components now in the Division of Clinical Research and the Division of Biometry and Applied Sciences—of the NIMH, Rockville, MD. The NIMH *Principal Collaborators* are Darrel A. Regier, MD, Ben Z. Locke, MSPH, William W. Eaton (1978–1983), and Jack D. Burke, Jr, MD (1983–); the NIMH *Project Officers* are Carl A. Taube, PhD (1978–1985) and William Huber (1985–). The *Principal Investigators and Co-Investigators* from the five sites are: Yale University, New Haven, Conn, U01 MH34224—Jerome K. Myers, PhD, Myrna M. Weissman, PhD, and Gary L. Tischler MD; Johns Hopkins University, Baltimore, MD, U01 MH33870—Morton Kramer, DSc, Ernest Gruenberg, MD, and Sam Shapiro, MS; Washington University, St. Louis, U01 MH33883—Lee N. Robins, PhD, and John Helzer, MD; Duke University, Durham, NC, U01 MH35386—Linda George, PhD, and Dan Blazer, MD; UCLA, U01 MH35865—Marvin Karno, MD, Richard L. Hough, PhD, Javier I. Escobar, MD, M. Audrey Burnam, PhD, and Dianne M. Timbers, PhD.

Contributors

JAMES C. ANTHONY, Ph.D.
Johns Hopkins Medical Institutions
Department of Mental Hygiene
Baltimore, MD

DAN G. BLAZER, M.D., Ph.D.
Duke University Medical Center
Department of Psychiatry
Durham, NC

RICHARD BOYER, Ph.D.
Psychiatric Research Unit
Montreal, Quebec, Canada

MARTHA LIVINGSTON
  BRUCE, Ph.D.
Yale University School of Medicine
Depression Research Unit
Department of Psychiatry
New Haven, CT

AUDREY BURNAM, Ph.D.
The Rand Corporation
Santa Monica, CA

AMY DRYMAN, Sc.D.
Johns Hopkins Medical Institutions
c/o Department of Mental Hygiene
Baltimore, MD

WILLIAM W. EATON, Ph.D.
Johns Hopkins Medical Institutions
Department of Mental Hygiene
Baltimore, MD

JAVIER ESCOBAR, M.D.
Veterans Administration Medical
  Center
Newington, CT

LOUIS P. FLORIO, M.S.
Yale University School of Medicine
Depression Research Unit
Department of Psychiatry
New Haven, CT

LINDA K. GEORGE, Ph.D.
Duke University Medical Center
Department of Psychiatry
Durham, NC

JACQUELINE M. GOLDING,
  Ph.D.
Western Consortium for Public
  Health
Berkeley, CA

JOHN E. HELZER, M.D.
University of Vermont College of
  Medicine
Department of Psychiatry
Burlington, VT

CHARLES HOLZER, III, Ph.D.
University of Texas
Department of Psychiatry
Galveston, TX

DANA HUGHES, Ph.D.
Duke University Medical Center
Department of Psychiatry
Durham, NC

MARVIN KARNO, M.D.
University of California
Neuropsychiatric Institute
Los Angeles, CA

SAMUEL J. KEITH, M.D.
National Institute of Mental Health
Division of Clinical Research
Rockville, MD

RICHARD LANDERMAN, Ph.D.
Duke University Medical Center
Department of Psychiatry
Durham, NC

PHILIP J. LEAF, Ph.D.
Yale University School of Medicine
Health Policy Research Unit &
  Depression Research Unit
Department of Psychiatry
New Haven, CT

BEN Z. LOCKE, M.S.P.H.
National Institute of Mental Health
Epidemiology and Psychopathology
  Branch
Division of Clinical Research
Bethesda, MD

LAWRENCE T. McEVOY, M.A.
Washington University School of
  Medicine
Department of Psychiatry
St. Louis, MO

JEROME K. MYERS, Ph.D.
Yale University
Department of Sociology
New Haven, CT

THOMAS PRZYBECK, Ph.D.
Washington University School of
  Medicine
Department of Psychiatry
St. Louis, MO

DONALD S. RAE, M.S.
National Institute of Mental Health
Epidemiology and Psychopathology
  Branch
Division of Clinical Research
Rockville, MD

DARREL A. REGIER, M.D.,
  M.P.H.
National Institute of Mental Health
Division of Clinical Research
Rockville, MD

LEE N. ROBINS, Ph.D.
Washington University School of
  Medicine
Department of Psychiatry
St. Louis, MO

MARVIN SWARTZ, M.D.
Duke University Medical Center
Department of Psychiatry
Durham, NC

JAYSON TIPP, M.A.
Washington University School of
  Medicine
Department of Psychiatry
St. Louis, MO

MYRNA M. WEISSMAN, Ph.D.
New York State Psychiatric
  Institute
Department of Clinical
  Genetic Epidemiology
Columbia University
Department of Psychiatry
New York, NY

1 Introduction

DARREL A. REGIER / LEE N. ROBINS

Mental illness is a reality that penetrates the national consciousness in many forms including experiences of one's own or a family member's distress, more detached but nevertheless disconcerting street encounters with the homeless mentally ill, and almost daily news reports of devastation wrought by alcoholism and drug abuse. Mental health practitioners share those images and experiences with the lay public and add their own more extensive and sharper impressions. But even those who work with the mentally ill on a professional clinical basis cannot form an accurate picture of the scope and nature of various symptoms and disorders in our nation or even within our own communities. For such a perspective, we need scientific surveys of large samples of the population that are beyond the limitations of either personal or professional clinical experience.

Thanks to an unprecedented study started by the National Institute of Mental Health (NIMH) over a decade ago, we are now able to present the most comprehensive report ever assembled on the prevalence rates of mental disorders in the United States. This report from the Epidemiologic Catchment Area (ECA) program fills a void that was identified during the late 1970s by the President's Commission on Mental Health (1978) in its comprehensive review of the state of American mental health research and services.

To put the President's Commission in context, it is important to recognize that major advances in the understanding and treatment of mental disorders had been made since the previous national review by the Joint Commission on Mental Illness and Health (1961). Even the definitions of mental disorders such as schizophrenia, depression, anxiety disorders, and substance abuse had changed as diagnostic criteria used for research evolved into the official nomenclature of the American Psychiatric Association, published as the *Diagnostic and Statistical Manual of Mental Disorders, Third Edition* (1980). Before the ECA study, there had been no information on the prevalence of these newly defined disorders in the general population, and none on what proportion of individuals with these disorders received mental health services.

To provide such information, all fields of medicine rely on the research disciplines of epidemiology and health services research. Epidemiological studies are used to define the scope and characteristics of illness as part of a total research, clinical service, and prevention strategy. Such definitions are essential to improve our understanding of the causes of illnesses as well as their clinical course, appropriate treatments, and the community services needed because of them. There are generic objectives of epidemiological studies (Morris, 1964) as well as applications more specific to the field of mental disorders (Regier & Burke, 1989). These scientific objectives formed the framework for the current study.

The first objective of epidemiological studies is a community diagnosis to estimate the rates of illness in a defined population. This estimate provides a baseline for understanding the mix of disorders present and the extent to which untreated cases exist in the population. Basic prevalence rates are important for health planners, who must provide for the types of treatment services that will be needed if currently untreated cases are to be brought into the health care system. Likewise, the rate at which new cases of a disorder appear in the population (the incidence rate) is important to assess. The total number of individuals with a disorder during any period of time is the sum of cases present at the beginning of that period plus new (incident) cases appearing during the period. High rates result both from the occurrence of new cases and the failure of earlier cases to recover.

In 1961, the Joint Commission on Mental Illness and Health drew upon mental hospital census data from the NIMH National Reporting Program and counts of treated persons from such studies as *Social Class and Mental Illness* (Hollingshead & Redlich, 1958) to recommend the Community Mental Health Centers program as a means of decreasing the high rate of institutionalization for patients with mental illness (Redick et al., 1983). In addition, it was hoped that the provision of public mental health outpatient treatment would provide care to the poor, who appeared to have especially high rates of severe mental disorder and institutionalization.

Almost 20 years later, the President's Commission on Mental Health reviewed available epidemiological data as part of its program to assess the scope of mental illness in the population, determine the number served, and identify those who were not being served. Given the recent changes in diagnostic criteria and the absence of prevalence data on specific mental disorders, it was not possible for the NIMH to provide the information on rates of the more severe disorders, likely to be seen in clinical settings, requested by the President's Commission at the level of detail needed (Regier et al., 1978).

Furthermore, the NIMH was unable to complete the full clinical picture of specific disorders. In all branches of medicine, the identification of mild or subclinical conditions provides great potential for early intervention and prevention of the disability associated with the full-blown illness. Information on the full range of clinical conditions existing in the population also makes it possible to identify new syndromes or modify existing criteria to define syndrome subtypes for which more specific effective treatments may be possible. The ECA surveys, designed to fill these knowledge gaps, began in the same year that the DSM-III criteria were published (1980). They remain the only large-scale population-based study that applies these criteria to patients and nonpatients.

After identifying base rates of illness, the ECA study was to identify high-risk subgroups within the population, those with unusually high rates of illness as well as groups with unusually low rates. In addition to providing profiles of individuals at unusually high risk for developing an illness, such a strategy allows testing of causal hypotheses. While it is unlikely that a single cause of mental disorders will be found, just as no single cause explains cancer or heart disease, the eventual aim of epidemiological research is to identify specific components in a causal chain of factors that produce an illness. For those factors that are amenable to change, direct interventions may be designed as a means of reducing rates of illness in a population.

The first step in discovering the causal chain to be interrupted is the demonstration of higher rates of illness in a particular group. The next step, identification of specific causal factors, is more difficult. For example, there is still no consensus regarding the reasons for the higher rate of schizophrenia among lower socioeconomic groups that was demonstrated in the 1930s (Faris & Dunham, 1939). Some view the higher rate as evidence that poor living conditions can provoke mental disorder, perhaps through exposure to poor nutrition, or through toxic or infectious agents affecting fetal development, or through the stress of living in unsafe and crowded neighborhoods. Others speculate that the association between schizophrenia and poverty results from the inability of persons with schizophrenia to work, which leads to downward social mobility. Another theory is that the parents of persons with schizophrenia often themselves had mental disorders that interfered with their performance as breadwinners, and so reared their children in poverty. Similarly, a wide range of hypotheses, including various types of social and psychological environmental exposures and biological variations, have been postulated to explain the higher rates of depression found among females in comparison to males. However, these hypotheses have not yet been scientifically validated.

In keeping with one of the major requests of the President's Commission, the ECA study sought to assess how well the health service delivery system responded to the needs of individuals with these disorders. The rates of attendance in specialty mental health, general medical, and other human services settings were determined at the same time as the diagnostic assessments were made. Thus, the ECA study tells us who seeks help for what disorders. This linkage of epidemiological and health services research makes it possible to identify diagnostic and sociodemographic groups who are least adequately served.

Data from the ECA can provide a baseline against which to measure the effectiveness of new programs of treatment, such as the Depression Awareness Recognition and Treatment (D/ART) program, intended to reduce the prevalence of mood disorders by early identification and treatment just as the National Institutes of Health programs have reduced hypertension in the population (Regier et al., 1988b).

The ECA study provided limited information about changes in rates of disorder over time, since only a single follow-up examination was carried out one year after the initial interview. Nonetheless, a comparison of results for different birth cohorts suggests that changes have occurred. For example, Klerman et al. (1985) have suggested that rates of depression appear to have been rising in Western society. They have postulated that exposure to some unspecified environmental stress associated with modern living conditions has contributed to higher rates of depression in individuals now in their twenties and thirties. Historical differences detected by the ECA or similar studies in the future may help to identify the factors that have contributed to higher or lower rates of depression and other disorders.

The current interest in and study of many of these epidemiological questions is very much rooted in America's wartime and immediate postwar experience. The experience of World War II created considerable public concern about the higher-than-expected prevalence of mental disorder detected at initial screening examinations for military recruits. In addition, the psychiatric casualties of that war were studied by leading American psychiatrists. The identification and treatment of battlefield stress-induced disorders led to a general interest in hypotheses about the role of social stress as a cause of mental disorders in the general population.

As a result of the post–World War II focus on mental health, which stimulated the creation of NIMH, researchers undertook several large-scale community surveys of mental disorder, some of which attempted to test causal social stress hypotheses. These surveys included the Stirling County study of 1,010 subjects (Leighton et al., 1963), the Midtown Manhattan study of 1,660 subjects (Srole et al., 1962), and the Baltimore Morbidity study, which examined 809 persons (Commission on Chronic Illness, 1957).

These studies used sophisticated sampling methods and employed trained interviewers, using highly structured interview protocols. They undertook the measurement of the true prevalence of psychological symptoms, syndromes, and the level of impairment in communities rather than in treatment settings. Psychiatrists reviewed summaries of the interviews conducted to make final determinations regarding the presence of psychopathology. Both the Stirling County and the Midtown Manhattan studies tested associations between measures of social stress, including social disintegration, and higher rates of psychological symptoms, disorders, or disability. The Baltimore study was part of a general medical and mental disorder morbidity survey, which was designed to produce prevalence estimates but not to test etiologic hypotheses.

In the Stirling County study, the lifetime prevalence of any mental disorder defined by the first edition of the *Diagnostic and Statistical Manual* (DSM-I) (American Psychiatric Association, 1952) was 57%, with significant impairment found in 24% of subjects. Current rates were estimated at 90 percent of the lifetime rates. In the Midtown Manhattan study, no specific mental disorders were assessed, but 23% of the respondents were considered to have significant current impairment from psychiatric symptoms. This latter study received considerable, and often skeptical, press coverage at the time for identifying up to 81% of the population as having at least some mild degree of impairment. In contrast, the Baltimore study used a more restrictive definition of psychopathology and found only 11% of the population as qualifying for a current DSM-I psychiatric diagnosis, with less than 2% having moderate-to-severe impairment.

The wide disparity in prevalence rates produced by these studies may have resulted from differences in diagnostic criteria and assessment procedures, rather than from differences between the population groups. They heightened scientific concerns about the absence of clear diagnostic criteria. The importance of agreement on diagnostic criteria was underscored by the finding of substantial differences in the rates at which schizophrenia and depressive illnesses were being diagnosed in the United States and United Kingdom psychiatric hospitals (Kramer, 1969). The U.S./U.K. study of psychiatric diagnosis demonstrated that similar diagnostic rates could be achieved when common diagnostic criteria and a standardized assessment instrument were used (Cooper et al., 1972).

The standardized assessment instrument developed for the U.S./U.K. study, the Present State Examination, was later used in a wide range of epidemiological studies of mental disorder, primarily in Europe. Representative community surveys include those in London (Bebbington et al., 1981); Canberra, Australia (Henderson et al., 1979); Athens, Greece (Mavreas et al., 1986); and Edinburgh, Scotland (Dean, Surtees, & Sashidharian, 1983). One month's current prevalence rates from these studies ranged from 9% to 16%, with a median rate of 11% found in the London study. While this narrowed range of variation was encouraging, it is important to note that this assessment instrument did not diagnose substance abuse, severe cognitive impairment, or any personality disorders. In addition, the total number of subjects from the studies ranged from 157 to 576, numbers too small to provide reliable estimates for most of the specific disorders covered or for total disorder within age/sex groups.

Within the United States, substantial progress was made during the

1970s in the development of specific diagnostic criteria. This began with the development of the St. Louis Criteria (Feighner et al., 1972), followed by the Research Diagnostic Criteria (RDC) (Spitzer, Endicott, & Robins, 1978). The latter criteria were incorporated into a standardized psychiatric interview, the Schedule for Affective Disorders and Schizophrenia (SADS) (Endicott & Spitzer, 1978), used in several large clinical research studies, as well as in the New Haven community study of mental disorders (Weissman, Myers, & Harding, 1978).

An essential element for conducting any epidemiological study is a diagnostic method appropriate for use with the study population. With relatively small samples, it may be possible to use methods and interviews identical to those available in clinical practice settings. However, when large samples are needed to achieve study objectives, clinical methods must be adapted to allow nonclinician interviewers to interview respondents in their homes. Nonclinicians need clear and highly structured interviews because they cannot be expected to explain psychiatric concepts to puzzled respondents or to interpret replies to open-ended questions with respect to their clinical significance. In some mental health epidemiological studies, a two-stage procedure has been used in which the population is initially screened by means of brief symptom questionnaires (Bebbington et al., 1981). Then, more intensive clinical interviews are given to all or most of those with high symptom scores, along with a representative sample of those with low scores. One significant drawback of this method is the inevitable attrition that occurs when multiple interviews are used—a drawback that led the ECA investigators to choose a single-stage examination procedure.

The Stirling County and Midtown Manhattan studies had demonstrated that lay interviewers can reliably collect symptomatic information in large-scale surveys. In addition, the New Haven study had demonstrated the feasibility of using clinical interviewers who were not psychiatrists to collect symptom information with a standardized interview that could be scored to produce specific diagnoses according to well-specified criteria, in this case the Research Diagnostic Criteria. However, at the time of the President's Commission on Mental Health, no interview was available that was suitable for a large scale survey using lay interviewers and could also incorporate the newly developing DSM-III criteria. Hence, it was necessary to develop a new diagnostic instrument that would meet these two criteria and could be scored by a computer to expedite analysis.

NIMH staff coordinated a series of national and international consultations to review available instruments. As a result of these consultations, the NIMH selected the Renard Diagnostic Interview (Helzer et al., 1981) as an instrument written in the style needed for an epidemiological survey of specific disorders. This interview had initially been designed to operationalize the St. Louis (Feighner) criteria. After modification by its developers to assure coverage of DSM-III diagnoses, the revised instrument was designated as the NIMH Diagnostic Interview Schedule (DIS) (Robins et al., 1981b).

Since the ECA study would be a groundbreaking investigation in psychiatric epidemiology, it required the highest possible level of research expertise to develop and modify assessment instruments, to address the complex sampling problems of combining community and institutional populations, and to develop data collection and analysis plans that would assure a high quality and yet affordable research program.

Guided by these requirements, the NIMH staff decided against using a single contractor for a national sample survey, and instead chose a multisite collaborative approach. This accomplished several critical objectives. First, it permitted the issuing of multiple requests for applications, resulting in competitive research applications from many distinguished investigators. Second, the approach took advantge of different investigators' interest in and access to special populations, including blacks, Hispanics, the aged, urban, and rural populations. Third, it allowed the five sites to be treated as replications. If a surprising finding occurred across all sites, this would lay to rest suspicions that it was a chance occurrence caused by some methodological flaw, and greatly strengthen its credibility. Finally, investigators could conduct surveys in areas where they were familiar with local institutions and service availability to facilitate close coordination between their prevalence and service-use assessments.

Since the ECA was to be a multisite study, the protocol was designed for epidemiologic surveys in geographically defined "catchment areas." These catchment areas were to contain population groups of at least 200,000 residents.

NIMH's objective for the ECA study was an estimate of the prevalence of mental disorders in both treated and untreated populations. This would allow estimating prevalence rates of both the severe mental disorders typically found in institutions and the less severe disorders that typify disorders in the community. By not limiting the sample to those in treatment settings, it was also possible to study the factors that might contribute to seeking mental health services in multiple sectors of the "defacto U.S. mental health services system" (Regier et al., 1978).

To determine sample sizes needed for the ECA projects, estimates of the probable prevalence rates of specific disorders were garnered from earlier, more limited studies. Discovering risk factors for disorders as rare as schizophrenia, which occurs in about 1% of the community population, was found to require approximately 3,000 interviews per site. It was also necessary to determine appropriate sampling rates for the institutional population. A survey of the number of beds in local long-term institutions in the St. Louis site indicated that a simple random sample of 3,500 would yield only 50 institutional residents, too few to study in any detail. Therefore, it was decided to sample from institutions at about ten times the rate as from households. Thus, the final requirement was set for samples of 3,000 household residents and 500 institutional residents. This sample size, required to assess prevalence rates of specific disorders and to study institutional as well as household residents, was much larger than that evaluated in any previous epidemiological survey of mental disorders. In fact the three earlier North American surveys in Stirling County, Manhattan, and Baltimore together totaled about 3,500 subjects—the number required in the ECA study from each site.

The study design, along with essential qualifications for applicants, was released by NIMH in the form of a request for contract proposals (RFP). The peer review process was used to select the investigators and also to assess the soundness of the protocol developed by NIMH and the budgetary support needed and to review progress periodically throughout the data collection and data analysis phases of the study. Yale University was the first successful applicant, in September 1978, with a proposal to study New Haven and surrounding communities. Two additional rounds of applications were requested in 1979 and 1980 to reach the full complement of research sites that eventually participated in the study. In 1979, Johns Hopkins and Washington University were selected to study, respectively, areas of Baltimore and St. Louis, and in 1980, Duke University and UCLA were selected to study Durham, North Carolina, and parts of Los Angeles, respectively. Together, personnel at these five sites conducted interviews with about 20,000 respondents. Initially it was hoped that additional sites would be added; this did not happen because of funding limitations.

Such a complex multisite research project required an extensive administrative effort. An NIMH steering committee consisting of Ben Locke, Carl Taube, Jack Burke, Jeffrey Boyd, William Eaton, and Lawrence Kessler, chaired by Darrel Regier, coordinated the overall project. A scientific advisory committee representing the government and the principal investigators for each project met regularly to review and reach consensus on issues of data collection, instruments, analysis, and publication. A methods committee was responsible for assuring the use of comparable sampling and assessment procedures across all five sites, as well as for developing appropriate scoring procedures and computer programs to analyze the mass of data produced. In addition, each site developed its own administrative structure to coordinate interviewer training, data collection, quality control mechanisms, and data analysis. All interviewer trainers participated in a common training program at Washington University, St. Louis, to maximize the comparability of the interviews conducted at the five sites. After data had been collected, entered on a computer tape and cleaned, tapes containing those data common to all sites were submitted to the NIMH for editing, scoring, and consolidation into a single core data tape that was then distributed to all the sites. The results presented in this volume are based on the tape for the first ECA interview. This data tape is also now available for public use through the National Technical Information Service.

CONCLUSION

After more than ten years of sustained effort on the part of ECA investigators, it is now possible to present the most comprehensive report on psychiatric disorders in America ever assembled. The sample size of approximately 20,000 people in five different areas across the country dwarfs those in all prior epidemiological studies directed at the full range of mental disorders. This volume draws together the results from the five sites and projects them from the study sample to represent the entire U.S. population with respect to age, sex, and racial/ethnicity groups.

In the following pages, you will find detailed descriptions of the types of disorders we encountered in the study and descriptions of population groups in which they tend to be concentrated. Offering the first comprehensive presentation of findings from both the community and institutionalized sectors of the general population, we review various characteristics, including age, gender, race/ethnicity, level of education, income, rural or urban residence, and employment status, as they relate to the prevalence of each type of disorder.

We rely throughout on diagnostic criteria in the American Psychiatric Association's *Diagnostic and Statistical Manual, Third Edition* (1980). A modification of those criteria has already been published (*DSM-III-Revised*, 1987). Further changes in diagnostic criteria are anticipated as more information on mental disorder subtypes accumulates and as new syndromes are identified. Accordingly, along with diagnoses according to DSM-III criteria, prevalence rates for specific psychiatric symptoms are included in many of the chapters. These symptoms, along with measures of their clustering in time, their duration, and the disability they produce, are the building blocks of mental disorders. The building blocks are unlikely to change over time, although they will be reassembled in different patterns to create new diagnoses. The availability of data for the prevalence of specific symptoms makes it possible to use results from this study to determine prevalence rates and associated characteristics of newly defined disorders. Thus, the ECA study can be expected to be a prime source of psychiatric epidemiological information for years to come.

By shedding scientific light on mental disorders that have so often been shrouded by shame and stigma, we hope to make possible a more objective and optimistic approach to mental illness. Fear of an illness is increased by our ignorance of its essential characteristics, boundaries, and clinical course. New information relating to each of these issues is provided in this volume. As these data are combined with those generated by synergistic research efforts in molecular genetics, neurosciences, psychopharmacology, and behavioral sciences, we will not only be able to secure more accurate counts of how many people suffer from mental disorders, we will make progress toward being able to intervene more effectively to reduce their suffering.

2 Procedures Used in the Epidemiologic Catchment Area Study

PHILIP J. LEAF / JEROME K. MYERS / LAWRENCE T. McEVOY

The success of the ECA project depends on the application of two procedures: (1) highly structured interviews suitable for administration by lay interviewers that allow the identification of individuals with psychiatric disorders and the recognition of specific psychiatric disorders, and (2) the use of survey sampling procedures that allow the generalization of results to a defined population, such as individuals living in the sample area or in the United States as a whole.

CONDUCTING THE INTERVIEW

The interview designed for the ECA has two standard sections, a diagnostic section, the Diagnostic Interview Schedule (DIS), which assesses the presence or absence of specific diagnoses, and a Health Services Questionnaire, which encompasses questions about the utilization of both general medical facilities and those in the mental health sector. There was also a third section devoted to questions of special interest to the local site. This section will not concern us in the present volume; we only present results based on the two sections that were shared across sites.

DIAGNOSTIC INTERVIEW SCHEDULE

As noted in chapter 1, the ECA took advantage of the acceptance of DSM-III as the standard nomenclature of the United States to devise an interview carefully matched to its criteria. This made it possible to combine

11

responses to its questions according to the algorithms specified in DSM-III to make specific diagnoses. This interview, the DIS, is a fully structured interview schedule developed for use by nonclinicians that employs the same diagnostic criteria used by clinicians (Anthony et al., 1985; Helzer et al., 1985; Robins et al., 1985; Robins et al., 1981a; Robins et al., 1982).

To be used in a large community survey, the DIS had to be written so that it could be administered by individuals without clinical training. Among the most important requirements were questions simple enough to be understood regardless of respondents' educational level; examples meaningful enough to trigger memories or appropriate experiences and symptoms; and questions that did not offend or embarrass respondents. Extensive pretesting was done to achieve these goals, and the evidence that they were met is convincing. Interviewers were given the opportunity to note refusals to answer or failure to understand in some sites; notations of either occurrence were few. Less than 1% of the respondents who agreed to be interviewed initially failed to complete the interview. The great majority enjoyed it and gave evidence of this enjoyment by willingly completing a brief follow-up interview on health services utilization 6 months later and a repeat of the full interview in person 12 months later.

Willingness to answer interview questions is no guarantee, of course, that they are being answered honestly. Unfortunately, there are no clear criteria by which to judge the accuracy of answers. A number of studies related to validity have been carried out by the ECA researchers themselves and by other users of the interview. Among the measures used have been a second DIS given by a psychiatrist; a clinical interview given by a psychiatrist; reliablity of questions in the first interview at the time of the last interview one year later; and prediction of treatment contacts in the year following the interview. All of these measures showed agreement or prediction very much better than chance. Problems in interpreting the meaning of these tests have been intensely discussed in a number of publications (Anthony et al., 1985; Burke, 1986; Dohrenwend, 1989; Helzer et al., 1985; Robins, 1985, 1989).

The DIS does not require the interviewer to make any decisions concerning the existence or nonexistence of a psychiatric disorder. The interviewer reads specific questions and follows positive responses with additional prescribed questions. Each step in the sequence of identifying a psychiatric symptom is fully specified and does not depend upon the judgment of the interviewers.

The DIS utilizes a process similar to that employed by a doctor interviewing a patient and assessing the nature and cause of a problem. First the instrument attempts to identify whether a symptom has been experienced, and next whether it was of clinical significance. Clinical significance is ascertained by asking whether the individual has talked to a health professional about the symptom, has taken medication because of it, or feels that it has interfered substantially with his or her activities.

The interviewer then goes on to determine whether the symptom always had a physical explanation (that is, was caused by a medical illness, an injury, a physical condition—such as pregnancy, or was a side effect of the consumption of alcohol or drugs). It is only after the severity of the symptom has been established and possible physical causes ruled out that it is considered as possibly indicating the existence of a psychiatric disorder. Qualifying symptoms plus other items such as duration and frequency of appearance of symptoms and age of onset required for the diagnosis are evaluated by a computer program to determine whether all diagnostic criteria have been met. It is through the use of this computer program that the reports which follow in this book are made possible.

All the symptom questions are asked of all respondents. There was no skipping out of a section after a few negative answers suggested that the person would not meet diagnostic criteria. This made it possible to study patterns of symptoms even in persons whose problems did not constitute a diagnosable syndrome.

The DIS does not attempt to cover all 122 adult diagnoses in DSM-III. It covers disorders of greatest frequency for which diagnostic criteria are explicit in DSM-III and which can be evaluated on the basis of a personal interview alone (see Table 2–1). Disorders difficult to identify in the absence of a medical history or examination, such as delirium or organic hallucinosis, were omitted. In addition, in the interest of keeping the interviews to a reasonable length, some disorders assessed by the DIS were not covered in all sites. Omitted disorders include postramatic stress syndrome, tobacco use, psychosexual dysfunction, transsexualism, egodystonic homosexuality, bulimia, and pathological gambling. One disorder assessed at all five of the ECA sites, anorexia nervosa, is omitted because the number of cases identified was extremely small.

The DIS allows reporting the prevalence of psychiatric disorders according to different time frames. In this book, the relationship of psychiatric disorder to transient experiences like unemployment, income, or use of treatment services is reported for *active* illnesses, defined as disorders that meet two conditions: (1) criteria have been met at some time in the person's life, and (2) there has been some sign of the disorder within the year before interview. A count of active disorders is useful information for purposes such as the development of annual budgets for the provision of mental health services and looking for possible social consequences of illness. However, because long-lasting disorders are more likely to be active then those of brief duration, association of active disorders with possible predictors of occurrence ("risk factors") is confounded with their association with possible predictors of duration, and the two cannot be teased apart.

TABLE 2–1 Psychiatric Disorders Covered by the Diagnostic Interview
Schedule (DIS)

Affective disorders:
    Major depressive disorder
    Dysthymia
    Bipolar
    Atypical bipolar

Schizophrenia and schizophreniform

Substance use disorders:
    Alcohol abuse or dependence
    Sedative, hypnotic abuse or dependence
    Opioid abuse or dependence
    Amphetamine abuse or dependence
    Cocaine abuse
    Hallucinogen abuse
    Cannabis abuse or dependence

Anxiety disorders:
    Obsessive compulsive
    Agoraphobia
    Social phobia[a]
    Simple phobia
    Panic
    Generalized anxiety[a]
    Post-traumatic stress disorder[b]

Anorexia nervosa[c]

Somatization

Antisocial personality

Tobacco use disorder[b]

Psychosexual dysfunction[b]

Transsexualism[b]

Egodystonic homosexuality[b]

Pathological gambling[b]

Cognitive impairment[d]:
    Severe
    Mild

---

[a]Data from this volume included even though disorder was not assessed at all five ECA sites.

[b]Not included in data presented in this report although data are available at some sites.

[c]Not included in this volume because the low prevalence resulted in few observed cases in the five ECA sites.

[d]Not a DSM-III diagnosis.

"Lifetime" disorders do not have this problem. A disorder is considered as having occurred during the respondent's lifetime if criteria for it have ever been met, whether or not there are recent symptoms of the disorder. Duration has no effect in principle, although we must recognize that longer lasting disorders may be better recalled and thus less subject to reporting error. Because duration is not confounded with occurrence for lifetime disorders, they are preferable when considering relationships with risk factors. In a cross-sectional study like the ECA, however, there are three complications. Because members of the population are of varying ages, they have had different lengths of time in which to develop a disorder. Obviously, young respondents have many years ahead of them in which to develop disorders, and the effect of a risk factor may not yet be revealed. Second, respondents available for interviews do not include those who have died before the date of the survey. Young deaths have been shown to be higher in persons with psychiatric disorder (Tsuang & Woolson, 1978). These two losses mean that lifetime prevalence rates of psychiatric disorder found in a survey are lower than they would be if a cohort was selected at birth and followed to death. A third problem is that except for factors present at birth, such as sex and ethnic group, a cross-sectional study cannot be certain whether a correlate of a lifetime disorder is a potential cause of the disorder or its consequence. If, for example, many alcoholics are bachelors, should this be interpreted to mean that absence of a close, confiding relationship leads to excessive drinking or that alcoholics are perceived as undesirable marriage partners?

While answering such questions in a fully satisfactory fashion requires longitudinal studies, nonetheless a survey of psychiatric disorders in those alive at any given moment suggests many hypotheses about the possible causes and consequences of psychiatric disorders, hypotheses that can be tested later with other designs, as well as generating information needed to estimate need for services.

DIAGNOSTIC ALGORITHMS

DSM-III criteria for diagnoses include both positive criteria and exclusionary criteria. The latter usually stem from the presence of another disorder thought to explain the disorder of interest. Other exclusions are full recovery for schizophrenia and recent bereavement for depressive episodes. Computer programs for the DIS were constructed to allow looking at disorders with or without exclusions. Other options were also provided, such as whether or not to require impairment in functioning for depression, drug abuse, and mania, and whether cognitive impairment is assessed only at the clearly clinically significant level or in a milder form. Because these options exist, it is important to specify exactly the rules being used in presenting prevalence data. In each chapter, the authors give the rules used in that chapter. But there was an overall decision to ignore exclusions by coexisting disorders. The problem with excluding one diagnosis if another disorder is present is that one cannot then learn empirically how much overlap there is between the two. Having dropped these diagnostic exclusions, we are able to present information about the frequency with which disorders co-occur. In addition, an initial investigation showed that there is not always greater overlap between disorders when one is excluded by another according to DSM-III criteria than when there is no exclusion rule (Boyd et al., 1984). Further, the DSM-III exclusion rules are often incomplete, with statements like "Not due to another mental disorder such as— —." A few disorders are listed, but the statement implies that other unspecified disorders also qualify; further, no rules are offered for deciding when one disorder is "due to" another.

SELECTING SAMPLES

The ECA funded investigators at five sites to estimate the prevalence of psychiatric disorder by interviewing samples of residents in selected mental health catchment areas, whether they resided in households or institutions (see chapter 1). In all cases, investigators elected to survey areas that were near the universities in which they worked, because they were well informed about local institutions and their university affiliation helped them to get cooperation from both potential research subjects and local institutions. These sites taken together are, of course, not necessarily representative of the country as a whole.

Institutional residents were expected to account for a disproportionate share of those with psychiatric disorders. Prisons were expected to provide cases of substance abuse and antisocial personality, nursing homes to provide many cases of dementia, and psychiatric hospitals to provide a variety of the more severe psychiatric disorders.

As explained in chapter 1, because a very small proportion of the total population is institutionalized, even a very large study like the ECA would provide too few institutionalized cases to compare disorders by type of institution unless institutions were sampled more heavily than households. Therefore it was decided to use a sampling fraction for institutions about ten times that for households. Thus, applicants were asked to propose a design that would yield 3,000 household members and 500 institutional residents.

The only location requirement by NIMH was that the boundaries of the sampled areas coincide with official Mental Health Catchment areas and that they contain a minimum population size to avoid oversaturating the area with interviews. The proposals were also to include a plan to reinterview respondents twice, after six and twelve months.

To make results from the five sites as good an estimate for the whole United States as possible, this report has weighted the respondents so that their age, gender, and racial structure is the same as that found in the whole of the U.S. in 1980. These adjustments were found to make surprisingly little difference in estimates of mental disorder. Although there was no effort at representing the nation, the five sites taken together have demographic distributions much like the country as a whole.

Nonetheless there are some limitations that should be noted. None of the sites included many Asian-American or American Indian respondents. As a result there were too few to study either ethnic group separately, and in analyses, they are combined with whites. There is a substantial Hispanic sample, but because most of these reside in Los Angeles, they are largely of Mexican heritage; Cubans and Puerto Ricans are underrepresented. Blacks came predominantly from areas to which they had migrated from the rural and urban south, and consequently, blacks of West Indian origin are few.

The five ECA sites differ considerably in size and characteristics of their residents (see Table 2–2).

New Haven. The New Haven ECA corresponded with the service area for the Connecticut Mental Health Center in 1980, and approximates the New Haven–West Haven Standard Metropolitan Area, as defined by the census. It consists of 13 towns with a population of 420,021 in 1980. The city of New Haven contains approximately one-third of the population of the area, with the remaining area primarily urban (three smaller cities) and suburban. The smallest town, Bethany, contained only 4,330 residents in 1980. Only a very small segment of this catchment area could be considered rural in character and even this is relatively close to an urban area. Almost one-third of the population of the city of New Haven is black, while none of the other 12 towns was more than 9.2% black. Hispanics (primarily Puerto Rican in origin) made up 2.0% of the adults in the catchment area.

Eastern Baltimore. The Eastern Baltimore ECA conformed to the Eastern Health District of the city of Baltimore. This area consisted of approximately one-third of the city of Baltimore and included the catchment areas of three mental health centers, Johns Hopkins Hospital, Baltimore City Hospital, and Harbel Mental Health Center. Included in the area were government offices, an inner city component inhabited primarily by blacks, and an area of the city adjacent to the county consisting of detached houses. Approximately one-third of the catchment area was black. The population in 1980 was 268,000.

St. Louis. The St. Louis ECA consisted of three areas of the Eastern Missouri Mental Health District. These areas were not contiguous; they were selected for their socioeconomic dispersion and because together their populations had much the same demographic and socioeconomic

TABLE 2–2 Overview of ECA Sites

Characteristic[a]	New Haven	Baltimore	St. Louis	Durham	Los Angeles
Area (square miles)	300	50	1,600	2,002	35
Total households	150,371	93,000	141,460	101,895	128,706
Total population	420,021	268,000	401,264	269,863	335,941
Population 18+	300,110	175,206	279,907	196,790	245,855
Age 18-64	248,833	143,999	235,643	166,542	215,640
Age 65+	51,227	31,207	44,264	30,248	30,215
Percent 65+	12.1	11.6	11.0	11.2	9.0
Ethnicity percent:					
White (and other)	87.8	65.0	80.3	63.0	52.1
Black	10.2	34.3	19.0	36.4	4.5
Hispanic	2.0	0.8	0.7	0.5	43.3
Percent institutional[b]	3.4	2.3	1.6	2.0	2.2
Data collection period	7/80–7/81	1/81–11/81	4/81–3/82	6/82–5/83	1/83–8/84
Response rate in community survey	77%	78%	79%	79%	68%

[a]Data from *U.S. Census of Population* (1980).
[b]Census definition of institutional not exactly comparable to criteria used in the ECA project.

characteristics as the state of Missouri and the United States, except for a higher proportion of blacks (19% versus 10.4% for the U.S.). One segment of the ECA was in the city of St. Louis and was the most disadvantaged catchment area in the state. A second segment was a section of northeastern St. Louis County bordering on the city of St. Louis. The third segment was a three-county area, St. Charles, Lincoln, and Warren counties, containing suburban communities, small towns, and rural areas. The 1980 population of this ECA was 401,264.

Durham. The Durham ECA consisted of five counties in North Carolina: Durham, Vance, Franklin, Granville, and Warren. In 1980, this catchment area had a population of 269,863. The catchment area consisted of a diverse population including some of the poorest communities in the study as well as a substantial number of individuals working in major research institutions in the Research Triangle Area. Durham County was primarily urban, but much of the remainder of the catchment area was rural. One of the counties, Warren, had a black majority, and almost one-third of the population of this county lived below the poverty level. One of the counties was one of the fastest growing communities in the country. The Durham

ECA site contained the largest percentage of blacks (36%) of the five ECA sites.

Los Angeles. Los Angeles was the largest city in the ECA, and only a small part of the city was selected for survey. The selected sections were two noncontiguous areas served by different mental health centers. One area, 83% Hispanic, included East Los Angeles, Montebello, and part of Pico Rivera. The second segment of the ECA, primarily white, consisted of Culver City, Venice, Mar Vista, Marina del Rey, Fox Hills, Ladera Heights, Windsor Hills, and part of West Los Angeles. The 1980 population of the selected areas was 335,941.

SAMPLING COMMUNITY POPULATIONS

Each of the five research teams faced the task of obtaining a sample that was representative of the individuals living in the catchment areas selected in a cost effective manner (Holzer et al., 1985). Several of the teams also wanted to ensure that they interviewed enough members of specific sub-populations such as the elderly, blacks, or Hispanics to be able to estimate their rates of mental disorder. Therefore, in Los Angeles a predominantly Hispanic catchment area was selected, and in St. Louis, blacks were over-sampled by stratifying blocks by estimated racial mix. The New Haven, Baltimore, and Durham sites all developed procedures for oversampling elderly individuals, those over 65 in New Haven and Baltimore, and those over 60 in Durham. Because oversampling of some groups meant respondents varied in their probability of being selected for interview, responses had to be weighted to make them representative of the resident populations. These procedures will be described.

COMMUNITY RESPONDENTS

Each individual residing in a selected catchment area had a known probability of being invited for interview. In simple random samples, all individuals have the *same* probability of selection, but this was not the case in the ECA study. Since these procedures used in the selection of the ECA samples have been described in detail elsewhere (Holzer et al., 1985; Leaf et al., 1985a), we will present only a brief overview of the strategies used. Traditionally, census data are used to select blocks for sampling. However, this was not feasible for the first two sites because sampling had to be done before 1980 census data became available and when 1970 data were grossly out of date.

The household sample in New Haven was drawn primarily from listings obtained from three electrical utility companies. This list was augmented by using the city directory to identify households in public and other apartment complexes whose households would not be individual customers of the utility companies. Commercial and vacant units were eliminated during the field operations. Households were sampled in clusters of eight using a random start. Two of these eight units were included in the general survey and the six remaining units were included only if they contained at least one individual age 65 or older (who constituted the elderly oversample).

The Baltimore ECA used the Real Property File of the Baltimore Department of Planning, a file containing a list of all physical structures in the city and the number of housing units contained in each structure. Blocks were selected at random, based on the expected number of households. Next, all blocks selected were reenumerated to include buildings erected since the Real Property File was created and eliminate those torn down or vacant.

The St. Louis site had access to preliminary 1980 census listings for enumeration districts, which provided number of households but no information about the racial distribution. These census data were augmented by using vital statistics data on births by race and interviewers' estimates of proportions black by block, based on visual survey. Standard sampling procedures were used to select blocks, and households within blocks, with an oversampling of blocks predicted to contain black residents.

The procedures used in Durham were similar to those used in St. Louis with the exception that, by then, 1980 census data allowed stratification by racial composition and poverty status. Both St. Louis and Durham had to use enumeration districts in the rural areas for sampling purposes since rural areas are not composed of city blocks.

The Los Angeles ECA selected sample blocks based on 1980 census data with dwellings in the selected blocks reenumerated prior to sampling households.

Using the enumeration procedures described above, each research team selected a random sample of households sufficient to obtain 3,000 to 5,000 respondents after loss by refusal or failure to contact.

Eligibility of Respondents. All individuals age 18 and older residing in the selected five catchment areas were eligible for the study. Members of dwelling units within the catchment area were eligible even though they might be traveling, in an acute general hospital, or away at school when the residents of the household were enumerated. Institutions located both inside and outside catchment areas borders could provide catchment area residents. Institutions serving catchment area residents were surveyed to decide which of their residents qualified as residents of the area, and so were eligible as respondents.

A very small proportion of individuals living in the ECA sites are missing from the study, those with no usual household. Group quarters, such as communes, convents, and residential hotels, were eligible for survey, but not transient facilities such as commercial hotels and temporary shelters, even though persons in these facilities may have had no more permanent address. It is likely that including the homeless would have had only a small impact on results because they constituted a small part of the overall population, although recent studies show them to be growing in size and to have a high rate of psychiatric disorder (Institute of Medicine, 1988).

SELECTION OF HOUSEHOLD RESPONDENTS

From each household selected using the survey procedures outlined above, one individual was selected to be asked to respond to the survey. All the sites used the same general procedures for selection of a single respondent within a household, except in the process of oversampling the elderly. In the Baltimore site all persons in a household over 65 were interviewed, while in New Haven and Durham, extra households were selected in which only elderly residents were eligible for interview.

In each household, all the residents ages 18 and over were first enumerated and a list of the residents was made, sorted by sex and age. Procedures described by Kish (1965) selected one individual from that list at random, so that the probability of choosing was inversely proportional to the size of the household.

SAMPLING INSTITUTIONAL RESIDENTS

The combining of residents in households with those residing in institutions heralds a new era in psychiatric epidemiology, and thus there are no established methods for generating institutional samples. Furthermore, 1980 census data on institutions were not yet available at the time these samples were drawn.

The ECA teams jointly developed methods for sampling individuals living in institutions based on three components: location of the institution, last community address of the resident, and the length of time since an individual resided in a household (Leaf et al., 1985a). If an individual had been residing continuously for more than one year in institutions, his or her address was considered to be that of the current institution of residence. These long-stay subjects, therefore, were residents of the ECA area if their institution was within its boundaries. Individuals residing in institutions for less than one year prior to the time of the survey were considered to have the address from which they entered the institution. They were eligible for inclusion in the sample if their last community residence was within the catchment area, whether the institution was inside or outside its boundaries.

The one-year residency criterion was selected to allow individuals to maintain a community residence despite a limited period in a nursing home or prison outside of the catchment area. But a longer period was not desirable because the character of neighborhoods change over time, and eventually those who left them for institutions ceased to be representative of their current residents.

Procedures used to identify and survey individuals living in institutions varied from site to site. Where the catchment areas covered large independent communities, as in New Haven and Durham, a large proportion of the institutionalized residents lived in institutions physically within the geographic boundaries of the ECAs. Where the catchment areas were parts of the metropolitan areas, the probability that residents would be institutionalized outside of the catchment area increased. The size and the location of the catchment areas also influenced the types of institutions to be surveyed.

Table 2–3 presents the number of interviews collected at each site listed by type of institution. In New Haven, the sampling procedures differed by type of institution. Twenty-one nursing homes were selected at random within the New Haven catchment area and six residents chosen from each.

TABLE 2–3 Institutional Residents by Site[a]

	New Haven N	Baltimore N	St. Louis N	Durham N	Los Angeles N	Total N
Residence:						
Household	4,872	3,227	2,956	3,801	2,947	17,803
Nursing home[b]	37	146	115	138	107	543
Prison[c]	97	153	115	119	192	676
Psychiatric hospital	54	34	14	43	15	160
Total	5,060	3,560	3,200	4,101	3,261	19,182

Note. All numbers exclude individuals with missing information on race or age.
[a]Includes only in-person interviews conducted during the first wave of the ECA project.
[b]Includes chronic hospitals.
[c]Includes residential alcohol and drug treatment settings, since many in such settings are referred from prison or are offered residential treatment as an alternative to incarceration.

Administrators in three homes denied investigators access. Four psychiatric facilities were included in the survey, two state hospitals, a Veterans Administration hospital, and a private psychiatric hospital. In each, 50% of eligible residents were randomly selected. In the State's correctional facilities, a one in six sample of eligible residents was obtained.

The Baltimore ECA used the same three sampling strata: mental hospitals; nursing, convalescent, and rest homes; and state-operated correctional facilities. Only 7 nursing homes were located within the ECA, while an additional 21 nursing homes located outside the ECA contained ECA residents. One of these homes refused to participate in the study. In the 27 participating nursing homes, all eligible residents with lengths of stay of less than one year were included in the survey. In the seven facilities located inside the ECA, one-third of the residents eligible because they had been there more than one year were included in the survey. Four mental hospitals were surveyed, including a state mental hospital, two private psychiatric hospitals, and a short-term mental health facility serving as the admission unit for the state mental health hospital. The central filing system of the Maryland State Division of Corrections was accessed to identify residents of the catchment area in prison. However, because the state penitentiary was located within the catchment area boundaries, the large number of prisoners serving sentences of more than one year would all have been eligible for inclusion. It was decided not to interview any of these long-term prisoners because of the difficulty of interpreting data from these respondents in the context of prevalence rates and risk factors. Fifty percent of the male prisoners and all the female prisoners who were eligible for inclusion on the basis of incarceration of less than one year and prior residence in the catchment area were selected.

In St. Louis, the sampling frame consisted of 93 long-term institutions in a 5 county region including 64 nursing or boarding homes, 4 jails, 10 state prisons, 3 chronic hospitals, 5 mental hospitals, 5 residential treatment centers for alcohol or drugs, the State School and Hospital for the mentally retarded, and one halfway house. A list of individuals within each institution was developed. Segments of size eight were selected from this list using a random start. Residents in nursing homes, chronic hospitals, and the State School and Hospital were selected at one-fourth the rate of residents in other institutions to reduce the number of respondents too ill to be personally interviewed.

In the Durham ECA project, all eligible institutions in the catchment area were included in the study with the exception of two nursing homes that refused access to their residents. Interviews were obtained from residents in 5 psychiatric facilities, 25 long-term care facilities, 2 halfway houses from the nursing home stratum, and 10 correctional facilities. The federal prison located within the catchment area was excluded from the study because this facility is used for psychiatric testing of federal prisoners suspected of having psychiatric disorders. Its inclusion would have led to an overestimate of the prevalence of psychiatric disorder among prisoners. In Durham, individuals who had entered an institution less than 30 days before enumeration were declared ineligible because many of them had been household residents during the earlier phase of the study and had already had an opportunity for selection. Residents were not sampled from institutions directly in proportion to size since there was an interest in making between facility comparisons.

Interviewing institutional residents presented a particular problem for the Los Angeles ECA project because of the city's large size. In order to identify institutions in which catchment area residents might be found, a survey was first conducted of all psychiatric hospitals and psychiatric wards in Los Angeles County and a one-sixth sample of nursing homes, board and care group homes, and substance abuse units in the county. This survey was used to identify facilities that included more than one resident of the Los Angeles ECA. A list was developed of institutions predicted to contain residents, and clusters of institutions were selected from the list. Prisons surveyed were limited to those in the southern part of the state, and thus relatively near Los Angeles.

The varying patterns of selection reflected differences in the kinds of facilities in each area and the extent to which each site was a self-contained geographical unit. Through these varying methods, each site managed to randomly select catchment area residents who were institutionalized in state-operated correctional facilities, nursing homes and board and care homes, and psychiatric hospitals according to common definitions.

WEIGHTING THE DATA

In selecting its sample, each of the ECA sites had adopted a method that gave each resident of the catchment area a known probability of selection, but none had used a simple random sample. This was a consequence of the need to interview efficiently (in geographic clusters), to guard against effects of within household similarities by selecting only one individual per household, and to get sufficient representation of groups of special interest, the aged, blacks, and the institutionalized. It was necessary, therefore, to adjust variance estimates to account for these deviations from selecting a simple random sample. These *selection biases* were corrected for by *weights* inversely proportional to the respondent's relative chance of selection.

A second problem in every site was that some households were not enumerated and so no respondent was identified, and in some where enumeration took place, the selected respondent could not be contacted or refused to be interviewed. Errors due to failure to complete an interview were overcome by a second weight multiplied by the selection bias weight to make the interviewed sample equivalent to census figures for that area with respect to age, sex, and ethnicity. Because failure to interview was not very biased by age, sex, or ethnicity, this weight had little effect on results.

These two weights made the ECA samples representative of the population of the catchment areas from which the samples were selected. However, in this volume we are interested in generalizing to the United States rather than to these specific ECA sites. We accomplish this task by a third weight, which adjusts the sample to the age, sex, and racial distribution of the whole United States as of 1980.

By weighting the total sample to give it the characteristics of the nation as a whole in terms of 36 age-sex-ethnic categories (with 2 sexes; 6 age brackets; 18–24, 25–34, 35–44; 45–54, 55–64; 65 +; and 3 ethnic groups: black, Hispanic and others), we attempt to generalize from these 5 areas to the nation. This weight, like our second weight, actually made very little difference in our prevalence estimates because the 5 sites together had much the same age and sex characteristics as the nation, and ethnicity, as we shall see, was not a very powerful correlate of psychiatric morbidity.

For a few of our estimates, we have had to exclude information on respondents from one or two sites because of minor differences that crept into our supposedly identical interviews. Further, proxy interviews (conducted in a small number of cases where the designated respondent was too ill for interview) were not used at all sites, and where used, diagnoses often could not be made because the informants had insufficient information about the symptoms and problems. In this volume, diagnostic information is restricted to that collected by personal interview. A diagnosis is assessed only if a respondent answered at least two-thirds of the symptom questions pertaining to it. In a few cases, it became clear to the interviewer early in the interview that a respondent was not capable of answering the questions. In such a case, the interviewer went directly to the section assessing cognitive impairment, which consisted of the Mini-Mental State Exam (Folstein, Folstein, & McHugh, 1975). If the respondent could not pass the Mini-Mental State Examination, the interview with the respondent was terminated, with assessment completed for only one diagnosis, cognitive impairment. In some sites, a collateral informant was interviewed to complete the assessment. In this volume, however, only diagnoses obtained from interviews with the original respondent are reported.

Table 2–4 presents the age, sex, and racial/ethnic characteristics of each ECA site and of the nation. Under each site the actual number of interviews collected is shown as well as the percentage of each catchment area with a specific characteristic. The second to last column shows the number of unweighted cases available for analysis for each age/sex/race and site category when all five sites are taken together, and the final column shows the percentage each of those sex/age/ethnic groups constitutes of the nation's adult population.

If we use the rule of thumb that no results should be reported based on

TABLE 2–4 Demographic Characteristics of the ECA Sample: Actual Number of Interviews and Weighted Percent[a]

	New Haven		Baltimore		St. Louis		Durham		Los Angeles		Total U.S.	
	N	%	N	%	N	%	N	%	N	%	N	%
White and Others												
Men												
18–29	320	11.6	245	8.6	276	11.6	240	9.0	259	8.0	1,340	12.6
30–44	338	10.8	203	6.9	219	10.2	267	8.8	256	6.9	1,283	10.9
45–64	312	12.6	227	9.7	225	11.2	311	8.5	163	7.2	1,238	11.4
65+	917	5.9	262	5.0	158	5.1	256	3.5	103	3.2	1,696	5.4
Women												
18–29	358	12.0	272	9.1	285	11.6	240	9.1	208	7.1	1,363	12.4
30–44	403	11.5	250	6.8	239	11.0	274	8.5	297	7.6	1,463	11.3
45–64	404	14.5	352	11.3	285	11.7	423	9.5	175	7.6	1,639	12.4
65+	1,440	8.9	444	7.7	277	7.9	576	6.2	185	4.6	2,922	7.8
Black												
Men												
18–29	90	1.6	223	6.2	158	3.0	159	5.8	33	0.9	663	1.8
30–44	53	1.5	124	3.9	135	2.9	142	4.2	30	0.7	484	1.4
45–64	36	1.1	72	3.4	77	1.7	137	3.8	11	0.4	333	1.1
65+	44	0.3	68	1.4	84	0.7	157	1.9	3	0.1	356	0.5
Women												
18–29	82	2.2	294	7.8	235	4.0	167	7.0	21	0.7	799	2.0
30–44	62	1.8	234	5.5	255	3.4	213	5.4	36	0.8	800	1.6
45–64	51	1.3	168	4.5	150	2.2	236	5.3	16	0.7	621	1.4
65+	70	0.5	96	1.7	123	1.2	286	3.1	7	0.2	582	0.7
Hispanic												
Men												
18–29	28	0.6	4	0.1	5	0.3	5	0.2	299	9.0	341	1.2
30–44	10	0.3	4	0.1	2	0.0	4	0.1	260	6.0	280	0.8
45–64	5	0.2	2	0.1	4	0.0	2	0.0	124	4.7	137	0.6
65+	3	0.02	2	0.0	0	0.0	0	0.0	55	1.5	60	0.2
Women												
18–29	18	0.5	1	0.02	1	0.1	3	0.1	251	8.4	274	1.1
30–44	8	0.2	5	0.2	1	0.01	2	0.1	233	6.3	249	0.9
45–64	4	0.2	5	0.2	4	0.2	0	0.0	139	5.1	152	0.6
65+	4	0.03	3	0.1	2	0.04	1	0.0	97	2.4	107	0.2
Total	5,060		3,560		3,200		4,101		3,261		19,182	

[a]Total weighted to U.S. population. Site data weighted to population in catchment areas sampled at each site.

fewer than 30 individuals, we noted the following limitations: we cannot report on black males or females over 45 in Los Angeles or on Hispanics of any specific age sex group *outside* of Los Angeles. However, when sites are combined, no very small cells remain, although results for older Hispanics may be unstable. This "rule of 30" will be used throughout the volume to avoid emphasizing findings based on few cases.

TABLE 2-5 Summary of Age, Race, and Sex Distributions by Site[a]

	New Haven N	New Haven %	Baltimore N	Baltimore %	St. Louis N	St. Louis %	Durham N	Durham %	Los Angeles N	Los Angeles %	Total U.S. N	Total U.S. %
White	4,492	87.8	2,255	65.0	1,964	80.3	2,587	63.0	1,646	50.5	12,944	84.1
Black	488	10.2	1,279	34.3	1,217	19.0	1,497	36.4	157	4.8	4,638	10.4
Hispanic	80	2.0	26	0.8	19	0.7	17	0.5	1,458	44.7	1,600	5.5
Men	2,156	46.5	1,436	45.4	1,343	46.7	1,680	45.8	1,596	48.5	8,211	47.7
Women	2,904	53.5	2,124	54.6	1,857	53.3	2,421	54.2	1,665	51.5	10,971	52.3
18–29	896	28.5	1,039	31.8	960	30.6	814	31.2	1,071	33.9	4,780	31.0
30–44	874	26.1	820	23.5	851	27.5	902	27.0	1,112	28.4	4,559	26.8
45–64	812	29.9	826	29.1	745	26.9	1,109	27.1	628	25.7	4,120	27.5
65+	2,478	15.6	875	15.7	644	14.9	1,276	14.7	450	12.0	5,723	14.7
Total	5,060		3,560		3,200		4,101		3,261		19,182	

Note. All numbers exclude individuals with missing information on race or age.
[a]Weighted to population in catchment areas sampled at each site.

The need for the weighting procedures can be seen clearly in the summary data in Table 2-5. Because of the deliberate oversampling of the elderly and blacks mentioned above, the unweighted percent of respondents aged 65 and older (which can be calculated from the last column labeled "N") greatly exceeds their percentage after weighting to their proportion in the country as a whole (5,723/19,182 or 30% unweighted vs 15% after weighting) and the unweighted percent of blacks (4,638/19,182 or 24%) exceeds their weighted percent (10.4%). The selection of a heavily Hispanic catchment area in Los Angeles has also resulted in a larger proportion Hispanic in our sample than in the country as a whole (8.3% versus 5.5%).

CONDUCTING STATISTICAL ANALYSES

Weighted data constitute a problem for estimating whether two samples differ. Standard statistics to test significance of difference assume the data come from simple random samples. The weighting procedures that we described and the clustering procedures used in the selection of respondents violate this assumption. Weighted and clustered samples have larger variances than do simple random samples. Without adjusting for this, the precision of estimates is exaggerated, and differences can appear statistically significant when they are not.

In previous reports of the ECA projects, we have used a variety of procedures to compensate for weighting and clustering when conducting statistical analyses: Taylor series linearization, balanced repeated replication, and jackknife repeated replication. These procedures all produce similar results but all are costly to implement. In addition, they cannot be used to test differences that include relatively small subsamples, such as Hispanics or prison inmates.

The statistical adjustment we shall use to compensate for our weighted sample was developed by Max Woodbury at Duke University. It downweights the sample to the size of a simple random sample with the same variance. One can then use standard tests of significance. We have tested its results against the three more complex methods used previously and find it comparable and, if anything, somewhat more conservative.

The formula for calculating the reduced sample size is $\Sigma W_s / \Sigma W_s^2$ where W_s equals the poststratification weights developed to multiply each individual's scores proportionate to the frequency of his or her age/sex/ethnic category in the total population. We calculated this adjusted weight for each respondent. The effect of the correction is to reduce the 19,182 persons actually interviewed to the equivalent of 9,239 selected as a simple random sample. Ordinary t-tests can then be used to detect significance of differences for this downweighted sample. Although this procedure does not specifically address deviations from simple random sampling introduced by clustering, its use produces results that tend to overcompensate rather than undercompensate for artifacts produced by stratification. Given the large samples used in this study, the resulting conservative estimate of statistical significance exempts from discussions small differences that may in fact be statistically significant but are too small to have substantive interest. Because the correction is a constant applied to each respondent's weighted values, it has no effect on estimates of prevalences or their relationships, but affects only tests of statistical significance.

Throughout the volume, results presented are statistically significant for two-tailed tests at $p < .01$ using the Woodbury downweight, unless specifically stated otherwise. This conservative level was chosen because of the large sample size that, even after applying the downweight, produced statistical significance for clinically trivial differences. When discussing smaller subpopulations, however, less stringent p values appear appropriate, and are discussed in the text.

DESCRIBING THE CORRELATES
OF PSYCHIATRIC DISORDER

So far we have described how data concerning the existence of specific psychiatric disorders over the lifetime and over the last year are collected and scored, the selection of the sample to which these procedures were applied, how we extrapolated results found in the sample to the nation, and the procedures used to compare differences between prevalences in different groups. In addition to describing the prevalence of specific disorders, the following chapters assess their course, their co-occurrence, and their correlates. We now describe the correlates available in the ECA. The correlates presented are demographic variables, treatment experiences, and other disorders.

Demographic correlates that are determined at birth may well be indicators of factors that directly contribute causally to disorders because they clearly precede the occurrence of the disorder. Such factors are sex, ethnicity, and age at time of interview. Another possible causal factor is final educational level, because education typically ends before many, but not all, disorders begin. The following chapters will relate these early variables to occurrence of disorder ever in the respondent's lifetime.

Other correlates of disorder describe the respondent's life situation as of the time of interview. For example, at interview respondents may or may not be employed, married, institutionalized, or living in a rural area. Because these statuses may be of long duration or a recent change, we cannot be sure whether they began before or after onset of the disorder with which they are associated, and thus whether they are more likely to be its cause, its consequence, or perhaps only a correlate of the disorder. We can best relate such variables to active disorders since at least they occupy the same time span—close to the time of interview.

Use of mental health services (including treatment for alcohol and drug abuse) was assessed over the prior year for inpatient care and over the prior six months for outpatient mental health services received from mental health specialists, general medical physicians, psychologists, and social workers. Because the treatment was recent, it should be most closely associated with active disorders, and so treatment is presented as a correlate of active disorder. However, respondents suffering from each disorder were also asked whether they had *ever* discussed the symptoms of that disorder with a physician. Since their response covered discussion at any time in their lives, it is best associated with a history of the disorder at any time in the past.

Because these correlates will appear throughout all the chapters to follow, we provide, in Appendix A, the numbers of cases available with each characteristic by age, sex, and ethnic group (Table A-1). We also show (Table A-2) how many persons whose diagnostic status was ascertained are available for studying each possible correlate. These tables can be consulted to learn what the base number is on which percentages in the later chapters are calculated. Some variables can be studied in only parts of the population. For example, use of medical services was not asked of those institutionalized, because such services are usually provided through the institution of residence. Income and occupation were asked only of those currently employed. Because rural samples were available in only two sites, Durham and St. Louis, rural–urban comparisons are restricted to household residents in these two sites. In addition to reductions because some respondents were ineligible to be asked some questions, there are also reductions because of minor differences in the interview instruments used at the five sites. Where differences occur, analyses are limited to sites that share a common pattern of questioning. Affected is information about personal earnings, which was not asked in St. Louis, and about unemployment in the last five years, which was asked in New Haven and Baltimore of only a subset of respondents. Total numbers also vary slightly because of occasional missing data for some respondents, although more than a minimal rate of refusals to answer was obtained only for questions about income.

Tables generally show results for all sample members who answered the pertinent questions from all five sites combined, weighted to national distributions of age, sex, and ethnic group. Where some sites or categories of subjects are excluded, this is noted in the table. Thus, when there is *no* notation, the results are based on sample members in all five sites weighted to represent the nation. Results are presented as percentages, followed by their standard error in parentheses: % (SE). The significance of differences is reported as *p* values.

It will be noted that despite the large sample, some risk factors are rare in some age/sex/ethnic groups. This explains why many of the results reported in future chapters are not presented in as much detail as in the Appendix tables. As noted, where the number is below 25, percentages will ordinarily be omitted in subsequent chapters, and where the number is 25–29, percentages will be bracketed to remind the reader that they are unstable.

A strong association found between psychiatric disorder and a demographic factor may or may not be helpful in explaining the frequency of a disorder in the general population, depending on whether that demographic factor is common or rare. For example, even if every prisoner were an alcoholic, prisoners would account for little of the alcoholism in the population because only .10% of the adult population are prisoners (Table 2–6). To assist in interpreting the importance of the various variables associated with psychiatric disorder in possibly accounting for its frequency in the population, we present the frequency of each of these correlates for reference in Table 2–6.

Clearly high rates of disorder in the institutionalized or in those earning more than $35,000 in the year before interview or in those who cohabited for a year or more without every marrying, or in farmers can have little impact on rates in the country as a whole. Elevated rates of disorder in larger groups will have relatively greater impact on the public health of the nation.

TABLE 2-6 Frequency of Demographic Groups in the Population
(After Weighting)

	%		%
Sex, Age, Ethnicity		*Residence*	
Men	47.7	Any institution[a]	1.05
Women	52.3		
		Nursing home	.79
Age <30	30.6	Psychiatric hospital	.16
30–44	26.4	Prison	.10
45–64	27.3		
65+	15.7	Household	98.95
Black	10.5	*Household Size*	
White/Other	84.2	Alone	12.5
Hispanic	5.3	Two persons	30.8
		Three persons	19.8
Education		Four persons	18.5
<8 grades	8.6	Five or more	18.4
<8 grades	8.6		
8 grades	7.0	*Marital History*	
9–11 grades	18.3	Married and never	
12 grades	28.0	divorced/separated	49.5
13–15 grades	20.6	Divorced/separated once	15.2
16+ grades	17.5	Divorced/separated	
		twice or more	11.5
Employment and Dependency		Single, never cohabited	
Working full time	55.1	for a year	20.4
Not full time	44.9	Cohabited for one year	
Welfare or disability	10.0	or more, never married	3.4
Last Year's Earning If		*Medical and Health Services*	
Working Full Time		*If in Household*	
Less than $5,000	9.9	None	42.0
5,000 − <10,000	18.3	Any medical services	58.0
10,000 − <15,000	22.5	Medical hospitalization	
15,000 − <20,000	17.1	(1 yr)	13.0
20,000 − <25,000	12.5	Mental health outpatient	
25,000 − <35,000	11.3	(6 mo)	7.6
35,000 − <50,000	5.0	Mental hospitalization	
50,000+	3.4	(1 yr)	0.9
Of Those Working Full Time			
Managers or professionals	28.7		
Technical or sales	29.6		
Farmers	1.5		
Skilled	13.7		
Unskilled	16.4		
Service	10.1		

[a]Because census data were not available at the time of these analyses, the institutional population was not independently reweighted to 1980 census figures. A special subsequent calculation from census data shows that the correct percentage is 1.3%.

CONCLUSION

The Epidemiologic Catchment Area Projects consisted of five independent surveys that have been combined in this volume to produce estimates of our nation's mental health. Deciding how to put these data together has been a complex enterprise, carried out jointly by the authors. We have attempted to be explicit about the methods we have used to translate clustered, weighted data from five sites into estimates of the nation's psychiatric well-being in order to open our methods to discussion and replication.

We also note that we cannot vouch for the accuracy with which respondents answered because we obtained no information except through interview. However, both internal evidence and comparable earlier studies indicate that survey methods obtain reasonably accurate information even about items as personal and potentially embarrassing as psychiatric symptoms.

The evidence internal to the interviews includes the high level of consistency of patterns of symptoms across sites. Such stability is not imaginable if denial or random inaccuracy were common. Previous epidemiologic studies where various types of external records were available such as drinking diaries, diaries of spontaneous abortion, arrest records, military records of drug use, psychiatric hospital records, and results of urine screening for drugs immediately after the interview (Huizinga & Elliott, 1983; Maddux & Desmond, 1975; Robins, Davis, & Nunco, 1974; Wilcox & Horney, 1984) have found impressively high rates of honesty in surveys of general population samples.

While any large-scale epidemiological effort suffers from imperfections and uncertainties, the ECA Project presents the most comprehensive investigation of psychiatric disorders yet undertaken. Much remains to be done before we understand the processes that produce variations in rates of disorder and use of health services; this volume reflects the initial phase of our study, not our ultimate understanding of the problems that increase or decrease an individual's chance of having a psychiatric disorder.

3 Schizophrenic Disorders

SAMUEL J. KEITH / DARREL A. REGIER /
DONALD S. RAE

For many years, our understanding of the prevalence and course of schizophrenia has depended on observations from the clinical literature or from clinically derived "samples of convenience." As a result of this limited data base, a range of clinical assumptions about schizophrenia has been developed with far-reaching implications for our understanding of the extent of the illness and our planning for its treatment. Until recently we have not had the capacity to examine fully the validity of our assumptions and their implications. However, with the completion of the ECA study, we can now examine previous hypotheses using adequate population-based data.

Of particular significance for the study of schizophrenia is the availability of information on both community and institutional populations. Because of the severity of this illness, it has often been assumed that all patients with this illness will eventually come into treatment. This assumption made access to community populations appear less urgent and thus deprived us of opportunities to examine the full range of severity levels associated with this disorder. A broader population base can offer a more complete understanding of this illness and its course. In addition, deinstitutionalization of psychiatric patients over the past 30 years and strict legal restrictions on involuntary commitment have made obsolete the assumption that most individuals with schizophrenia will be found in treatment settings. Hence the opportunity to look at differences in symptom patterns and prevalence rates for different types of institutional and household settings has greatly assisted our ability to "complete the clinical picture" (Morris, 1964) of this disorder.

Schizophrenia has been described as a disorder that drastically alters the expectations of approximately 1% of the population during the course of a lifetime (Babigian, 1985; Jablensky, 1986; Yolles & Kramer, 1969). In the United States this has been translated into an estimate that 2 to 4 million people will experience the onset of schizophrenic symptoms at just the time when those affected may be trying to complete an education or select

33

a career. Clinical descriptions have further postulated that for between a fourth to a third of patients, the course of the illness is unrelenting from the very first episode (Strauss & Carpenter, 1981). For an additional 50% disabling symptoms are expected to appear intermittently throughout life, spawning further social and occupational diabilities. Although the available treatments for schizophrenia are effective in reducing the psychotic symptoms of the disorder, they frequently fail to provide protection from the pattern of repeated relapse and functional decline that is a clinical hallmark of the illness.

Small wonder that the economic burden posed by schizophrenia is so severe. Patients with the disorder occupy over 30% of the nation's mental hospital beds—more than 100,000 beds on any given day (Manderscheid & Barrett, 1987). Treatment costs alone exceed $7 billion annually, and indirect costs—for example, of social services, loss of productivity, and premature mortality—account for at least double that figure, making the financial burden of schizophrenia in the United States approximately equal to that of all cancers combined (Gunderson & Mosher, 1975; Hall, Goldstein, et al., 1985). The demoralizing effects of this devastating illness are partly revealed by the exceptionally high suicide attempt and completion rate of its victims. Past clinical studies have estimated that one in four patients with schizophrenia will attempt suicide and one in ten will succeed in the first ten years of the illness (Roy, 1986; Winokur & Tsuang, 1975). Further, compared to the general population, persons with schizophrenia have a twofold increase in overall mortality, with excess mortality particularly likely to be caused by "unnatural death" (Allebeck & Wistedt, 1986). Schizophrenic patients at the greatest risk for premature death are those younger than 40 years (Black & Winokur, 1988).

In this chapter we use the recent data from the five-site ECA study to examine a number of specific issues critical to our understanding of schizophrenia. In so doing, we can assess the validity of the clinical assumptions about the severity of the illness as well as describe its manifestations and course and their correlates.

DIAGNOSTIC CRITERIA

Schizophrenia in DSM-III is an illness defined by six sets of inclusion and exclusion criteria (Table 3–1). The first set (A criteria) are the characteristic psychotic ("positive") symptoms of schizophrenia, derived in large part from the first rank symptoms defined by Kurt Schneider (1959). Criterion B, the deterioration from a previous level of functioning, exemplifies the negative symptoms of schizophrenia. Criterion C defines the duration required —at least six months of some signs of the illness (C2)—and re-

Table 3-1 Lifetime Prevalence of Schizophrenia Diagnostic Criteria in Household and Institutional Populations

Criteria	Lifetime Prevalence in % (SE)	
	Household Residents	Institutional Residents
Any of A criteria (at least one psychotic symptom)	3.3 (0.2)	8.5 (1.3)
A_1 Bizarre delusions	1.6 (0.1)	6.6 (1.0)
A_2 Other delusions	0.1 (0.0)	1.3 (0.2)
A_3 Persecutory delusions with hallucinations	0.7 (0.1)	4.8 (1.0)
A_4 Auditory hallucinations: voices converse/ commentary	0.6 (0.1)	5.1 (1.0)
A_5 Auditory hallucinations: more than one or two words	1.7 (0.1)	6.4 (0.9)
A_6 Loose associations with inappropriate affect or catatonia	0.2 (0.0)	2.7 (0.6)
B. Deterioration in function	1.8 (0.1)	5.6 (0.9)
C_1 Current symptoms	3.7 (0.2)	12.4 (0.7)
C_2 6-mo active, 2-yr prodrome, or 6-mo residual A symptoms	2.9 (0.2)	7.2 (0.9)
D. Any affective disorder present was after psychotic symptoms	100.0 —	99.1 —
E. Onset before age 45	4.5 (0.2)	6.7 (0.6)
F. No retardation or organic mental disorder	99.2 (0.1)	80.5 (1.1)

quires that some signs of the illness be current (C1). It is the C2 criterion of six months' duration that separates schizophrenia from schizophreniform disorder, which requires only two weeks to six months of illness, and serves in many cases as a provisional or "holding pattern" diagnosis (Keith & Schooler, 1989). The duration requirement may be met in one of three ways—a six-month duration of active symptoms, a two-year prodrome, or six months of residual impaired function. The C1 requirement for current symptoms is determined in the DIS by asking whether the person has ever been back to normal for a full year since onset of symptoms. A negative answer meets the C1 criterion.

In this chapter, the requirement for current symptoms has been dropped. This decision was made because there is an inconsistency between the DSM-III criteria and text, the latter stating that there is no absolute requirement for current symptoms. The text was thought more authoritative, since this requirement has been dropped in the DSM-III revision (American Psychiatric Association, 1987). Criterion D excludes the diagnosis if an affective syndrome developed before the first psychotic symptoms unless it was very brief. Criterion E requires an age of onset before 45, a requirement that is under considerable investigation currently; the difference between those with onset after age 45 and those who meet this criterion appears less substantial than originally thought (Harris & Jeste, 1988). Criterion F requires that the illness not be due to any organic disorder. It is expected that this criterion will also receive much attention over the next decade as investigations into the etiology and pathophysiology of schizophrenia continue.

In the household population the prevalence of each individual schizophrenia criterion is relatively low. Positive symptoms (delusions or hallucinations) had been experienced by 3.3% of the household population and 8.5% of the institutional population (Table 3-1). Only two of these positive symptoms, bizarre delusions and auditory hallucinations, were reported by more than 1% of the household population.

The B criterion, which requires deterioration from a previous level of functioning after the onset of the illness, was found in 1.8% of the household population and 5.6% of the institutional population. The other inclusion criteria, C1, C2, and E, occur among the household population at rates of 3.7% (C1—current symptoms), 2.9% (C2—six months active, two years of prodrome, or six months of residual symptoms), and 4.5% (E—onset before age 45).

As might be expected, higher percentages of the institutional than household population met some or all of the criteria for schizophrenia. In the institutional sample, 7.2% had symptoms of six months' duration, 12.4% had current symptoms, and 6.7% had onset before age 45. Less than 1% were excluded because their psychotic symptoms followed the onset of an affective disorder.

Although 3.3% of the household population and 8.5% of the institutional population met the A criteria (psychotic symptoms), the prevalence of the full diagnosis of schizophrenia was only 1.4% and 5.6% in the household and institutional populations, respectively (Table 3-2). Absence of criterion B, deterioration from a previous level of functioning, appears

Table 3–2 Prevalence of Schizophrenic Disorders by Place of Residence

	Prevalence in % (SE)			
Resident Status	One-Year		Lifetime	
Household population (98.7%)	1.0	(0.1)	1.4	(0.1)
Institutional population (total) (1.3%)	4.5	(0.6)	5.6	(0.1)
Mental hospitals (0.1%)	16.7	(4.9)	20.4	(5.8)
Nursing homes (0.9%)	3.0	(0.5)	3.8	(0.7)
Prisons (0.3%)	5.4	(1.6)	6.7	(1.9)

mainly responsible for the failure of persons with psychotic symptoms to qualify for the diagnosis. Among persons in institutions, the prevalence of meeting criterion B (5.6%) is identical to the prevalence of schizophrenia. Among the household population, the prevalence of schizophrenia (1.4%) is lower than the proportion meeting the B criterion (1.8%), which indicates that some additional people are screened out of this diagnosis by too short a duration (C), an age of onset after 45 (E), or a prior history of an organic mental disorder (F).

The clinical and older epidemiologic literature has generally estimated that schizophrenia affects 1% of the adult population. In the ECA data (shown in Table 3–3) a slightly higher percentage, 1.3% of the population, was identified as having had a diagnosis of schizophrenia at some time in their lives. Schizophreniform disorder, which differs only in a shorter duration of the symptoms, was found in about 0.2% of the population. Hence

Table 3–3 Prevalence of Schizophrenic Disorders by Disorder Subtype

	Prevalence in % (SE)				
Disorder	Active (One-Year)		Lifetime		Remission[a,b]
Schizophrenia	0.9	(0.1)	1.3	(0.1)	33%
Schizophreniform	0.1	(0.0)	0.2	(0.0)	28%
Schizophrenic disorders—total	1.0	(0.1)	1.5	(0.1)	32%

Note. Combined 5-site data, standardized to U.S. adult (age 18+) population

[a]Lifetime prevalence (Lt) minus one-year prevalence (1 yr) divided by lifetime prevalence (Lt), or (Lt − 1 yr)/Lt.

[b]Remission rates are calculated on the basis of exact point estimates of prevalence—not equal to ratios calculated with rounded rates in the table.

the overall lifetime rate for the schizophrenic disorders was approximately 1.5% of the adult population—slightly higher than previous estimates. With a remission rate of 32%, this would mean that in any given year approximately 1% of the population suffers from schizophrenia. The one-month point prevalence rate of 0.7% is also somewhat higher than European rates, which range from 0.25 to 0.53% (Jablensky, 1986). Hence, despite the changes in diagnostic criteria that have occurred over the last few years, the overall lifetime prevalence rate of approximately 1% of the population is remarkably consonant with the earlier literature. In the remaining analyses, we will combine schizophrenia and schizophreniform disorder and refer to the two as the schizophrenic disorders.

With an adult population in the United States of 165,000,000 a prevalence rate of 1.5% for these disorders means that 2,400,000 people will have warranted a diagnosis of either schizophrenia or schizophreniform disorder at some time. At this rate, the schizophrenic disorders are five times more common than multiple sclerosis, six times more so than insulin-dependent diabetes, and sixty times more so than muscular dystrophy.

HOUSEHOLD AND INSTITUTIONAL PREVALENCE

Prevalence rates are provided for those living in households and in three types of institutions: mental hospitals, nursing homes, and prisons. These samples are combined and standardized to the 1980 census of the U.S. population to estimate national rates (Table 3–2).

The one year prevalence of schizophrenia in the household sample is 1.0% and the lifetime prevalence is 1.4%. For the institutional population, which includes about 1.3% of the total U.S. population, the one year prevalence of schizophrenia is 4.5% and the lifetime prevalence is 5.6% (see Table 3–2). This means that less than 6% of those actively (within one year) schizophrenic are currently institutionalized. As would be expected among institutions, mental hospitals had the highest schizophrenia prevalence rate; 17% of their patients received a one-year and 20% a lifetime diagnosis. However, because mental hospital patients constiute only 0.1% of the total population, only 1.3% [(0.1% × 20%)/1.5%] of those with a lifetime diagnosis of schizophrenia are currently in mental hospitals. A larger proportion of persons with a lifetime diagnosis of schizophrenia (2.3%) are now in nursing homes than mental hospitals. Nursing homes received a substantial influx of mentally disordered patients during the process of deinstitutionalization (Redick et al., 1974).

A somewhat surprising finding was the relatively high prevalence of schizophrenia in the prison population. Prison population prevalence rates were 5.4% for one-year and 6.7% for lifetime, about one-third the rates for mental hospitals. Since there are about three times as many prisoners as mental hospital residents, the proportion of all schizophrenics in prison (1.34%) is about the same as in long-term mental hospitals. This is clearly a finding that deserves more careful study to determine the proportion of these schizophrenic individuals who may have additional diagnoses of substance abuse or antisocial personality that lead to contact with the criminal justice system rather than the health care system.

We compared the community and institutional prevalence rates of schizophrenia to rates for two other major mental illness syndromes—affective disorders (mania, dysthymia, and major depression) and anxiety disorders (phobia, panic disorder, and obsessive-compulsive disorder). The corresponding lifetime prevalence figure for affective disorders was 8.3% overall, but 12% in nursing home residents; 21% among prisoners, and 30% among patients in mental hospitals. For anxiety disorders, the lifetime prevalence figure was 15% overall; 16% in nursing home residents, 28% in prisoners, and 51% in patients in mental hospitals.

Although only a small minority of schizophrenics are in mental hospitals, more of them are hospitalized than are persons with affective disorder or anxiety disorder. Schizophrenia is 14 times more prevalent in psychiatric hospitals than in the community; affective disorder and anxiety disorder are each only 3.5 times more prevalent in psychiatric hospitals than in the community.

CORRRELATES OF SCHIZOPHRENIA

AGE

The age groups with the highest concentrations of schizophrenia are the 18–29 year olds, with a one–year rate of 1.2%, and the 30–44 year olds, with a one-year rate of 1.5% (Table 3-4). For the group 45–64 years, the rate falls to about one-half that found in the younger age groups—0.6%. There is a still greater drop among those aged 65 years and older, who have a one-year rate of 0.2% and a lifetime rate of 0.3%. This pattern of higher rates for the younger than older cohorts holds when sex and ethnic group are controlled (Table 3–13).

GENDER AND DEMOGRAPHIC DIFFERENCES

There is no significant difference between men and women in one-year or lifetime prevalence rates, but there is a trend toward a higher rate for women (Table 3–5).

Table 3-4 Prevalence of Total Schizophrenic Disorders by Age Group

Age Group	Prevalence in % (SE)				Remission[a]
	One-Year		Lifetime		
Total	1.0	(0.1)	1.5	(0.1)	32%
18–29	1.2	(0.2)	1.7	(0.2)	28%
30–44	1.5	(0.2)	2.3	(0.3)	35%
45–64	0.6	(0.2)	1.0	(0.2)	34%
65+	0.2	(0.1)	0.3	(0.1)	36%

[a]Lifetime prevalence minus one-year prevalence divided by lifetime prevalence.

The higher rate in women may not indicate that women are more susceptible to schizophrenia than men. Women have lower socioeconomic status (SES) and higher rates of separation and divorce than men—factors that are independently associated with significantly higher schizophrenia prevalence rates. As we shall see later (Table 3–13), when these factors are controlled in a logistic regression there is not a significantly higher rate of schizophrenia among women.

When compared to men, women seem to have their initial symptoms later and have a briefer course. This may in part explain the frequent finding in treatment studies of a two to one ratio of men to women. Gender differences need to be explored with respect to treatment seeking and the effectiveness of treatment.

Table 3-5 Prevalence of Schizophrenic Disorders by Gender

Gender	Prevalence in % (SE)				Remission
	One-Year		Lifetime		
Total	1.0	(0.1)	1.5	(0.1)	32%
Male	0.9	(0.1)	1.2	(0.2)	24%
Female	1.1	(0.1)	1.7	(0.2)	37%

RACE–ETHNICITY

The lifetime rate for blacks (2.1%) is significantly higher than that found for both white/Anglo (1.4%) and Hispanic (0.8%) groups (Table 3–6). When

Table 3-6 Prevalence of Schizophrenic Disorders by Ethnic Group

| Ethnic Group | Prevalence in % (SE) | | Remission |
	One-Year	Lifetime	
White and other	0.9 (0.1)	1.4 (0.1)	34%
Black	1.6 (0.2)	2.1 (0.2)	25%
Hispanic	0.4 (0.2)	0.8 (0.3)	46%

age and sex groups are compared (Table 3-7), a higher black rate was found for all age/sex groups except men 45–64. Of particular note is the low rate among Hispanics, particularly Hispanic males (0.3%). Virtually no Hispanic males aged 30 and over were found with a one-year diagnosis and only 0.2% were found with one-year diagnosis in the 30–44 year age group.

Controlled for age, gender, marital status and, most importantly, SES level (see below, Table 3-13), the significant difference between black and white prevalence rates disappears. Hence the higher rates which appear for the black population may well be explained by the confounding variables of lower socioeconomic status and higher rates of marital separation or divorce, which are independently associated with higher rates of schizophrenia. Of course, in a cross-sectional study such as this one, it is not possible to state definitively that current marital status and socioeconomic status explain the relation between race and disorder, because schizophrenia can lead to poor job status and marital breakup.

MARITAL STATUS

The lifetime prevalence for the schizophrenic disorders is two to three times higher among the never married (2.1%) and divorced/separated (2.9%) groups than among the married (1.0%) or widowed (0.7%) (Table 3-8). In light of the great difficulty in maintaining interpersonal relationships that accompanies schizophrenia, one may hypothesize that the onset of schizophrenia often prevents marriage. If it begins after marriage, the consequent difficulty in maintaining interpersonal relationships could lead to separation or divorce. Alternatively, the stress associated with the loss of social supports following separation or divorce might trigger an onset in those vulnerable to this disorder.

Another perspective is obtained by looking at marital status for persons with schizophrenia. The current marital status of men and women with schizophrenia is similar; 41% of both sexes are married and 4% widowed.

Table 3-7 Prevalence of Schizophrenia/Schizophreniform in Detailed Demographic Groups

	1-Month		6-Month		1-Year		Lifetime	
	Prevalence in Percent (SE)							

	1-Month		6-Month		1-Year		Lifetime	
All Ethnic Groups								
Both Sexes:								
All ages	0.7	(0.1)	0.9	(0.1)	1.0	(0.1)	1.5	(0.1)
18–29	0.9	(0.2)	1.2	(0.2)	1.2	(0.2)	1.7	(0.2)
30–44	1.1	(0.2)	1.4	(0.2)	1.5	(0.2)	2.3	(0.3)
45–64	0.5	(0.1)	0.6	(0.2)	0.7	(0.2)	1.0	(0.2)
65+	0.1	(0.0)	0.1	(0.0)	0.2	(0.1)	0.3	(0.1)
Male:								
All ages	0.7	(0.1)	0.8	(0.1)	0.9	(0.1)	1.2	(0.2)
18–29	0.9	(0.2)	1.1	(0.3)	1.1	(0.2)	1.4	(0.3)
30–44	1.0	(0.3)	1.1	(0.3)	1.2	(0.3)	1.6	(0.4)
45–64	0.6	(0.1)	0.7	(0.3)	0.7	(0.3)	0.9	(0.3)
65+	0.1	(0.0)	0.1	(0.0)	0.1	(0.0)	0.2	(0.1)
Female:								
All ages	0.7	(0.1)	1.0	(0.1)	1.1	(0.1)	1.7	(0.2)
18–29	0.9	(0.2)	1.3	(0.3)	1.4	(0.2)	2.0	(0.3)
30–44	1.2	(0.3)	1.6	(0.3)	1.8	(0.3)	3.0	(0.4)
45–64	0.3	(0.1)	0.6	(0.2)	0.6	(0.2)	1.1	(0.3)
65+	0.1	(0.1)	0.2	(0.1)	0.3	(0.1)	0.3	(0.1)
White								
Both Sexes:								
All ages	0.6	(0.1)	0.9	(0.1)	0.9	(0.1)	1.4	(0.1)
18–29	0.8	(0.2)	1.1	(0.2)	1.2	(0.2)	1.7	(0.3)
30–44	1.0	(0.2)	1.4	(0.3)	1.5	(0.3)	2.3	(0.4)
45–64	0.4	(0.2)	0.6	(0.2)	0.6	(0.2)	1.0	(0.2)
65+	0.1	(0.0)	0.1	(0.0)	0.2	(0.1)	0.3	(0.1)
Male:								
All ages	0.7	(0.2)	0.8	(0.2)	0.9	(0.2)	1.1	(0.2)
18–29	0.8	(0.3)	1.0	(0.3)	1.0	(0.3)	1.3	(0.4)
30–44	1.0	(0.4)	1.2	(0.4)	1.3	(0.4)	1.7	(0.5)
45–64	0.7	(0.3)	0.7	(0.3)	0.8	(0.3)	0.9	(0.3)
65+	0.1	(0.0)	0.1	(0.0)	0.1	(0.0)	0.2	(0.1)
Female:								
All ages	0.6	(0.1)	0.9	(0.1)	1.0	(0.1)	1.7	(0.2)
18–29	0.8	(0.2)	1.3	(0.3)	1.4	(0.3)	2.0	(0.4)
30–44	1.0	(0.3)	1.6	(0.4)	1.7	(0.4)	3.0	(0.5)
45–64	0.2	(0.1)	0.5	(0.2)	0.5	(0.2)	1.1	(0.3)
65+	0.1	(0.1)	0.1	(0.1)	0.2	(0.1)	0.3	(0.1)

Table 3-7 continues

Males remain single (40%) more frequently than females (29%), while females (26%) are significantly more likely to be divorced or separated than males (13%). Although more women than men with schizophrenia marry, their marriages are much more likely to end in divorce.

Table 3–7 continued

	1-Month		6-Month		1-Year		Lifetime	
	Prevalence in Percent (SE)							

	1-Month		6-Month		1-Year		Lifetime	
Black								
Both sexes:								
All ages	1.3	(0.2)	1.5	(0.2)	1.6	(0.2)	2.1	(0.2)
18–29	1.6	(0.4)	1.9	(0.4)	2.0	(0.5)	2.5	(0.5)
30–44	1.7	(0.4)	1.8	(0.5)	2.1	(0.5)	2.9	(0.5)
45–64	0.8	(0.4)	0.9	(0.4)	0.9	(0.4)	1.3	(0.4)
65+	0.3	(0.2)	0.3	(0.2)	0.3	(0.2)	0.6	(0.2)
Male:								
All ages	1.2	(0.3)	1.3	(0.4)	1.4	(0.4)	2.0	(0.4)
18–29	1.5	(0.6)	2.0	(0.7)	2.1	(0.7)	2.9	(0.8)
30–44	1.5	(0.8)	1.6	(0.8)	1.6	(0.8)	2.1	(0.9)
45–64	0.6	(0.5)	0.6	(0.5)	0.6	(0.5)	1.1	(0.6)
65+	0.2	(0.1)	0.2	(0.1)	0.2	(0.1)	0.2	(0.1)
Female:								
All ages	1.4	(0.3)	1.6	(0.3)	1.7	(0.3)	2.2	(0.3)
18–29	1.7	(0.6)	1.9	(0.6)	1.9	(0.6)	2.1	(0.6)
30–44	1.8	(0.5)	1.9	(0.6)	2.5	(0.6)	3.5	(0.9)
45–64	1.0	(0.6)	1.2	(0.6)	1.2	(0.6)	1.5	(0.6)
65+	0.4	(0.3)	0.4	(0.3)	0.4	(0.3)	0.8	(0.4)
Hispanic								
Both sexes:								
All ages	0.4	(0.2)	0.4	(0.2)	0.4	(0.2)	0.8	(0.3)
18–29	0.5	(0.3)	0.5	(0.3)	0.5	(0.3)	1.0	(0.5)
30–44	0.4	(0.3)	0.4	(0.3)	0.4	(0.3)	0.8	(0.4)
45–64	0.4	(0.4)	0.4	(0.4)	0.4	(0.4)	0.4	(0.4)
65+	0.0	(—)	0.4	(0.4)	0.4	(0.4)	0.4	(0.4)
Male:								
All ages	0.3	(0.2)	0.3	(0.2)	0.3	(0.2)	0.3	(0.2)
18–29	0.6	(0.5)	0.6	(0.5)	0.6	(0.5)	0.6	(0.5)
30–44	0.0	(—)	0.0	(—)	0.0	(—)	0.2	(0.2)
45–64	0.0	(—)	0.0	(—)	0.0	(—)	0.0	(—)
65+	0.0	(—)	0.0	(—)	0.0	(—)	0.0	(—)
Female:								
All ages	0.5	(0.3)	0.6	(0.3)	0.6	(0.3)	1.2	(0.5)
18–29	0.3	(0.3)	0.3	(0.3)	0.3	(0.3)	1.5	(1.0)
30–44	0.7	(0.7)	0.7	(0.7)	0.7	(0.7)	1.3	(0.8)
45–64	0.8	(0.8)	0.8	(0.8)	0.8	(0.8)	0.8	(0.8)
65+	0.0	(—)	0.7	(0.7)	0.7	(0.7)	0.7	(0.7)

Note. No standard error calculated when the prevalence is zero.

EDUCATION

We noted that schizophrenia frequently interrupts the chance to complete an education or select a career. The ECA data show that up to the start of college there is no significant difference between education levels achieved

Table 3-8 Prevalence of Schizophrenic Disorders by Marital Status

Marital Status	Prevalence in % (SE)			
	One-Year		Lifetime	Remission
Married	0.6	(0.1)	1.0 (0.2)	45%
Single	1.5	(0.3)	2.1 (0.3)	27%
Widowed	0.6	(0.2)	0.7 (0.2)	22%
Separated/Divorced	2.4	(0.4)	2.9 (0.5)	19%

by those with schizophrenia compared to the entire population. However, a nonsignificantly higher proportion of schizophrenics did not complete their final level of schooling, whether it was elementary school, high school, or college. While the percentage with a high school diploma is the same for those with schizophrenia as for the general population, this does not mean schizophrenia has no effect on education. If schizophrenia was unrelated to education, there should be a *higher* percentage of high school graduates among schizophrenics than others because schizophrenics tend to be young, and younger age groups contain more high school graduates. In any case, persons with a diagnosis of schizophrenia do show a substantial disadvantage in completing college: 4.8% hold a college degree compared to 17% in the total population (Table 3-9). This is significant in light of the fact that those with schizophrenia are slightly overrepresented among college entrants. The often reported clinical pattern of a psychotic breakdown

Table 3-9 Educational Levels of Those with Lifetime Schizophrenic Disorders Compared with the U.S. Population as a Whole

Years of Education	Total U.S. Population		With Schizophrenic Disorders	
	%	(SE)	%	(SE)
0-7	9.1	(0.2)	13.2	(2.6)
8	7.2	(0.3)	7.5	(2.1)
9-11	18.0	(0.4)	21.9	(3.4)
12 (h.s. graduate)	28.3	(0.5)	27.8	(4.2)
13 – 15 (some college)	20.3	(0.4)	24.8	(4.0)
16 + (college graduate)	17.2	(0.5)	4.8	(1.7)
	100.0		100.0	

in the early college years is supported by the ECA data. Clearly, by the early twenties when one would expect to graduate from college, the cognitive and other disabilities associated with schizophrenia have had a devastating negative effect on the capacity of a student to perform competently.

EMPLOYMENT HISTORY

The employment pattern for those with schizophrenia reveals substantial problems with this area of social functioning. Our data show that 43% of people with schizophrenia were currently working compared to 56% of the total population (Table 3–10). Of males with schizophrenia, 54% were working compared with 70% of nonschizophrenic males. Indeed, among those with a diagnosis of schizophrenia, 43% last worked over a year ago compared to 34% of the total population—figures which indicate significantly longer periods of unemployment for those with this disorder. Income levels for people with schizophrenia are also low—55% earn less than $15,000, compared to 35% of the rest of the population. Since individuals with schizophrenia tend to be young, the differences in employment levels would be even more dramatic if the employment rates were adjusted by age.

FINANCIAL ASSISTANCE

Public financial assistance plays a substantial role in the life of people with schizophrenia in the community. Fourteen percent of persons with schizophrenia receive disability income compared with 5.0% of the total popula-

Table 3–10 Employment History of Those with Schizophrenic Disorders (Lifetime) Compared with the U.S. Population as a Whole

Employment Status	Total Population		Schizophrenic Disorders	
	%	(SE)	%	(SE)
Currently employed	56.3	(5.4)	42.8	(4.1)
Unemployed 1–6 months	6.4	(0.3)	10.1	(2.7)
Unemployed 6–12 months	3.0	(0.2)	3.6	(1.4)
Unemployed > 1 year	34.3	(0.5)	43.5	(4.4)
	100.0		100.0	

tion (Table 3–11). Disability benefits are particularly common for schizophrenic males, 20% of whom qualify for benefits compared to 6% of nonschizophrenics; for females the rate is 9.7% compared to 4.0% without this disorder.

In addition to receiving disability assistance, a relatively high proportion (14%) receive welfare payments, compared to the general population (3.1%). However, the male and female rates (4.9% and 20% respectively) differ in the opposite direction from disability payments because females receive more family assistance benefits. With regard to social security income, however, persons with schizophrenia are less likely to receive payments than the average for the population (5.9% versus 17%).

Since individuals with schizophrenia are young, few have reached the retirement ages when most people receive social security payments. However, they may also less often receive social security payments after age 65 because of their lower employment rate during the normal working ages when contributions to the social security system are made.

SOCIOECONOMIC STATUS (SES)

A dramatic difference in prevalence of schizophrenia emerges between the lowest and the highest socioeconomic classes (using the Nam criteria for SES: Nam & Powers, 1965). The difference is consistent across all time intervals (one month, six months, one year, and lifetime diagnosis) and for schizophrenia, schizophreniform disorder, and the combined diagnoses. The lifetime prevalence of the combined diagnosis for the lowest SES group (level V) is 2.5%; for the highest (level I), 0.5%; thus, schizophrenia is almost five times more common at the bottom of the socioeconomic ladder than it is at the top (Table 3–12).

With respect to the socioeconomic status prevalence data, the findings

Table 3–11 Current Financial Assistance Received by Those with Schizophrenic Disorders (Lifetime)

Financial Assistance Status	Total Population		Schizophrenic Disorders	
	%	(SE)	%	(SE)
Disability income (SSI)	5.0	(0.2)	13.7	(3.0)
Welfare income	3.1	(0.1)	14.3	(2.6)
Social Security income	16.8	(0.3)	5.9	(1.4)
Unemployment compensation	2.2	(0.1)	2.7	(1.5)

Table 3-12 Prevalence of Schizophrenic Disorders by Socioeconomic Status (SES) Group

SES Group[a]	Prevalence in % (SE)				Remission
	One-Year		Lifetime		
Level I (High)	0.4	(0.2)	0.5	(0.2)	24%
Level II	0.8	(0.2)	1.2	(0.3)	28%
Level III	0.9	(0.2)	1.4	(0.2)	39%
Level IV	1.3	(0.2)	1.9	(0.2)	31%
Level V (Low)	1.9	(0.4)	2.5	(0.4)	24%

[a]In Nam & Powers (1965) quintiles.

are consistent with studies done 50 years ago, showing that schizophrenia was overrepresented in the lowest classes (Faris & Dunham, 1939; Hollingshead & Redlich, 1958). While the debate between the "downward drift" hypothesis and the psychotogenic property of lower class life seems to have become muted over the past decade, the finding of increased prevalence in the lower classes persists. Cause or effect resolution must await further research.

COMBINING CORRELATES

To learn the relative importance of age, sex, ethnic background, marital status, and socioeconomic status in describing persons with schizophrenic disorders, these variables were combined in a logistic regression (Table 3-13). Being older than 65 and Hispanic were associated with a significantly low rate of schizophrenic disorder; being single, divorced or separated, aged 30-44, and at lower socioeconomic levels were associated with a significantly high rate. Neither being female nor black was significant when other variables were controlled. The most potent correlates were age and socioeconomic status. Schizophrenics were 15 times more likely to be between 30 and 44 than over 65 and 10 times more likely to be in the lowest than in the highest economic stratum.

USE OF MENTAL HEALTH
AND OTHER MEDICAL AND HUMAN SERVICES

For individuals with such severe disorders, it might be expected that virtually all would be receiving some type of outpatient or inpatient mental health treatment. In fact, however, among those with symptoms in the six

Table 3-13 Demographic Variables Associated with Schizophrenic Disorders: Odds Ratios for Lifetime Prevalence, Controlling for Age, Sex, Race, Marital Status, and SES Level

Demographic Variable	Odds Ratio	p-Value
Age:		
18–29	1.00	
30–44	1.81	.0091
45–64	0.62	.0927
65+	0.12	.0000
Gender:		
Male[a]	1.00	
Female	1.32	.1694
Race/Ethnicity:		
Non-black/Non-Hispanic[a]	1.00	
Black	0.82	.2219
Hispanic	0.27	.0009
Marital status:		
Married[a]	1.00	
Single	1.88	.0128
Separated/Divorced	2.18	.0008
Widowed	1.20	.6699
SES level (Nam quintiles):		
Level I (highest)[a]	1.00	
Level II	2.35	.0737
Level III	3.03	.0147
Level IV	5.02	.0008
Level V (lowest)	9.65	.0000

[a]Reference group for logistic regression odds ratio comparison.

months prior to interview, only 57% had received some form of outpatient mental health service in that time or inpatient hospitalization within the prior year (Table 3–14). The majority (70%) of those treated were seen by mental health specialists such as psychiatrists, psychologists, psychiatric social workers, or other professionals in mental health facilities. The remainder received their only mental health treatment from general medical physicians or human service professionals such as the clergy or non-mental health social service agencies. Indeed, although schizophrenia is often said to be an illness that eventually requires hospitalization, only 40% of people with a lifetime diagnosis of schizophrenia state that they have ever been admitted to a mental hospital and only 13% reported an admission during the past year.

Table 3–14 Mental Health Visits—Outpatient (Six-Months) and/or Inpatient (One-Year)—by Those With Schizophrenia Within Six Months

Mental Health (MH) Service Type	Among Those with Schizophrenic Disorders	
	% Using	(SE)
Any MH service	57	(5.1)
Specialty MH service	40	(5.4)
General medical MH	17	(4.1)
Gen medical MH only	12	(3.7)
Other human MH services	14	(3.6)
Human service MH only	6	(2.8)

CHARACTERISTICS OF PEOPLE WITH SCHIZOPHRENIA

PSYCHOTIC SYMPTOMS AND SUICIDE ATTEMPT RATES

Among people who met the full diagnostic criteria for schizophrenia, the most common symptoms in those living in households were bizarre delusions and auditory hallucinations of more than one or two words—found in 58% and 54% respectively. Persecutory delusions accompanied by hallucinations were somewhat less commonly reported (34%); as were voices commenting or conversing (13%). Somatic, grandiose, religious, or nihilistic delusions (4.2%), which were reported only if volunteered, and thought disorder (4.3%), judged by the interviewer on the basis of the respondent's behavior during the interview, were rare. The symptom patterns among those with schizophrenia and schizophreniform disorder considered separately were similar to the combined category.

In contrast to those living in private homes, there were significantly higher rates of all psychotic symptoms except "other delusions" in the institutionalized schizophrenics (Table 3–15). Bizarre delusions and auditory hallucinations of more than one to two words were found in more than 70% of patients or inmates. Persecutory delusions and auditory hallucinations with voices conversing were found in more than half. The rate of current formal thought disorder (21%) detected by the interviewer was more than five times as great as that found in the household population. Hence, it is clear that the institutionalized are affected by much higher psychotic symptom levels, which at least partially accounts for their institutionalization.

As indicated earlier, other studies have revealed relatively high rates of

Table 3–15 Schizophrenia Diagnostic Symptoms Ever Experienced by Persons
with Lifetime Diagnosis of a Schizophrenic Disorder

	Prevalence in % (SE)			
Symptom Criteria	Household		Institution	
Meet A criterion: at least one psychotic symptom	100[a]	(—)	100[a]	(—)
A$_1$ Bizarre delusions	58	(4.1)	74	(5.8)
A$_2$ Other delusions	4	(1.6)	2	(1.2)
A$_3$ Persecutory delusions with hallucinations	34	(2.4)	57	(5.0)
A$_4$ Auditory hallucinations, voices converse/comment	13	(2.4)	52	(6.4)
A$_5$ Auditory hallucinations of more than one or two words	54	(3.5)	72	(5.1)
A$_6$ Loose associations with inapprop. affect or catatonia	4	(1.4)	21	(5.9)

[a]By definition, anyone with schizophrenia *must* have at least one psychotic symptom.

both suicide attempts (one in four attempting) and completed suicides (one in ten) during the first ten years of the illness (Roy, 1986; Winokur & Tsuang, 1975). The ECA investigation, which used a lifetime rather than ten year time frame, also found a relatively high lifetime prevalence of suicide attempts. Suicide attempts had occurred in 28% of schizophrenics, with lower rates among males (20%) than females (32%). There has been no longitudinal followup of the ECA subjects to document suicide completion rates.

REMISSION RATES

We defined the remission rate as the percent of those with a lifetime diagnosis of schizophrenia whose most recent symptom occurred more than one year ago. For the combined diagnoses of schizophrenia and schizophreniform, the findings are remarkably close to the common clinical rule of "thirds." The remission rate for this combined category was 32%, with nonsignificant differences between the two subtypes (Table 3–3). The stability of the remission rate across all age groups in the combined diagnosis category (Table 3–4) suggests that remission, as defined by at least one year without symptoms, does not necessarily occur with aging—approximately two-thirds, regardless of age, reported symptoms within the past year.

Because of the relatively low base rates for these disorders, very few of the differences in remission rates reach statistical significance and should be viewed as trends deserving future clinical study. For example, the higher rate of remission among women (37%) compared with men (24%) does not reach statistical significance but suggests that the slightly higher prevalence rate among women may include a less severe and transient subtype of the illness (Table 3-5).

For the sociodemographic groups defined by race/ethnicity (Table 3-6) and socioeconomic status (Table 3-12), there was no significant difference in remission rates. Nonetheless, the remission rates by socioeconomic class reveal an interesting pattern of low remission rates in both the highest and the lowest classes (24% for both class I and for class V), with the highest remission rate (39%) in class III.

The only significant predictor of a high remission rate (45%) is being currently married (Table 3-8). The rate for the married is significantly higher than the 19% rate for the separated/divorced category and nonsignificantly higher than that found among the single (27%) and the widowed (22%). This suggests that continuing symptoms play an important role in the high divorce and separation rates of schizophrenics who marry.

AGE OF ONSET

It has frequently been stated that most schizophrenic patients had their initial episode by the age of 25 (Klorman, Strauss, & Kokes, 1977). Our data indicate that this clinical observation applies to the total population of schizophrenics as well: 71% of those who have either schizophrenia or schizophreniform illness had their first symptom by age 25. The mean age of onset is 19.9 years old. The age of onset for women appears to lag some three to four years behind the age for men through age 37 (Figure 3-1).

In DSM-III-R, the requirement for onset before age 45 has been dropped because of the debate over whether the appearance of a "schizophrenia-like" syndrome in later life indicates a distinct illness or merely an unusually late onset of schizophrenia. That such late appearances do happen is shown by the fact that 5.2% of the ECA cases of schizophrenia had onsets after the age of 40 (but before age 45, since DSM-III diagnostic rules were followed).

DURATION OF SYMPTOMS

The mean duration of the illness calculated for cases not active in the last year was 15.5 years. However, this calculation was based on small numbers, since two-thirds had had symptoms in the past year.

We compared men and women with a lifetime diagnosis of schizophrenia with respect to their reporting a symptom within the last year. Sixty-three

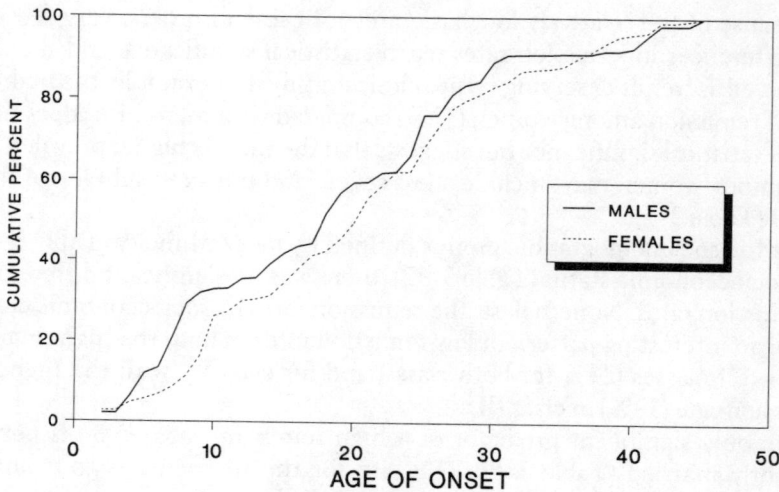

Figure 3–1 Cumulative Age of Onset, Schizophrenia/Schizophreniform

percent of females and 76% of males reported symptoms within the past year. When symptoms began less than four years prior to the interview, 86% of women reported symptoms in the past year, compared with 62% of men. As the time from onset of the illness was extended to more than ten years prior to the interview, however, the pattern was reversed. Sixty-three percent of females who had onset more than ten years prior to the interview reported symptoms in the past year compared with 82% of males. This pattern suggests a more intense, yet compact type of illness in females, and a longer, more chronic one in males.

CONCLUSION

We have found a somewhat higher rate of schizophrenia in the U.S. population than rates found in community studies in Europe (Jablensky, 1986), although rates are not grossly different. We can have considerable confidence in these rates because of the large sample, the relatively complete ascertainment, the adjustment for nonresponse, and the careful application of standard diagnostic criteria. Beyond the probable accuracy of the estimates, this study provides rich sociodemographic, service use, and symptomatic correlates.

The clinical follow-up of cohorts from these studies over several years would be of particularly great value for assessing the clinical course and remission rates on a prospective basis. We look forward to future investigations utilizing the rich baseline data collected at the five sites involved in this historic study.

4 Affective Disorders

MYRNA M. WEISSMAN /
MARTHA LIVINGSTON BRUCE /
PHILIP J. LEAF / LOUIS P. FLORIO /
CHARLES HOLZER, III

The affective disorders are a group of mental conditions characterized by disturbances of mood, primarily depression and mania. The depressive and manic syndromes each consist of characteristic symptoms that tend to occur together and persist for weeks to years. Transient moods of sadness or elation occur frequently in the general population and are considered normal. Depressive symptoms also occur in a variety of medical and mental illnesses. However, here we are concerned with affective disorders as clinical syndromes codified in DSM-III. The syndromes we will describe include major depression, dysthymia, and bipolar disorder.

The major depression syndrome, by DSM-III criteria, includes an episode of depression defined as persistent (for at least two weeks), mood disturbance, plus at least four of the following: sleep disturbance, changes in psychomotor activity, loss of ability to experience pleasure and interest, fatigue, feelings of worthlessness or guilt, difficulty in concentrating, and preoccupation with death or a wish to die. Major depression is associated with impairment in social functioning. If criteria for major depression have been met but in addition an episode of mania has ever occurred, then the diagnosis is excluded in favor of a diagnosis of bipolar disorder. Table 4-1 juxtaposes the DSM-III criteria for a depressive episode against their operationalization by the DIS.

Major depression is believed by many to be a clinical syndrome made up of multiple disorders with different etiologies (Goldin & Gershon, 1988; Klerman et al., 1985). Some forms of major depression may have a larger genetic component; others a larger environmental component; while still others may be primarily the consequence of medical illness or changes in central nervous system biochemistry, perhaps consequent to taking drugs to treat a medical condition such as hypertension.

TABLE 4–1 DIS Questions to Evaluate DSM-III Criteria for Major Depressive Episode

DSM-III Criteria	DIS Questions
A. Dysphoric mood or loss of interest in all or almost all usual activities and pastimes.	In your lifetime, have you ever had two weeks or more during which you felt sad, blue, depressed, or when you lost all interest and pleasure in things that you usually cared about?
B. At least four of the following symptoms have each been present nearly every day for a period of at least two weeks:	Has there ever been a period of two weeks or more when you:
1. Poor appetite or significant weight loss (when not dieting), or increased appetite, or significant weight gain	Lost your appetite? Lost weight without trying to—as much as two pounds a week for several weeks? Your eating increased so much that you gained as much as two pounds for several weeks?
2. Insomnia or hypersomnia	Had trouble falling asleep, staying asleep, or with waking up too early? Were sleeping too much?
3. Psychomotor agitation or retardation	Talked or moved more slowly than is normal for you? Had to be moving all the time— that is, you couldn't sit still, and paced up and down?
4. Loss of interest or pleasure in usual activities, or decrease in sexual drive	Your interest in sex was a lot less than usual?
5. Loss of energy, fatigue	Felt tired out all the time?
6. Feelings of worthlessness, self-reproach, or excessive or inappropriate guilt	Felt worthless, sinful, or guilty?
7. Complaints or evidence of diminished ability to think or concentrate, such as slowed thinking, or indecisiveness not associated with marked loosening of association or incoherence	Had a lot more trouble concentrating than is normal for you? Your thoughts came slower than usual or seemed mixed up?
8. Recurrent thoughts of death, suicidal ideation, wishes to be dead, or suicide	Thought a lot about death—either your own, someone else's, or death in general? Felt like you wanted to die? Felt so low you thought of committing suicide? Attempted suicide?

Dysthymic disorder is a chronic (of at least two years' duration) disturbance of mood involving either depressed mood or loss of interest or pleasure in most usual activities along with some of the symptoms used to diagnose major depression. While the depressed mood may be interrupted by periods of normal mood for a few days to a few weeks, the essential feature is chronicity. Many patients have an acute depression superimposed upon dysthymia, termed "double depression" (Keller & Shapiro, 1982). The natural history, clinical course, and treatment of dysthymia has been less well described than the same features of major depression. There is some evidence that dysthymia occurs with increased frequency among the biological relatives of patients with major depression, suggesting that dysthymia may be part of the spectrum of major depression (Akiskal, 1981; Weissman et al., 1984). In the DIS, the operationalization of DSM-III dysthymia included the eight symptoms for major depression (Table 4-1), plus the additional symptoms of tearfulness and hopelessness. Criteria for five of the eight symptoms of major depression were modified to omit oversleeping as a sign of sleep disturbance, weight gain as a sign of appetite disturbance, moving all the time as a sign of psychomotor activity disturbance, slowed thinking as a sign of difficulty in concentration, and suicide attempts as a sign of preoccupation with death. Respondents met criteria for dysthymia if their depressed mood lasted over two years but they had too few associated symptoms to meet criteria for major depression, and if they had no psychotic symptoms such as delusions or hallucinations.

Bipolar disorder is diagnosed if an episode of mania occurs during the individual's life whether or not depression has ever been diagnosed. Most commonly, individuals with a manic episode also experience a period of depression. The essential feature of mania is a distinct period when the predominant mood is either elevated, expansive, or irritable, and there are associated symptoms including hyperactivity, pressure of speech, flight of ideas, inflated self-esteem, decreased need for sleep, distractibility, and excessive involvement in activities that have a high potential for painful consequences. Often the activities are flamboyant, bizarre, or disorganized. Table 4-2 compares DSM-III criteria for a manic episode with the DIS.

Hypomania is used to describe a condition that is similar to mania but not as severe. Persons who meet criteria for major depression and have hypomania as well are classified as bipolar II (or atypical bipolar disorder).

In cyclothymia there are symptoms characteristic of both depression and mania but they are of insufficient severity and duration to meet criteria for either a depressive episode or a manic episode. This diagnosis is not made in the ECA.

These bipolar disorders have dramatic clinical manifestations. There is evidence for a strong genetic contribution. Family, twin, and adoption studies, and preliminary linkage studies identifying chromosomal location

TABLE 4–2 DIS Questions to Evaluate DSM-III Criteria for Manic Episode

DSM-III Criteria	DIS Questions
A. One or more distinct periods with a predominantly elevated, expansive, or irritable mood.	Has there ever been a period of one week or more when you were so happy or excited or high that you got into trouble, or your family or friends worried about it, or a doctor said you were manic? When you were feeling that way (i.e., experiencing symptoms 1-7 in B), were you unusually irritable or likely to fight or argue?
B. Duration of at least one week during which at least three of the following symptoms have persisted (four if mood is only irritable):	Has there ever been a period of a week or more when you:
1. Increase in activity (either socially, at work, or sexually) or physical restlessness	Were so much more active than usual that you or your family or friends were concerned about it? Your interest in sex was so much stronger than is typical for you that you wanted to have sex a lot more frequently than is normal for you or with people you normally wouldn't be interested in?
2. More talkative than usual or pressure to keep talking	Talked so fast that people said they couldn't understand you?
3. Flight of ideas or subjective experience that thoughts are racing	Thoughts raced through your head so fast that you couldn't keep track of them?
4. Inflated self-esteem	Felt that you had a special gift or special powers to do things others couldn't do or that you were a specially important person?
5. Decreased need for sleep	Hardly slept at all but still didn't feel tired or sleepy?
6. Distractibility, i.e., attention is too easily drawn to unimportant or irrelevant external stimuli	Easily distracted so that any little interruption could get you off the track?
7. Excessive involvement in activities that have a high potential for painful consequences which is not recognized	Went on a spending spree—spending so much money that it caused you or your family some financial trouble?

of markers of putative genes support a genetic basis for some forms of bipolar disorder (Egeland et al., 1987). Family and linkage studies suggest that bipolar II and cyclothymia may be part of the bipolar spectrum (Gershon et al., 1982).

In the 1987 revision of DSM-III (DSM-III-R), these disorders identified as the affective disorders in DSM-III have instead been called mood disorders. However, the changes in diagnostic criteria are minimal, and the findings for the disorders based on DSM-III should be applicable to DSM-III-R criteria. A criterion has been added for bipolar disorder; it now requires impairment in occupational or usual social function. For dysthymia, the number of persistent symptoms required has been reduced from three to two, and the exclusion criteria have been increased by adding the rule that there must not have been unequivocal evidence for major depression during the first two years of the disturbance, or any evidence of mania ever, or evidence for an organic etiology. Subtyping has been added to distinguish between dysthymias of late and early onset and to distinguish dysthymias secondary to a preexisting psychiatric or medical disorder from those that are primary. These changes should make ECA findings for dysthymia, which are based on DSM-III criteria, less generalizable to DSM-III-R.

The ECA represents the first epidemiologic data on the rate and risk for affective disorder derived from community samples in the United States using DSM-III criteria. Prior to the ECA, our understanding of affective disorders was based on data from patient samples (Boyd & Weissman, 1981), small or select community samples (Dean et al., 1983; Surtees, Sashidharan, & Dean, 1986; Weissman & Myers, 1978a; Wittchen, Semler, & von Zerssen, 1985), or were derived from efforts to translate data collected about symptoms into proxies for DSM-III diagnosis (Angst & Dobler-Mikola, 1984; Blazer & Williams, 1980; Murphy, 1980; Uhlenhuth et al., 1983). Moreover, with the exception of the Weissman and Myers (1978) study, which also assessed bipolar disorder and depressive personality (a condition similar to dysthymia), these studies reported on only major depression and not on the fuller range of affective disorders.

Reviews of cross-national studies prior to the ECA, undertaken to derive estimates of prevalence and incidence of the affective disorders (Boyd & Weissman, 1981), show that most of the variation in findings can probably be attributed to differences between studies in diagnostic procedures rather than real differences associated with the place in which the study was done or its era.

These reviews point to a major strength of the ECA data for understanding the affective disorders. Since the majority of persons with affective disorder do not seek treatment, clinical studies may distort estimates of prevalence, incidence, and risk factors in the population at large. The ECA derives estimates from a probability sample of the total adult population, avoiding this source of potential bias.

The reviews also suggest the importance of a family history of affective disorder as a risk factor. While the ECA provided data on some risk factors, a family history of psychiatric disorder was not routinely collected. Thus the demographic risk factors identified in the ECA should be considered within this context.

RATES OF ANY AFFECTIVE DISORDER

The prevalence of affective disorder is defined in the ECA studies as the proportion of persons who reported enough symptoms on the Diagnostic Interview Schedule (DIS) to meet the DSM-III requirement for major depression, dysthymia, bipolar I, or bipolar II disorder. Lifetime prevalence (ever meeting criteria for one of these disorders) is available for all these disorders. Because dysthymia is considered a chronic disorder, its recency was not assessed. One-month and one-year rates of affective disorders do not, therefore, include dysthymia.

The lifetime prevalence of any affective disorder was found to be 7.8% (Table 4-3). The rate is substantially higher in women than men for all three time periods, lifetime, one year, and one month, and for all ethnic groups. The ratio of females to males affected varies across these categories, but overall is approximately 2:1. While blacks have slightly lower rates than the other ethnic groups, for the most part, the similarity rather than the differences in rates across ethnic groups is striking.

The relationship between one-year and lifetime rates gives some estimate of the frequency with which the disorder remits or remains chronic. Remission rates are calculated excluding dysthymia because its one-year rate was not available. Although it must be acknowledged that recall bias (that is, better recall of events in the recent past than in the distant past) might reduce remission estimates, it is still striking that most people with a history of the disorder report a recent episode. Remission rates average only 39% (22%–42%). These seemingly low rates of remission reflect both recent first onsets and recurring episodes.

RATES IN EACH SITE

The data in Table 4-3 are aggregated across the five ECA study sites. We also disaggregated these data to examine regional differences in prevalence (Table 4-4). The similarity in prevalence rates between sites is notable; however, rates of affective disorder at the Durham and Baltimore sites are lowest for each time period. Their lower lifetime rates of affective disorders may reflect, in part, the large black populations (blacks, we observed earlier, have slightly lower lifetime rates of affective disorders than do whites or

TABLE 4-3 Affective Disorders Prevalence by Sex and Ethnicity

| | N | Prevalence in % (SE) | | | | | | Remission in %[a,b] |
		1-Month[a]		1-Year[a]		Lifetime		
Total	19,182	2.4	(0.2)	3.7	(0.2)	7.8	(0.3)	39
Ethnicity								
White	12,944	2.3	(0.2)	3.7	(0.2)	8.0	(0.3)	42
Black	4,638	2.9	(0.5)	3.5	(0.6)	6.3	(0.8)	26
Hispanic	1,600	2.7	(0.7)	4.1	(0.9)	7.8	(1.2)	27
Sex								
Men	8,311	1.7	(0.7)	2.3	(0.2)	5.2	(0.3)	38
Women	10,971	3.1	(0.3)	5.0	(0.3)	10.2	(0.4)	40
Ethnicity by Sex								
Men:								
White	5,557	1.6	(0.2)	2.2	(0.2)	5.2	(0.4)	42
Black	1,836	1.4	(0.6)	1.8	(0.6)	3.4	(0.9)	22
Hispanic	818	2.5	(1.0)	3.7	(1.2)	6.1	(1.5)	24
Women:								
White	7,387	3.0	(0.3)	5.1	(0.3)	10.5	(0.5)	41
Black	2,802	4.1	(0.9)	5.0	(1.0)	8.7	(1.2)	24
Hispanic	782	2.9	(1.0)	4.4	(1.3)	9.5	(1.8)	30

[a]Dysthymia is excluded.
[b]Lifetime prevalence (Lt) minus one-year prevalence (1 Yr) divided by lifetime prevalence (Lt): (Lt−1 Yr)/Lt.

TABLE 4-4 Site Differences in Prevalence of Affective Disorders

| | N | Prevalence in % (SE) | | | | | |
		1-Month[a]		1-Year[a]		Lifetime	
New Haven	5,063	2.8	(0.3)	4.7	(0.4)	9.0	(0.5)
Baltimore	3,560	2.1	(0.3)	2.8	(0.3)	5.8	(0.5)
St. Louis	3,200	2.9	(0.4)	4.1	(0.5)	7.9	(0.7)
Durham	4,101	1.6	(0.3)	2.3	(0.3)	5.7	(0.5)
Los Angeles	3,436	2.5	(0.3)	3.9	(0.4)	8.7	(0.6)

[a]Dysthymia not included.

Hispanics) in these two communities. The lower rates in Durham can also be accounted for by lower rates of major depression in the rural as compared to the suburban or urban areas (Blazer et al., 1985).

PREVALENCE BY AGE, SEX, AND ETHNICITY

Age has a very strong influence on the prevalence of affective disorders in both sexes and all ethnic groups (Table 4–5). Both one-year and lifetime rates of affective disorders decrease with age. Although there are slight variations in the age pattern of one-year and lifetime rates in the two younger age groups, the elderly consistently report the lowest rates. The decrease in lifetime prevalence rates with age is counterintuitive. As a person ages there would seem to be more opportunity just through the passage of time for new cases to develop. Thus, one would expect that lifetime rates should be higher in older persons. The higher lifetime prevalence in the younger age group may reflect an artifact of memory (older

TABLE 4–5 Prevalence of Affective Disorders by Age, Sex, and Ethnicity

	Men				Women			
	1-Year[a]		Lifetime		1-Year[a]		Lifetime	
	%	(SE)	%	(SE)	%	(SE)	%	(SE)
Age:								
18–29	3.1	(0.5)	6.4	(0.6)	5.8	(0.6)	10.6	(0.8)
30–44	2.7	(0.5)	6.6	(0.7)	7.9	(0.8)	15.3	(1.0)
45–64	1.7	(0.4)	3.6	(0.5)	3.6	(0.5)	9.3	(0.8)
65+	0.6	(0.3)	1.6	(0.5)	1.5	(0.4)	3.3	(0.6)
White:								
18–29	2.8	(0.5)	6.3	(0.7)	5.8	(0.7)	10.9	(0.9)
30–44	2.9	(0.5)	7.2	(0.8)	8.3	(0.9)	16.1	(1.1)
45–64	1.8	(0.4)	3.7	(0.6)	3.6	(0.6)	9.5	(0.9)
65+	0.6	(0.4)	1.5	(0.6)	1.4	(0.4)	3.4	(0.7)
Black:								
18–29	2.9	(1.3)	5.3	(1.8)	7.6	(2.0)	11.1	(2.3)
30–44	1.4	(1.1)	2.6	(1.4)	5.1	(1.8)	10.5	(2.5)
45–64	1.1	(1.0)	1.9	(1.4)	2.8	(1.5)	6.0	(2.1)
65+	0.2	(0.7)	1.9	(2.1)	1.8	(1.7)	3.4	(2.2)
Hispanic:								
18–29	6.3	(2.3)	8.2	(2.7)	2.5	(1.6)	5.9	(2.4)
30–44	2.1	(1.7)	4.1	(2.3)	7.3	(2.9)	13.6	(3.8)
45–64	1.8	(1.8)	4.9	(3.0)	4.3	(2.7)	12.7	(4.4)
65+	0.0	(0.0)	4.3	(5.1)	2.3	(3.2)	2.6	(3.4)

[a]Dysthymia not included.

persons may have greater difficulty recalling past symptoms), differential mortality (persons with past episodes of depression may be less likely to survive to older age), or real changes in rates (a birth cohort effect).

The higher rate of affective disorder in women than men found earlier for all ethnic groups also is found for every age group among blacks and whites; Hispanics show no clear gender difference, perhaps only because numbers are small.

The slightly lower rate for blacks found earlier is largely accounted for by people in the 30–64 age brackets. Blacks' rates are equal to rates for whites in the youngest and oldest groups.

Specific Affective Disorders

SYMPTOMS, EPISODES, AND DISORDERS

The task of the ECA was to determine who in the population met criteria for the specific affective disorders, including bipolar disorders I and II, major depressive disorder, and dysthymia. To do this, it had to determine how many persons had affective symptoms in sufficient quantity and for a sufficient duration to comprise an affective episode, and whether other conditions were present which ruled out those specific diagnoses. Thus, the task of differentiating subtypes of affective disorders involves determining not only which sets of symptoms a person has, but also those the person does not have.

Manic symptoms were found to be rare in the general population. Only 3% of the population reported the first necessary symptom for a manic episode: a one-week period or more of elevated, expansive, or irritable mood (Table 4-6). These rates exclude persons whose symptoms occurred only in response to medication, drugs, or alcohol. Rates for other manic symptoms occur more frequently, although none of the manic symptoms was reported by even 10% of the population. Younger adults were more likely to report manic symptoms than older adults. Among ethnic groups, blacks were the most and Hispanics the least likely to report them. Men were more likely than women to report periods of hyperactivity, inflated self-esteem, and risky behavior, while women were more likely than men to report symptoms of racing thoughts and distractibility.

Depressive symptoms occurred much more frequently than manic symptoms (Table 4-7). Almost 30% of the population report having experienced a period lasting at least two weeks when they felt sad or blue—a necessary criterion for a depressive episode. Other symptoms were less prevalent, although some (for example, two-week periods of increased or decreased

TABLE 4-6 Manic Symptoms: Lifetime Prevalence by Age, Sex, and Ethnicity

	Percentage Reporting This Symptom Lasting One Week or Longer							
	Irritability or Euphoria	Hyperactive	Overtalkative	Racing Thoughts	Inflated Self-Esteem	Decreased Need for Sleep	Distractibility	Risky Activities
Total	2.7	9.3	2.8	4.6	5.2	7.5	7.2	3.1
Age:								
18-29	4.5*	12.9*	4.1*	6.4*	6.8*	11.1*	9.8*	5.2*
30-44	3.3	12.0	2.9	5.3	6.2	8.0	9.1	3.7
45-64	1.1	5.7	2.0	3.1	3.5	4.7	4.7	1.2
65+	0.6	3.4	1.3	2.1	3.3	4.2	3.0	1.0
Sex:								
Men	2.9	11.2*	2.5	4.1*	6.5*	7.3	6.5*	3.4*
Women	2.4	7.5	3.1	5.0	4.0	7.7	7.8	2.8
Ethnicity:								
White	2.6	9.0*	2.5*	4.5*	5.2*	7.3*	7.3*	2.8*
Black	3.7	12.3	5.0	6.1	6.4	9.8	7.3	4.9
Hispanic	2.4	7.1	3.4	3.0	3.1	6.2	5.0	3.2

*Significant difference by this variable ($p < 0.05$).

TABLE 4-7 Depressive Symptoms: Lifetime Prevalence by Age, Sex, and Ethnicity

	Percentage Reporting This Symptom Lasting Two Weeks or Longer								
	Dysphoria	Appetite Change	Sleep Change	Psychomotor Change	Loss of Interest	Fatigue	Guilt	Diminished Concentration	Death Thoughts
Total	29.9	23.8	22.9	9.1	5.2	15.9	10.5	13.9	28.2
Age:									
18–29	30.7*	27.3*	24.2*	9.6	4.4	16.1*	12.1*	16.4*	30.2*
30–44	33.6	27.4	26.0	11.0	8.1	20.7	13.9	16.8	32.4
45–64	27.9	20.5	20.3	8.0	4.8	14.0	8.5	11.4	25.1
65+	25.0	16.2	19.4	6.6	2.2	10.6	4.7	7.8	21.6
Sex:									
Men	23.5*	18.8*	18.3*	7.9*	3.4*	11.6*	8.6*	10.8*	22.8*
Women	35.7	28.5	27.0	10.2	6.8	19.9	12.3	16.7	33.0
Ethnicity:									
White	30.6*	23.8*	23.4*	9.1*	5.2*	16.6*	10.9*	14.2*	28.9*
Black	24.7	25.4	19.0	9.9	5.3	13.1	7.5	12.2	24.0
Hispanic	28.9	21.2	22.9	7.2	4.3	11.1	9.8	12.5	24.9

*Significant difference by this variable ($p < 0.05$).

appetite, sleep disturbance, or thoughts about death and dying) occurred in approximately one-quarter of the population at some point when they were not explained by physical illness or ingestion of drugs, alcohol, or medications. Rarest symptoms were periods of loss of all interest and retardation or agitation. Women were more likely than men to report each of the depressive symptoms, and oldest adults were the least likely to report each. Ethnic groups were less consistent. Blacks were most likely to report changes in appetite and retardation or agitation; whites most likely to report dysphoria, fatigue, guilt, and thoughts of death.

Although some affective symptoms occur with surprising frequency in the adult population, it is less common that enough symptoms occur together to comprise a manic or depressive episode. Only 0.8% (8 persons per thousand) had ever experienced a manic episode (Table 4-8). Only 6% of the population had had sufficient depressive symptoms occurring together to meet criteria for a major depressive episode, including episodes engendered by bereavement. Episodes of both kinds occurred in only about one-third of those who reported the characteristic mood changes. Manic episodes were more common among adults under age 45, but did not vary by sex or ethnicity. Depressive episodes were most common among adults between the ages of 30 and 44, women, and nonblacks.

As noted earlier, meeting criteria for a manic or depressive episode is only the first step in obtaining a diagnosis of a specific affective disorder. Table

TABLE 4-8 Affective Episodes: Lifetime and One-Year Prevalence/100 by Age, Sex, and Ethnicity

	Manic		Depressive	
	Lifetime	One-year	Lifetime	One-Year
Total	0.8	0.6	6.3	3.7
Age:				
18–29	1.1*	0.9*	6.7*	4.2*
30–44	1.4	0.9	9.5	5.1
45–64	0.3	0.2	5.0	2.9
65+	0.1	0.1	2.0	1.4
Sex:				
Men	0.7	0.5	3.6*	2.2*
Women	0.9	0.7	8.7	5.0
Ethnicity:				
White	0.8	0.6	6.6*	3.7
Black	1.0	0.8	4.5	3.3
Hispanic	0.7	0.5	5.6	3.9

*Significant difference by this demographic variable ($p < .05$).

4–9 describes the distribution of disorders and conditions among the 1,244 ECA respondents who had ever experienced a depressive episode. Nine percent of them also experienced a manic episode at some point in their lifetime, and so were diagnosed as having bipolar I disorder. Another 7% did not meet criteria for a manic episode but experienced a period of euphoria or irritability as well as some other manic symptoms, and so were diagnosed with bipolar II disorder. For 7%, depressive episodes occurred only shortly after the death of someone close and lasted less than one year. These respondents were designated as having a grief reaction, not a psychiatric disorder. The remainder (77%), experienced no manic episode, few manic symptoms, and a depressive episode that was not related to bereavement. This group was diagnosed as having a major depressive disorder.

Our evidence confirms the heterogeneity of the affective disorders. Major depression is the most common affective disorder followed by dysthymia (lifetime rates, 5% and 3% respectively; Table 4–10). Bipolar disorders I and II are considerably less frequent, 0.8% and 0.5% respectively. The age pattern of lifetime rates in most of the subtypes reflects the aggregated patterns: rates are significantly higher in the younger age groups (ages 18–44) and decrease with age, with the lowest rates among those aged 65 or older. Dysthymia differs from the other subtypes in reflecting little variability in rates between ages 18–64 years and declining in prevalence only after age 65. While the rates of bipolar disorders are comparable in men and women, over twice as many women as men have major depression and dysthymia. Thus the sex difference in rates of affective disorders shown in Table 4–3 is accounted for primarily by major depression and dysthymia. These findings on sex differences are consistent with findings

TABLE 4-9 Affective Disorders or Conditions Among Individuals Experiencing a Depressive Episode in Lifetime, by Site[a]

	No. with Depressive Episode	Affective Disorders (%) Among Persons with a Depressive Episode				
		Bipolar I	Bipolar II	Major Depression	Short-Term Grief	Total Affected
Total	1,244	8.5	7.3	77.3	6.9	100
New Haven	370	9.9	5.9	74.6	9.7	100
Baltimore	191	7.3	13.3	68.9	10.5	100
St. Louis	229	11.5	8.3	76.9	3.3	100
Durham	172	7.9	7.8	77.4	6.8	100
Los Angeles	282	5.2	7.3	82.9	4.7	100

[a]Total weighted to U.S. population. Site data weighted to population of the catchment areas sampled at each site.

TABLE 4-10 Lifetime Prevalence of Affective Disorder Subtypes by Age, Sex, and Ethnicity

| | Lifetime Prevalence in % | | | |
	Bipolar I	Bipolar II	Major Depression	Dysthymia
Total	0.8	0.5	4.9	3.2
Age:				
18–29	1.1***	0.7**	5.0***	3.0***
30–44	1.4	0.6	7.5	3.8
45–64	0.3	0.2	4.0	3.6
65+	0.1	0.1	1.4	1.7
Sex:				
Men	0.7	0.4	2.6***	2.2***
Women	0.9	0.5	7.0	4.1
Ethnicity:				
White	0.8	0.4	5.1***	3.3
Black	1.0	0.6	3.1	2.5
Hispanic	0.7	0.5	4.4	4.0

Note. Significant variation within groups, adjusted for age, sex, or ethnicity: **p < .01, ***p < .001.

from many clinical and epidemiologic and family studies (Weissman & Klerman, 1982, 1985).

There is little ethnic variation in rates of bipolar disorder. The prevalence of major depression and dysthymia, however, is lower among blacks than among whites and Hispanics. This lower rate of depressive disorders in blacks is especially interesting since a number of studies have reported that blacks have more depressive *symptoms* (not syndromes as defined by DSM-III) than whites (Somervell et al., 1989). Perhaps blacks suffer more from mild forms of distress than whites, but less from clinical depression.

Bipolar I, bipolar II, and major depression are nonoverlapping disorders. Dysthymia, in contrast, can coexist with any of the three other affective disorders. Considerable comorbidity was found between dysthymia and other affective subtypes, especially major depression. Almost half (42%) of the respondents with chronic dysthymia have also experienced at least one full episode of major depression in their lifetime (Figure 4-1). As noted earlier, "double depression" (that is, meeting criteria for both major depression and dysthymia) is so common among dysthymics that to better differentiate the two disorders, DSM-III-R has added a requirement for dysthymia that no major depressive episode can occur during the first two years of the disturbance.

There are some regional differences in lifetime rates of specific affective

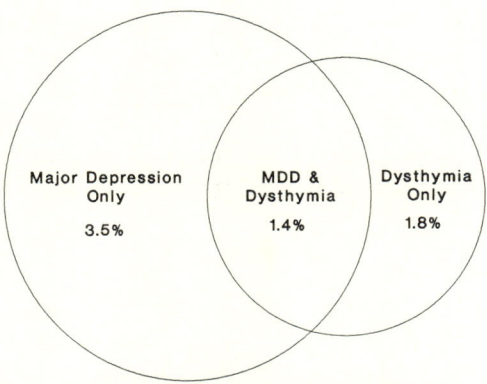

LIFETIME RATES IN POPULATION

(Among those with major depression, 28% also have dysthymia.
Among those with dysthymia, 42% also have major depression.)

Figure 4-1 Comorbidity Between Major Depressive
Disorder (MDD) and Dysthymia

disorder subtypes (Table 4–11). The rates of major depression are highest in
New Haven and Los Angeles. The rates of bipolar I disorder are highest in
New Haven and St. Louis, and the rates of dysthymia are highest in St. Louis
and Los Angeles. The prevalence of bipolar II disorder does not vary by site.

Within the year prior to interview, 0.7% of the respondents had experienced an episode of bipolar I disorder; 0.3%, of bipolar II; and 2.7%, of
major depressive disorder (Table 4–12). The risk factors for annual preva-

TABLE 4-11 Lifetime Prevalence of Affective Disorder Subtypes by Site[a]

	Lifetime Prevalence in % (SE)						
	Bipolar I		Bipolar II		Major Depression		Dysthymia
	%	(SE)	%	(SE)	%	(SE)	%	(SE)
New Haven	1.2	(0.2)	0.5	(0.1)	5.9	(0.4)	3.2	(0.3)
Baltimore	0.6	(0.2)	0.6	(0.2)	3.0	(0.3)	2.1	(0.3)
St. Louis	1.0	(0.2)	0.5	(0.2)	4.5	(0.5)	3.8	(0.5)
Durham	0.4	(0.1)	0.4	(0.1)	3.5	(0.4)	2.3	(0.3)
Los Angeles	0.6	(0.2)	0.5	(0.1)	5.6	(0.5)	4.2	(0.4)

[a]Weighted to population of the catchment areas sampled at each site.

lence are similar to those discussed for lifetime. Women and the young are at increased risk for major depression. One-year rates decrease with age for all the subtypes. The regional differences for one-year rates (Table 4–13) are similar to those observed for lifetime prevalence, with higher rates of major depression in New Haven and Los Angeles, lower rates of bipolar I in Durham and Los Angeles, and no significant variation by site in rates for bipolar II.

AGE OF ONSET

The ECA data confirm the clinical literature suggesting that bipolar disorder has an earlier age of onset than major depression (Goldin & Gershon, 1988). The mean age of onset for those reporting a history of bipolar I disorder is 18 years; for bipolar II, 22 years; and for major depression, 27 years (Table 4–14). For each of the disorders, the mean age of onset is lowest in the youngest age groups, almost by necessity since their current age is the maximum age at which their onsets can occur. If this sample were followed over time, numerous individuals in the younger age brackets would be found to experience a first episode sometime in the future, thus raising the mean age of onset.

TABLE 4–12 One-Year Prevalence of Affective Disorder Subtypes by Age, Sex, and Ethnicity

	One-Year Prevalence in Percent		
	Bipolar I	Bipolar II	Major Depression
Total	0.7	0.3	2.7
Age:			
18–29	1.0***	0.6	2.9***
30–44	1.2	0.3	3.9
45–64	0.2	0.2	2.3
65+	0.1	0.1	0.9
Sex:			
Men	0.6	0.3	1.4***
Women	0.8	0.3	4.0
Ethnicity:			
White	0.7	0.3	2.8
Black	0.9	0.5	2.2
Hispanic	0.6	0.2	3.3

Note. Significant variation within groups, adjusted for age, sex, and ethnicity: ***$p < .001$.

TABLE 4–13 One-Year Prevalence of Affective Disorder Subtypes by Site[a]

| | One-Year Prevalence in Percent (SE) | | | | | |
| | Bipolar I | | Bipolar II | | Major Depression | |
	%	(SE)	%	(SE)	%	(SE)
New Haven	1.0	(0.2)	0.2	(0.1)	3.4	(0.3)
Baltimore	0.5	(0.1)	0.4	(0.1)	1.9	(0.3)
St. Louis	1.0	(0.2)	0.4	(0.2)	2.7	(0.4)
Durham	0.3	(0.1)	0.3	(0.1)	1.7	(0.3)
Los Angeles	0.4	(0.1)	0.3	(0.1)	3.2	(0.4)

[a]Weighted to population of the catchment areas sampled at each site.

TABLE 4–14 Mean Age of Onset and Duration of Affective Disorders by Current Age

	N	Mean Age of Onset (Years)	Mean Years Duration[a]
Bipolar Disorder I			
Total	156	18.0	13.4
Current age:[b]			
18–29	68	14.8	7.7
30–44	65	17.7	16.5
Bipolar Disorder II			
Total	99	21.7	9.4
Current age:[b]			
18–29	44	18.6	4.6
30–44	35	24.9	7.4
Major Depression			
Total	914	26.5	8.7
Current age:			
18–29	264	18.1	4.9
30–44	369	26.2	7.8
45–64	184	34.9	13.8
65+	97	48.9	19.6

[a]Number of years between first and last reported episodes
[b]Too few cases over 45 to estimate their means

BIRTH COHORT AND MAJOR DEPRESSION

Previously, we showed that the lifetime prevalence rates were highest in the youngest age groups. This finding held for both men and women and at all five sites. This birth cohort effect has been reported in several previous clinical investigations (Klerman et al., 1985; Klerman, 1988; Rice et al., 1984) as well as in a small epidemiological survey conducted in 1975 in New Haven, Connecticut (Weissman & Myers, 1978) and in a 25-year longitudinal epidemiological survey in Sweden (Hagnell et al., 1982). Similar patterns have also been shown in two large family studies of the first-degree relatives of affectively ill probands (Price et al., 1985; Weissman et al., 1984). Although Murphy and associates (Murphy et al., 1984) have reported stable prevalence rates across cohorts, their study does not include the most recent cohorts, those who appear to be experiencing the greatest rise in rates. While other explanations (for example, memory effects, selective survival, changes in labeling of illness) could account for the apparent change in rates, the consistency of the findings suggests that the increase is real. When we examined age of onset by year of birth and by sex (see Figure 4–2a and 4–2b), we found that one reason for the increased lifetime prevalence appears to be that the age of onset of major depression is declining. Preliminary ECA results suggest that this decline in age of onset is consistent across all five sites.

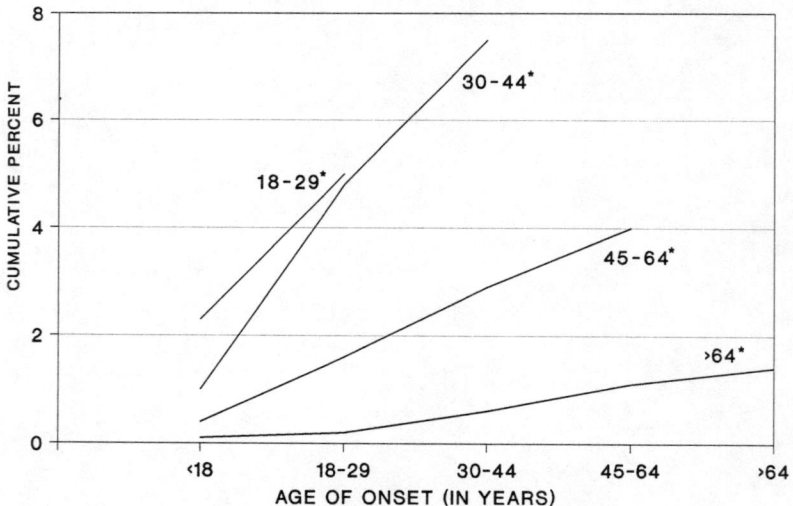

*Birth Cohort Defined by Age at Interview

Figure 4–2a Cohort Differences in Ages by Which Major Depressive Disorder Experienced

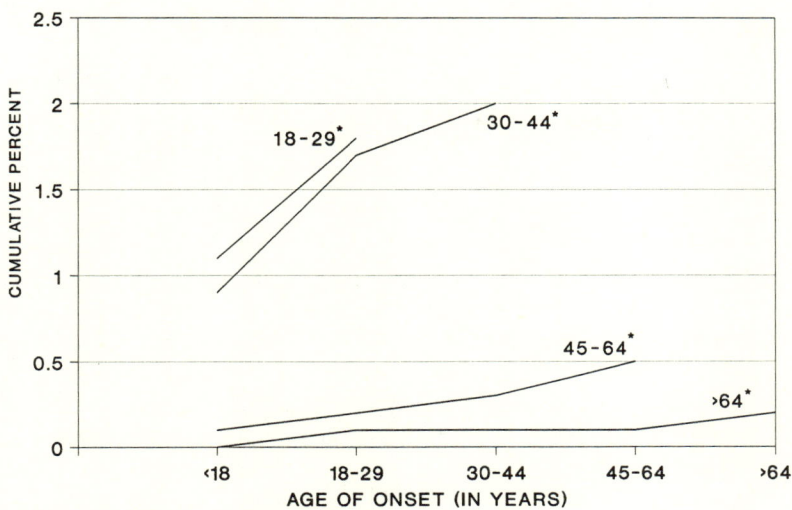

*Birth Cohort Defined by Age at Interview

Figure 4-2b Cohort Differences in Ages by Which Bipolar Disorder (I & II) Experienced

SOCIAL CORRELATES

We have already observed that the affective disorders are not uniformly distributed in the population but predominate among the young and, for major depression and dysthymia, among females and nonblacks. We now look at other social correlates of affective disorders.

MARRIAGE

Marital problems and depression have often been found to be closely associated (Briscoe & Smith, 1973). In the ECA study as well, marital history is strongly associated with affective disorder even controlling for sex, age, and race (Table 4-15). For bipolar disorders, the adjusted odds are higher for persons who are cohabiting, have a history of divorce (regardless of current marital status), or who have never married, compared to married or widowed persons without a history of divorce. A similar relationship, but not nearly so strong, holds for major depression.

When current marital status regardless of past history of divorce is considered (Table 4-16), the separated and divorced men and women have the highest rates of both disorders. Among adults over age 45, who are the

TABLE 4–15 One-Year Rates of Affective Disorder by Marital History

	Bipolar Disorder		Major Depression	
	One-Year Rate/100	Adjusted Odds Ratio[a]	One-Year Rate/100	Adjusted Odds Ratio[a]
Married (no divorces)	0.2	—	1.5	—
Never married	1.3	3.39**	2.4	1.62*
Divorced once	1.7	6.49***	4.1	2.61***
Divorced twice	2.1	7.46***	5.8	3.56***
Cohabiting	3.2	8.13***	5.1	3.19***

[a]Odds ratios adjusted for sex, age, and race/ethnicity versus the married, never divorced group.
*p < .05
**p < .01
***p < .001

group most likely to be widowed, widows have a risk of a bipolar episode as high as the separated or divorced do (results not shown).

The powerful relationship between marital status and affective disorders is reflected in correlations with household size. Major depression (but not

TABLE 4–16 One-Year Rates of Affective Disorder by Current Marital Status

	Bipolar Disorder		Major Depression	
	One-Year Rate/100	Adjusted Odds Ratio[a]	One-Year Rate/100	Adjusted Odds Ratio[a]
Married	0.7	—	2.1	—
Widowed	0.5	2.51	2.1	1.64
Separated/Divorced	1.7	2.20**	6.3	2.77***
Never married	1.6	1.55	2.8	1.38

[a]Odds ratios adjusted for sex, age, and race/ethnicity versus married.
**p < .01
***p < .001

bipolar disorder) is twice as common among people living alone as among others. Among people not living alone, rates of affective disorders do not vary by household size. But this seemingly strong effect of living alone is not the actual risk factor. When we look at *unmarried* adults, living alone is not significantly associated with affective disorders. It is the disruption of marital bonds that leads to living alone, rather than social isolation per se, which appears to increase the risk of an affective episode.

The strong protective effect of marriage against affective disorders is confirmed in much of the epidemiologic literature on subclinical depression as well as clinical research (Hirschfeld & Cross, 1982). Solid marital relationships may reduce exposure to stressors and provide a source of support during times of difficulties. Caution is necessary, however, before making assumptions about the causal direction in the relationships between marital status and affective disorders. A breakup of marriage may be a response by the well spouse to the stress of living with an ill person or may be brought about by the affected person's attributing his or her distress to failings in the spouse, as well as being a risk factor for an affective episode.

In the only longitudinal epidemiologic study attempting to sort out the timing of illness and the loosening or severing of close relationships like marriage, Henderson (1977) confirmed the association between weak social bonds and clinical neurosis (mostly depression). He also showed that weak social bonds were a risk factor for the onset of neurosis. However, the crucial aspect of social bonds was less their objective existence than how adequate the individual perceived them to be, suggesting that the personality and perception of the individual may be a more important determinant than the actual disruption of the close relationship. There are methodologic differences between Henderson's study and the ECA study which preclude direct comparability (for example, DSM-III diagnoses were not used; measures of marital discord were indirect). Nonetheless, Henderson's results should make us cautious in making assumptions about cause. Preliminary use of the longitudinal ECA data has provided evidence that the loss of a spouse—through divorce or widowhood—is associated with both new and recurring depressive episodes in all age groups and for both sexes (Bruce et al., in press), suggesting that the causal directions may be reciprocal.

EMPLOYMENT

Today, the majority of men and women under age 65 participate in the labor force. Rates of affective disorders, especially for major depression, tend to be lower for employed individuals compared to those not working (Table 4–17). Men and women who have been unemployed for at least six months in the last five years are more than three times as likely as others to

TABLE 4-17 One-Year Rates of Affective Disorder by Employment

	Bipolar Disorder		Major Depression	
	One-Year Rate/100	Adjusted Odds Ratio[a]	One-Year Rate/100	Adjusted Odds Ratio[a]
Currently unemployed				
No	1.0	—	2.2	—
Yes	1.1	1.36	3.4	1.48**
Unemployed 6 mo or more in last 5 yr				
No	0.8	—	2.0	—
Yes	1.9	1.86	6.1	3.25***
Wants a job				
No	0.8	—	2.2	—
Yes	1.6	1.38	5.6	2.70***

[a]Odds ratios adjusted for sex, age, and race/ethnicity versus "no" category.
**$p < .01$
***$p < .001$

have experienced a major depressive episode in the past year. Again, it is difficult to interpret the causal direction in these relationships. They can suggest both that men and women with a history of affective disorders have greater difficulty obtaining and maintaining employment, and that unemployed people are at greater risk of depressive episodes because they lack the sense of accomplishment, social bonds, time structure, and financial security provided by employment.

SOCIOECONOMIC STATUS

In contrast with some excellent epidemiologic research implicating low socioeconomic status in mental illness (Brown & Harris, 1978; Dohrenwend & Dohrenwend, 1969), the ECA data indicate that socioeconomic factors have little effect on the likelihood of experiencing an affective disorder (Table 4-18). The exception is a higher rate of bipolar disorder among adults with fewer years of education. The ECA study's finding of an absence of an association between socioeconomic status and affective disorders is not without support from other research. In Weissman and Myer's (1978) small community survey, current rates of major and minor depression were higher in the lower social classes, while lifetime rates were higher in the upper social classes. These findings may reflect a longer duration of symptoms in the lower social classes due to poorer access to treatment,

TABLE 4-18 One-Year Rates of Affective Disorder by Socioeconomic Status

	Bipolar Disorder		Major Depression	
	One-Year Rate/100	Adjusted Odds Ratio[a]	One-Year Rate/100	Adjusted Odds Ratio[a]
Occupation (if employed)				
White collar	1.0	—	2.5	—
Other	1.2	1.54	1.7	1.06
Income (annual)				
0 – $14,999	1.3	1.46	2.9	1.36
$15,000+	0.7	—	1.8	—
Education				
0 – 11 years	1.1	1.93**	2.6	1.19
12 years +	0.9	—	2.8	—

[a]Odds ratios contrast lower against higher socioeconomic groups and are adjusted for sex, age, and race/ethnicity.
**$p < .01$

rather than more episodes. In clinical studies, the prevalence of bipolar depressive disorder has been found to be higher among professional men and women and others of high educational and social achievement levels than among those of middle and lower levels (Welner et al., 1979; Winokur, Clayton, Reich, 1969; Woodruff et al., 1971).

More generally, the difference between our recent ECA findings and prior findings of more mental illness in low socioeconomic status adults speaks to the importance of the ECA study's ability to differentiate among types of psychopathology, including specific affective disorders, to distinguish diagnosable cases from subclinical conditions or depressive symptoms, and to eliminate the socioeconomic bias in clinic populations. The ECA study's epidemiologic data indicate that the risk of affective disorders cuts across socioeconomic boundaries and that low income, low status occupation, and little education do not make one more vulnerable to affective episodes.

URBAN-RURAL RESIDENCE

The apparent rise in affective disorders over the past century has sometimes been attributed to the fact that larger and larger proportions of the total population have been exposed to the stresses of urban life. To test this hypothesis, we can contrast rates of affective disorders in rural versus urban communities in two of the ECA sites, St. Louis and Durham. Our results differ in the two communities (Table 4–19). In St. Louis, rates of bipolar disorder are over two times higher, adjusting for age, race, and sex, in urban than rural areas, while major depressive disorder is less prevalent in the urban than the rural section of the community. In contrast, the urban areas of the Durham ECA have rates of bipolar disorder four times higher and major depressive disorders two times higher than the rural areas.

While the Durham rates confirm the hypothesis of urban/rural differences in affective illness, the St. Louis data are mixed. The geographic differences between the two communities are important. Many of the rural areas surveyed in the Durham ECA are substantially farther away from an urban center and less touched by suburban spread than those surveyed outside St. Louis. This more transitional quality of the St. Louis rural areas compared to Durham may explain the higher prevalence of major depression in them, relative to their respective urban centers.

FINANCIAL DEPENDENCY

Although low socioeconomic status among those employed has little influence on rates of affective disorder, individuals with bipolar disorders or major depression are approximately three times more likely than others to be financially dependent upon public aid (Table 4–20). This dependency

TABLE 4–19 Urban/Rural Differences in One-Year Rates of Affective Disorders (Data Weighted to Local Population)

	Bipolar Disorder		Major Depression	
	One-Year Rate/100	Adjusted Odds Ratio[a]	One-Year Rate/100	Adjusted Odds Ratio[a]
St. Louis:				
Rural	0.5	—	3.5	—
Urban	1.5	2.25***	2.5	0.63***
Durham:				
Rural	0.2	—	1.0	—
Urban	0.8	3.78*	2.3	2.25*

[a]Odds ratios contrast urban against rural groups and are adjusted for sex, age, and race/ethnicity.
*$p < .05$
***$p < .001$

TABLE 4–20 Financial Dependency of Persons with Bipolar or Major
Depressive Disorders in the Last Year

	Percent Financially Dependent	Adjusted Odds Ratio[a]
No affective disorder	9.2	—
Bipolar disorder	23.8	3.49***
Major depression	18.7	2.56***

[a]Odds ratios contrast affected with unaffected persons and are adjusted for sex, age, and race/ethnicity.
***$p < .001$

may reflect, in part, the higher rates of affective disorders observed among
the unemployed as well as the general impairment in social and occupational functioning characteristic of those with affective disorders. Previous
clinical research (Weissman & Paykel, 1974) has demonstrated the social
and interpersonal morbidity of depression in women, that is, the difficulty
depressed women have in caring for their children and in their marriages
and social life. The ECA study's data reveal the economic consequences as
well.

INSTITUTIONAL PREVALENCE

The rates of bipolar disorder and major depression are markedly higher
among individuals living in nursing homes or prisons than in private households. Rates in psychiatric inpatient facilities show the same trend, but
differences are not statistically significant (Table 4–21). The relatively low
proportion of people with affective disorders in psychiatric inpatient facilities may reflect the success of outpatient treatment and medication in
enabling them to function adequately outside of institutions. People in
nursing homes or prisons are, for the most part, confined to their institutions for legal or other medical reasons, and affective disorders may become
associated problems. It also sometimes happens that mania leads to violence or writing checks without sufficient funds in the bank. Such behavior
can eventuate in incarceration if the disorder is not recognized. Depression
may be missed in elderly persons, who are placed in nursing homes because
they seem to fail to recover from a physical illness or are misdiagnosed as
suffering from senile dementia.

TABLE 4–21 One-Year Rates of Affective Disorders by Place of Residence

Place of Residence	Bipolar Disorder		Major Depression	
	One-Year Rate/100	Adjusted Odds Ratio[a]	One-Year Rate/100	Adjusted Odds Ratio[a]
Households	1.0	—	2.7	—
Psychiatric facility	2.2	2.26	4.4	1.66
Prison	5.4	5.75*	9.2	3.63*
Nursing home	9.7	10.80*	16.2	6.96*

[a]Odds ratios contrast institutional residents with household residents and are adjusted for sex, age, and race/ethnicity.
*$p < .05$

USE OF HEALTH SERVICES

Persons with bipolar disorder and major depression are far more likely than those persons without these disorders to have used health services of all types over the course of six months to a year, including psychiatric in- and outpatient facilities and medical in- and outpatient facilities (Table 4–22). These figures confirm other ECA analyses (Leaf et al., 1985b, 1988) reporting the high use of both specialty and general medical services for affective disorders. This increased utilization may well reflect not only use in direct response to affective symptomatology, but also the substantial association between affective disorders and physical health problems. Nonetheless, these findings should be reviewed against the total picture of utilization: While persons with affective disorders make more use than others of health services, the majority of them still do not seek help (Shapiro et al., 1984). Moreover, the quality of the treatment they receive is unknown.

CONCLUSION

Among psychiatric disorders, the affective disorders are relatively common, having occurred in 8% of the adult population at some time in their lives. Severe and persistent affective symptoms are even more common, some of them occurring in close to a third of the adult population. The magnitude of the problem, then, underscores the importance of clinical and epidemiologic research in advancing our understanding of how to prevent affective

TABLE 4-22 Health Services Utilization by Persons with Bipolar or Major Depressive Disorders in the Last Year

	Psychiatric Outpatient (6 mo)		Psychiatric Inpatient (1 yr)		Medical Outpatient (6 mo)		Medical Inpatient (1 yr)	
	Rate of Use	Adjusted Odds Ratio[a]	Rate of Use	Adjusted Odds Ratio[a]	Rate of Use	Adjusted Odds Ratio[a]	Rate of Use	Adjusted Odds Ratio[a]
No affective disorder	6.4	—	0.6	—	56.7	—	12.2	—
Bipolar disorder	38.5	8.94***	9.6	18.36***	79.2	3.06*	29.5	3.35***
Major depression	38.3	7.77***	5.8	11.36***	77.1	2.39*	22.3	2.08***

[a]Odds ratios contrast affected with those without affective disorders and are adjusted for sex, age, and race/ethnicity.

*p < .05

***p < .001

episodes, how to treat individuals experiencing them more effectively, and how to encourage those likely to profit from currently available prophylaxis and treatment to avail themselves of it.

Not everyone is at equal risk of an affective disorder. The young are most likely to be experiencing an affective episode currently and to have had an affective disorder at some point in their lifetime. While the ECA study cannot definitively answer questions about causality, the association of affective disorders with lifestyle suggests that affective disorders may sometimes be triggered by a severing of intimate ties, unemployment, and urban living, all constant if not increasing forces in modern life.

The consequences of affective disorders to society include increased financial dependency and use of health services. While the past three decades have seen major advances in decreasing the suffering of individuals with affective disorders (through medication and other therapies) and preventing relapses, much remains to be done in these areas as well as in prevention of the first episode.

5 Alcohol Abuse and Dependence

JOHN E. HELZER / AUDREY BURNAM / LAWRENCE T. McEVOY

THE DIAGNOSIS OF ALCOHOLISM

A clear understanding of the prevalence and nature of alcoholism in the U.S. population has been frustrated by disagreement among researchers and clinicians as to how the variety of patterns of alcohol involvement should be classified and labeled. Broadly, these patterns are composed of three types of behaviors (Polich & Kaelber, 1985): (1) excessive consumption of alcohol; (2) the social and health problems that are a consequence of excessive consumption; and (3) alcohol dependence, characterized by impaired ability to regulate drinking and the development of physical tolerance and/or dependence. Alcohol dependence is central to many of the definitions of alcoholism (for example, Edwards et al., 1977). However, other definitions accept alcohol-related social and health problems as alternative indicators of alcoholism (Davies, 1976). Many practicing physicians use a variety of indicators in addition to dependence (Filstead, Goby, & Bradley, 1976).

The definition of alcoholism provided by DSM-III recognizes both dependence and negative social consequences as significant indicators of disorder. Two diagnoses are specified: Alcohol abuse requires a pattern of pathological (excessive or uncontrolled) alcohol use *plus* impairment in social or occupational functioning due to alcohol use. Alcohol dependence diagnosis requires *either* a pattern of pathological use *or* impairment in social or occupational functioning *plus* evidence of tolerance or withdrawal (physical dependence). Specific behaviors indicative of each of these criteria are given in DSM-III, and a summary of these criteria and symptoms as they are queried in the DIS is shown below in Table 5–14. According to DSM-III, abuse and dependence are independent; it is possible to diagnose abuse without dependence, dependence without abuse, or both dependence and abuse.

One advantage of the DSM-III criteria is that the focus is on specified patterns of behavior. Definitions that emphasize underlying constructs, such as the dependence syndrome (Edwards & Gross, 1976), are more difficult to utilize because the condition is not directly observable, nor easily inferred from observable behaviors. Perhaps as a result of this emphasis on specific behavior, the DSM-III definition of alcoholism has demonstrated a remarkably high degree of reliability and validity (Robins, 1982). Theoretical disagreements about the nature of alcoholism as a disorder have not been resolved. But DSM-III does provide a standard that can be used to identify, relatively consistently, those persons whose patterns of alcohol involvement are cause for concern.

The recently revised DSM-III criteria (DSM-III-R) include modifications in the alcohol diagnoses. According to these revisions, the central diagnosis is dependence, and alcohol abuse without dependence is defined only as a residual category, that is, evidence of continuing, but below threshold, problems with alcohol. These revisions reflect previous theoretical work and clinical experience suggesting that dependence represents a more severe stage of the disorder, preceded by abuse. The DSM-III-R revisions retain the emphasis on objective symptoms of pathological use, tolerance, and withdrawal, but change the emphasis on impairment in social/occupational functioning to continued use despite such impairment.

PREVIOUS EPIDEMIOLOGIC STUDIES

Most of what we know about the epidemiology of alcoholism in the United States from previous studies is based on rates of cirrhosis mortality, volume of alcohol beverage sales, and population surveys of drinking patterns. These studies, however, have provided information which is "fragmented, ambiguous, and often imprecise" with respect to the prevalence and incidence of alcoholism (Warheit & Auth, 1985).

A formula to estimate the number of alcoholics in the population from cirrhosis death rates (Jellinek, 1959) is inexact, both because of inaccuracies in recorded causes of death, and because there is no fixed ratio of alcoholism to liver cirrhosis, as the formula must assume. Alcohol beverage sales records can be used to calculate average per capita consumption of a population. But per capita consumption does not necessarily tell us about the prevalence of alcoholism. A given per-capita level, for example, could be associated with low rates of alcoholism in a population with a high proportion of moderate drinkers, or conversely with high rates of alcoholism in a population with a high proportion of abstainers.

Cirrhosis death rates and per capita consumption have another limitation. They are aggregate statistics, which can be used only to estimate overall rates in large populations. Aggregate statistics tell us nothing about the structure of alcoholism in the population, such as its severity, frequency of occurrence, or the relationships among its component symptoms. Aggregate statistics are also uninformative about personal characteristics associated with alcoholism or its risk factors such as age, sex, or the presence of other disorders. Such knowledge is obviously crucial to ultimately understanding causation and can inform efforts to develop appropriate health policies for prevention and treatment.

Given the weaknesses of such secondary indicators, the preferred, albeit more costly, way to study the epidemiology of a disorder has been to personally examine representative samples of the general population. Several epidemiologic surveys of alcohol use have been conducted in the United States. Typically, these surveys focus on drinking patterns (usually frequency of drinking and volume consumed per occasion) and on any number of a variety of alcohol-related problems or consequences. Most, however, have not attempted to define or assess prevalence of alcoholism as a specific disorder. This is perhaps not surprising given the predominant trend in this country since the early 1940s to characterize alcoholism as an underlying disease construct that eludes reliable measurement (Rohan, 1982).

Warheit and Auth (1985) have reviewed 12 of the most important of these surveys, all of which used samples representative of the national population. Taken together, they suggest that between 7 and 12% of adult, household residents are current heavy drinkers. Definitions of heavy drinking are necessarily arbitrary but include levels of drinking that are less than what is generally associated with alcoholism in clinical contexts (for example, having 5 drinks twice a month). The studies also suggest that between 5 and 10% of respondents currently have one or more alcohol-related problems, although the findings in this regard have been quite variable, ranging from 2 to 37% depending on the study.

The ECA study contributes in a number of ways to the wealth of information that has been collected in prior surveys on drinking patterns and problems. Most important is that the ECA is the first survey to assess alcoholism as a disorder in a large general population, using objective definitions that have been agreed upon for use in research and clinical practice by a significant portion of the medical community. Thus, this study represents an important link between what we know about alcoholism from our experience in treatment settings and the distribution of the disorder in the general population. Secondly, the study tells us much about the structure of alcoholism in the general population, including the frequency of specific symptoms and age of onset, and its distribution among particular subsamples. Finally, the study permits us to examine associated risk factors and the relationship of alcoholism or alcohol problems to the occurrence of other psychiatric disorders.

As we will see, DSM-III-defined alcohol disorder is one of the most prevalent of the lifetime disorders ascertained in the ECA survey. Alcoholism (a term of convenience we will henceforth use synonymously with alcohol abuse and/or dependence) is a major public health problem, both in the number of persons affected and in the damage it causes to the individual, his or her family, and society at large. In this chapter, we will discuss the prominence of alcohol disorders in the country as a whole, which symptoms are the most and least common, the age at which alcoholism begins, in which social groups it is most common, and inferences about its causes and consequences.

PREVALENCE FROM THE ECA STUDY

Prevalence is the proportion of persons who reported enough alcohol symptoms on the Diagnostic Interview Schedule (DIS) (Robins et al., 1981b) to meet the DSM-III (APA, 1980) requirements for an alcohol diagnosis. Lifetime prevalence counts symptoms occurring at any time in the individual's life, and for the DSM-III alcoholism criteria, symptoms need not be overlapping in time. The definition of current prevalence rates in the DIS (one-year; one-month) varies with the diagnostic category, but for the alcohol disorders the last appearance of at least one symptom defines whether the diagnosis is current, given that full criteria were met at some time.

Lifetime prevalence in the total ECA sample is 13.8% (Table 5-1); that is, one out of every seven persons meets the criteria. Lifetime prevalence for men is even more dramatic, with almost one-quarter (23.8%) meeting the criteria. The rate for women is much lower, 4.6%. Alcoholism is clearly a predominantly male disorder with a male:female ratio of over 5:1.

The huge lifetime prevalence for men strains credibility, but it is important to recognize what this represents. The DIS interview adheres strictly to the DSM-III criteria. For some disorders, like major depression and mania, DSM-III requires that the diagnosis be based on a cluster of symptoms occurring together. But for the alcohol disorders, a minimum of two symptoms is necessary and there is no requirement that they occur at about the same time. Therefore, a respondent can qualify for this diagnosis with one symptom in his youth an one in his middle years or old age. The occurrence at any time in the respondent's life of one symptom of pathological alcohol use and one of social or occupational impairment is sufficient for a DSM-III lifetime diagnosis of alcohol abuse. A minimum of one symptom of either of these along with some evidence of either tolerance or withdrawal is sufficient for a diagnosis of dependence. However, few of

Table 5–1 Alcohol Abuse and/or Dependence: Prevalence of Alcoholism by Sex and Ethnicity[a]

	Prevalence in Percent (SE)						Remission[a] (%)
	One-Month		One-Year		Lifetime		
Total	3.29	(0.18)	6.80	(0.26)	13.76	(0.36)	51
Ethnicity:							
Whites	3.17	(0.20)	6.69	(0.28)	13.58	(0.39)	51
Blacks	3.77	(0.61)	6.59	(0.80)	13.76	(1.11)	52
Hispanics	4.21	(0.89)	9.08	(1.28)	16.70	(1.66)	46
Men:	5.74	(0.35)	11.90	(0.49)	23.83	(0.64)	50
White	5.49	(0.37)	11.69	(0.53)	23.44	(0.69)	50
Black	6.68	(1.19)	11.51	(1.53)	23.71	(2.03)	51
Hispanic	7.39	(1.66)	15.97	(2.33)	30.02	(2.91)	47
Women:	1.06	(0.15)	2.16	(0.21)	4.57	(0.30)	53
White	1.03	(0.16)	2.11	(0.23)	4.52	(0.33)	53
Black	1.35	(0.50)	2.50	(0.68)	5.47	(0.99)	54
Hispanic	1.17	(0.67)	2.46	(0.97)	3.85	(1.20)	36

[a]Lifetime prevalence (Lt) minus one-year prevalence (1 Yr) divided by lifetime prevalence (Lt): (Lt − 1 Yr)/Lt.

those given the diagnosis of alcoholism have only the minimum number of symptoms.

Almost 7% of the total sample both met lifetime criteria and had at least one alcohol symptom during the past year, and about 3% have had a symptom in the past month (Table 5–1). The one-year:lifetime prevalence ratio (6.80/13.76) for the total sample is 0.49, that is, half of those who have ever met DSM-III criteria for alcoholism have had an alcohol-related problem in the past year. Similarly, a quarter (24%) of the lifetime cases report a problem in the last 30 days; 48% with a problem in the past year have had one in the past month. It is generally assumed that alcoholism is a chronic disorder, that is, those who have had serious difficulties at some point in their lives are likely to continue having them. However, those impressions about the chronicity and persistence of alcoholism are based largely on clinical samples—alcoholics who come to treatment for the disorder. Previous studies in the general population show turnover and recovery (Clark & Cahalan, 1976), consistent with our findings, suggesting that the disorder is not necessarily continuous. Even in samples drawn from treatment settings, alcoholism is known for remissions and relapse, "going on and off the wagon." At any one point in time, a large porportion of alcoholics can be expected to be sober. In our sample, 63% of those who met lifetime criteria for alcoholism and had been especially heavy consumers at some point in their lives (seven or more drinks daily for two weeks or more) told us that they had not had a period of drinking that heavily at any time in the past year.

There are few differences in rates between blacks and whites, either overall or by sex (Table 5-1). Blacks have only a slightly higher one-month prevalence than whites, and rates for lifetime and one-year prevalences are even more similar. (Recall that the "whites" category includes a few orientals and American Indians. Since these two nonwhite ethnic groups combined constitute only 2.5% of the total population, the category of "whites" is dominated by non-Hispanic Caucasians.)

Lifetime, one-year, and one-month prevalence rates for Hispanic men are higher than for the other two ethnic groups, although not significantly so, while rates for Hispanic women are more similar to rates for other ethnic groups but generally lower. Thus, the sex differential for Hispanics is particularly great.

Remission rates (defined as the proportion of lifetime cases that have had no alcohol problems in the past year) are quite consistent across the sex and ethnic groups. They are nearly identical for men and women and for blacks and whites. Remission rates are lower for Hispanics, especially Hispanic women, but again the difference is not statistically significant.

There is a significant variation in the lifetime prevalence rates among the five study sites (Table 5-2). Baltimore, St. Louis, and Los Angeles are similar to one another but have higher lifetime rates than New Haven and Durham. This pattern also holds for one-year prevalence, although Baltimore replaces St. Louis as the site having the highest rate. Remission rates at every site are in the range of 45-55%.

Table 5-2 Alcohol Abuse and/or Dependence: Site Differences[a]

	Prevalence in Percent (Se)						
	One-Month		One-Year		Lifetime		Remission (%)
New Haven	3.16	(0.33)	6.07	(0.45)	11.34	(0.60)	46
Baltimore	4.73	(0.41)	7.73	(0.53)	15.23	(0.72)	49
St. Louis	2.50	(0.38)	7.51	(0.64)	15.88	(0.89)	53
Durham	2.72	(0.34)	5.07	(0.46)	10.72	(0.64)	53
Los Angeles	3.71	(0.38)	6.98	(0.51)	14.96	(0.72)	53

[a]Weighted to population of the catchment areas sampled at each site.

PREVALENCE BY AGE, SEX, AND ETHNICITY

Lifetime prevalence rates are significantly higher among men and women under the age of 45 than among those older. For men, lifetime prevalence in the youngest age group (18–29 year olds) is 27%. It rises in the 30–44 year olds but falls in 45–64-year-olds, and is lowest of all (14%) in those 65 years and older (Table 5–3). Among women, the highest prevalence rate (7%) is found in the youngest age group, and it falls steadily to 1.5% in those 65 years and older. Possible reasons for this fall in lifetime prevalence with age include the artifact of recall, low survival rates among alcoholics, and response style as discussed in chapter 2, but we cannot dismiss the possibility that this is a reflection of a true cohort effect, that is, that alcoholism is more prevalent in younger generations of Americans. There has been a steady increase in per capita alcohol consumption in the United States since at least 1950 that has only begun to level off since 1981 (NIAAA, 1985), about the time the first ECA interviews were being conducted. In fact, in some areas, per capita alcohol consumption has almost doubled in the last 30 years (Wattis, 1983). Changes in societal drinking habits that might lead to increased rates of alcoholism are likely to affect younger adults more than older ones. As we will see below, alcoholism tends to have a youthful onset. Older persons were already beyond the major period of risk when recent changes in societal drinking patterns occurred.

Ethnic groups show strikingly different patterns of age-related lifetime rates of alcoholism (Table 5–3 and Figure 5–1). First, we contrast blacks and

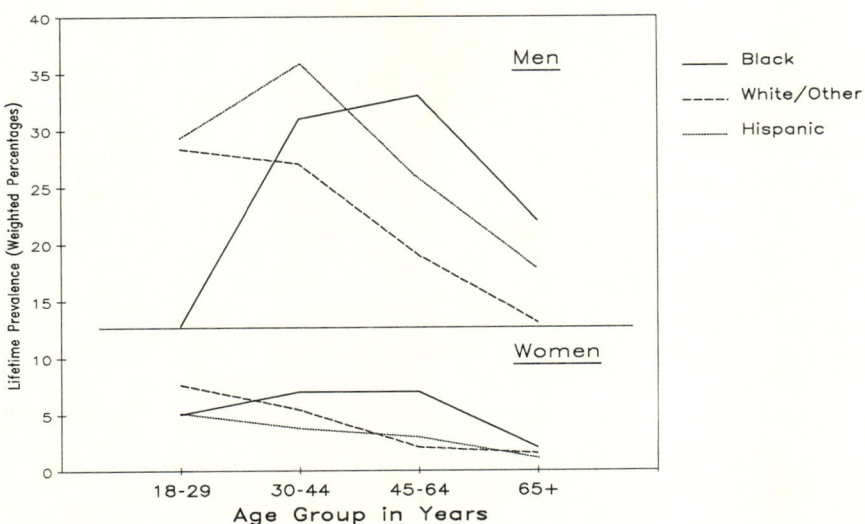

Figure 5-1 Alcohol Abuse/Dependence: Prevalence by Age, Sex, and Ethnicity

Table 5-3 Prevalence of Alcoholism by Age, Sex, and Ethnicity, in Percent (SE)

	Men				Women				Male to Female Ratio		
	One-month	One-Year	Lifetime	Remission	One-Month	One-Year	Lifetime	Remission	One-Month	One-Year	Lifetime
Total	5.74 (0.35)	11.90 (0.49)	23.83 (0.64)	50	1.60 (0.15)	2.16 (0.21)	4.75 (0.30)	53	5.4	5.5	5.2
Age:											
18–29	7.16 (0.67)	17.03 (0.98)	26.63 (1.16)	36	2.03 (0.37)	4.14 (0.53)	6.89 (0.67)	40	3.5	4.1	3.9
30–44	7.29 (0.75)	14.10 (1.10)	27.91 (1.29)	49	1.14 (0.30)	2.12 (0.40)	5.50 (0.64)	61	6.4	6.7	5.1
45–64	4.34 (0.58)	7.85 (0.77)	21.15 (1.17)	63	0.33 (0.16)	1.04 (0.28)	3.06 (0.47)	66	13.2	7.5	6.9
65+	1.93 (0.58)	3.10 (0.73)	13.52 (1.45)	77	0.40 (0.22)	0.46 (0.24)	1.49 (0.43)	69	4.8	6.7	9.1
Whites:											
18–29	7.63 (0.78)	18.10 (1.13)	28.31 (1.32)	36	2.22 (0.44)	4.54 (0.62)	7.50 (0.78)	39	3.4	4.0	3.8
30–44	6.46 (0.78)	13.52 (1.08)	27.00 (1.40)	50	1.04 (0.31)	1.96 (0.43)	5.47 (0.70)	64	6.2	6.9	4.9
45–64	4.02 (0.61)	7.20 (0.80)	19.75 (1.23)	64	0.20 (0.13)	0.81 (0.27)	2.60 (0.47)	69	20.1	8.9	7.6
65+	1.74 (0.59)	2.85 (0.75)	12.53 (1.49)	77	0.42 (0.24)	0.47 (0.25)	1.46 (0.45)	68	4.1	6.1	8.6
Blacks:											
18–29	4.03 (1.53)	7.92 (2.11)	12.61 (2.59)	37	1.11 (0.77)	2.37 (1.12)	4.19 (1.48)	44	3.6	3.3	3.0
30–44	11.04 (2.80)	16.30 (3.30)	31.33 (4.15)	48	2.08 (1.18)	3.37 (1.49)	6.88 (2.09)	51	5.3	4.8	4.6
45–64	8.17 (2.68)	15.24 (3.52)	32.99 (4.61)	54	1.34 (1.01)	2.56 (1.39)	7.33 (2.99)	65	6.1	6.0	4.5
65+	0.82 (1.36)	2.93 (2.55)	21.63 (6.21)	86	0.34 (0.72)	0.60 (0.96)	2.20 (1.82)	73	2.4	4.9	9.8
Hispanics:											
18–29	6.06 (2.30)	19.29 (3.81)	29.76 (4.41)	35	1.90 (1.38)	3.59 (1.87)	4.90 (2.17)	27	3.2	5.4	6.1
30–44	12.24 (3.86)	19.16 (4.63)	35.91 (5.65)	47	0.97 (1.10)	1.84 (1.51)	3.67 (2.11)	50	12.6	10.4	9.8
45–64	3.86 (2.65)	7.69 (3.67)	25.97 (6.03)	70	0.81 (1.20)	2.65 (2.15)	3.46 (2.44)	23	4.8	2.9	7.5
65+	5.47 (5.79)	6.57 (6.31)	18.10 (9.81)	64	0.00 —	0.00 —	0.79 (1.88)	100	—	—	22.9

whites. Among the youngest men (age 18–29), the lifetime prevalence rate of alcoholism in whites is over twice what it is in blacks. In the next age group, the rates are more similar, with a slight predominance in blacks. The black predominance becomes still greater in men 45–64, and in the oldest group (65 and over), the ratio of black to white rates is the reverse of what it was among the youngest group, that is, nearly twice as high in blacks compared to whites. The pattern for black and white women is similar to that for men.

In the two younger age groups, lifetime prevalence rates are higher for Hispanic men than for either black or white men, and Hispanics are intermediate in the older two groups. Hispanic men's rates exceed white men's in every age group, while Hispanic women's exceed whites' only in the 45–64 age group. Rates for elderly Hispanic women are the lowest found for any ethnic age group, less than 1%. None of these differences is statistically significant.

One-year prevalence rates are highest in the youngest ages and fall in each successive older group (Table 5–3). Further, in each successive age group, the current rates are a smaller proportion of the lifetime rates. Thus, not only have older persons had less alcoholism, but older alcoholics have recent problems less often. This is demonstrated by the remission rates, which rise consistently with age. The high rate of remission in the elderly is particularly notable among blacks. While elderly black men have rates of lifetime alcoholism almost double that in elderly whites, their one-year prevalence rates are about the same, and their one-month rates is less than half of that in whites. Only 14% of blacks 65 and older who have a lifetime diagnosis of alcoholism have had any problems in the last year and less than 4% in the last month. The corresponding figures for elderly whites are 23% in the last year and 14% in the last month.

While alcoholism is obviously a disorder predominant among males, there is evidence of convergence in the rates between sexes in the younger age groups. With only two exceptions, the male to female ratios in Table 5–3 are lowest in the 18–29 year olds for all prevalence periods and ethnic groups. Thus, alcoholism has become more prevalent in younger age groups for both men and women, but the increase is particularly great for young women.

SUBTYPES OF ALCOHOLISM

According to DSM-III, an individual can simultaneously meet DSM-III criteria for alcohol abuse and dependence. Of the total ECA sample, 1.6% met criteria for alcohol dependence but not abuse; 5.8% for abuse but not dependence, and 6.4% met criteria for both abuse and dependence. We will group together those who met criteria for dependence, with and without abuse in addition, transforming alcohol abuse into a residual category as it is in DSM-III-R. Alcoholism, as we use the term here, is the sum of the abuse only and dependence (with or without abuse) subgroups (columns 1 plus 4 and columns 6 plus 9, Table 5-4).

For the entire sample, the lifetime prevalence of total alcoholism is 13.8% and 7.9% have been dependent. The proportion of alcoholics who have been dependent rises with age (Table 5-4). Among men, 46% of those in the youngest age group met criteria for dependence; this proportion rises to 82% in those 65 and over. Among women, this rise is from 51% in the youngest group to 76% in the oldest. The increase with age in the proportion of alcoholics who have been dependent is consistent across ethnic groups. This indicates either that the relatively few older persons who have warranted a diagnosis of alcoholism are more likely than younger persons to have had the more serious form of the disorder, or perhaps this low rate is partly explained by poor recall for the less serious form that did not progress to dependency.

As we might expect, the symptom level for abusers (without dependence) is much lower than for those dependent, though criteria for either disorder requires only two symptoms. There is a wide range of severity, as measured by the number of reported lifetime symptoms, among those meeting criteria for either alcohol abuse or dependence (Figure 5-2). However, among those with abuse only, the modal number of lifetime symptoms is the minimum of two, and the mean number of symptoms is only 3.3. Among those diagnosed as alcohol dependent, the mode is 6, and the mean is 6.4.

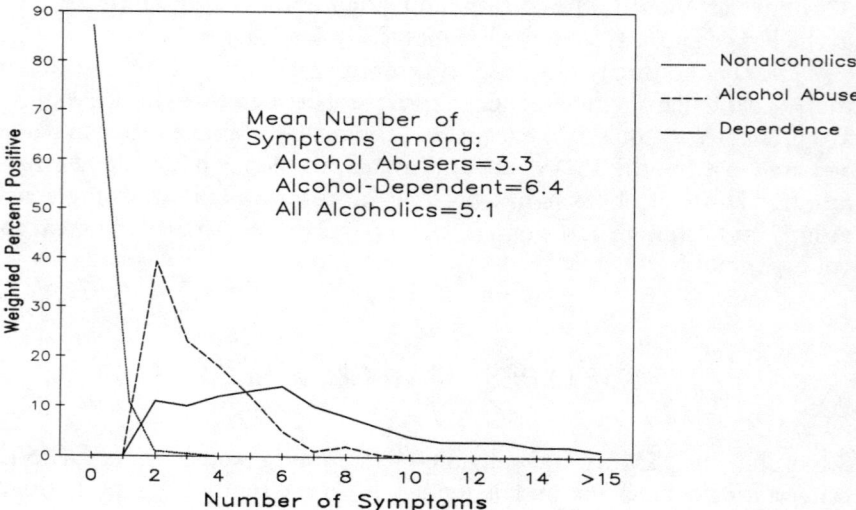

Figure 5-2 Number of Alcoholic Symptoms in Alcoholics and Nonalcoholics

Table 5–4 Prevalence of Lifetime Alcohol Abuse and Dependence by Age, Sex, and Ethnicity in Percent (SE)

	Men					Women				
	Abuse Only	Dependence Only	Abuse Plus Dependence	Dependence with/without Abuse	Proportion of All Alcoholics Who Have Been Dependent	Abuse Only	Dependence Only	Abuse Plus Dependence	Dependence with/without Abuse	Proportion of All Alcoholics Who Have Been Dependent
Total	10.30 (0.46)	2.69 (0.24)	10.84 (0.47)	13.53 (0.51)	57	1.76 (0.19)	0.51 (0.10)	2.31 (0.22)	2.82 (0.24)	62
Age:										
18–29	14.41 (0.92)	2.16 (0.38)	10.05 (0.79)	12.21 (0.86)	46	3.35 (0.47)	0.41 (0.17)	3.12 (0.46)	3.53 (0.49)	51
30–44	13.27 (0.97)	2.82 (0.48)	11.82 (0.93)	14.64 (1.02)	52	1.73 (0.36)	0.67 (0.23)	3.09 (0.48)	3.76 (0.53)	68
45–64	6.03 (0.68)	2.87 (0.48)	12.25 (0.94)	15.12 (1.03)	72	0.90 (0.26)	0.47 (0.19)	1.69 (0.35)	2.16 (0.40)	70
65+	2.43 (0.65)	3.42 (0.77)	7.66 (1.13)	11.09 (1.33)	82	0.36 (0.21)	0.48 (0.24)	0.66 (0.29)	1.14 (0.37)	76
Whites:										
18–29	15.66 (1.06)	2.09 (0.42)	10.56 (0.90)	12.65 (0.97)	45	3.76 (0.56)	0.31 (0.16)	3.43 (0.54)	3.74 (0.56)	50
30–44	14.10 (1.10)	2.76 (0.52)	10.13 (0.95)	12.90 (1.06)	48	1.76 (0.41)	0.63 (0.24)	3.08 (0.53)	3.71 (0.58)	68
45–64	5.61 (0.71)	2.56 (0.49)	11.58 (0.99)	14.14 (1.08)	72	0.73 (0.25)	0.38 (0.18)	1.49 (0.36)	1.87 (0.40)	72
65+	2.18 (0.66)	3.01 (0.77)	7.34 (1.17)	10.35 (1.37)	83	0.38 (0.23)	0.47 (0.26)	0.61 (0.29)	1.08 (0.39)	74
Blacks:										
18–29	5.33 (1.75)	2.05 (1.10)	5.23 (1.74)	7.28 (2.03)	58	1.19 (0.80)	0.75 (0.63)	2.25 (1.09)	3.00 (1.26)	72
30–44	8.64 (2.51)	3.33 (1.60)	19.37 (3.53)	22.69 (3.75)	72	1.92 (1.13)	1.41 (0.97)	3.55 (1.53)	4.96 (1.79)	72
45–64	9.09 (2.82)	5.75 (2.28)	18.16 (3.78)	23.91 (4.18)	72	2.37 (1.33)	1.26 (0.98)	3.70 (1.66)	4.96 (1.91)	68
65+	3.85 (2.90)	5.24 (3.36)	12.54 (5.00)	17.78 (5.77)	82	0.19 (0.54)	0.71 (1.04)	1.30 (1.41)	2.01 (1.74)	91
Hispanics:										
18–29	15.73 (3.51)	3.52 (1.78)	10.51 (2.96)	14.03 (3.35)	47	3.14 (1.75)	1.04 (1.02)	0.72 (0.85)	1.76 (1.32)	36
30–44	11.05 (3.69)	3.04 (2.02)	21.81 (4.86)	24.86 (5.09)	69	1.27 (1.26)	0.04 (0.22)	2.36 (1.70)	2.39 (1.71)	65
45–64	8.58 (3.85)	1.80 (1.83)	15.59 (4.99)	17.39 (5.22)	70	1.31 (1.52)	0.66 (1.08)	1.50 (1.62)	2.15 (1.94)	62
65+	7.28 (6.62)	3.90 (4.94)	6.92 (6.47)	10.83 (7.92)	60	0.11 (0.71)	0.00 —	0.68 (1.74)	0.68 (1.74)	86

Despite their lower number of lifetime symptoms, abusers are slightly *more* likely than those dependent to have experienced a symptom in the past year (54% versus 47%), showing that abuse is an early (or perhaps easily forgotten) form of the disorder.

CROSS-SECTIONAL ALCOHOLISM RATES

Since our measure of current prevalence can include persons with only a single current symptom, it does not tell us how many are experiencing enough symptoms close to the time of interview to meet full diagnostic criteria. However, in three of the ECA sites—Baltimore, Durham, and Los Angeles—respondents were asked to date the recency of last occurrence of every symptom they reported. By counting symptoms present within a specified recent period, we can determine what proportion of subjects meet "cross-sectional" criteria for various time frames including the past month and the past year (Figure 5–3).

It is interesting to contrast the cross-sectional rates (Figure 5–3) with rates in Table 5–1 where "current" prevalence requires the presence of only a single symptom. The latter are greater, but not strikingly so. One-month prevalence for the total sample is 3.3%, versus 2.2% for the one-month

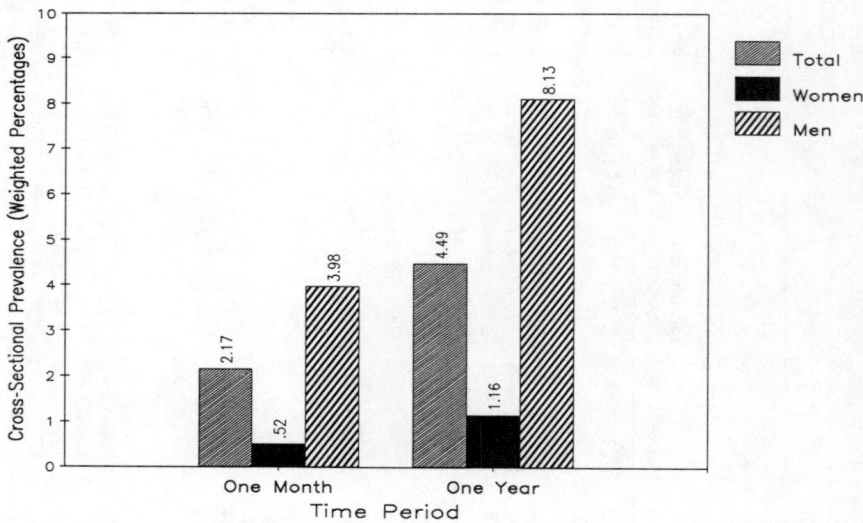

Figure 5–3 Cross-Sectional Prevalence of Alcohol Abuse/Dependence
Data from 3 ECA Sites—Baltimore, Durham, Los Angeles

cross-sectional diagnosis, and the comparable one-year figures are 6.8% compared to 4.5% cross-sectionally. By either estimate, alcoholism is a major problem, with 4.5 to 7% of the population being actively symptomatic in the past year, and 2 to 3% in the past month. The sex ratio heavily favors males for both one-month (7.7) and one-year (7.0) cross-sectional findings.

DRINKING PATTERNS

So far, we have been looking only at DSM-III-defined alcohol disorders. But substance abuse is unique among psychiatric disorders in that substance exposure is a prerequisite for illness development. Since differences in exposure will affect the frequency of disorder, it is interesting to examine alcohol consumption patterns by ECA site (Figure 5–4). The first category consists of those who have never taken a drink of alcohol, that is, lifelong abstainers. Next are social drinkers, those who do not deny drinking but do deny both heavy consumption and all of the alcohol-related problems we asked about. Heavy or problem drinkers are those who report consumption of seven or more drinks at least one evening a week for several months (or daily for two or more weeks) and/or one or more lifetime drinking problems, but fail to meet DSM-III criteria for alcohol abuse or dependence. It

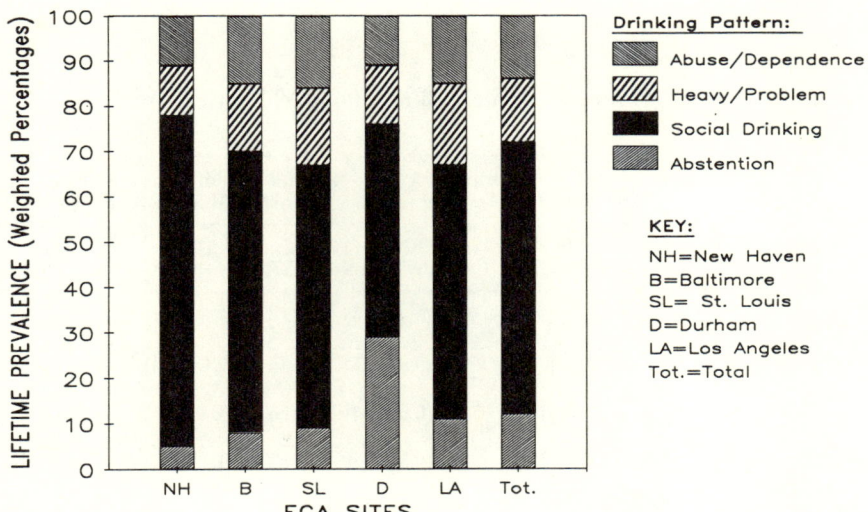

Figure 5–4 Lifetime Drinking Patterns by ECA Site
Site Data Weighted to Local Population; Total Weighted to National Demographic Distribution

is clear that the vast majority of people included in this survey have consumed alcohol in their lives; only 10% of the aggregate ECA sample are classified as lifelong abstainers.

More than two-thirds of those exposed to alcohol are social drinkers, while one out of six exposed have had enough problems to be considered alcoholic. But these rates vary by ECA site. New Haven and Durham, which have the lowest lifetime prevalence rates of alcoholism, also have the lowest rates of heavy or problem drinking; apart from this similarity, however, the drinking patterns in these two sites differ. New Haven has the lowest rate of abstinence, and the highest rate of social drinking. For Durham, a more rural region lying in the Bible Belt, the opposite is the case. Here, over a quarter (28%) of the population abstains from alcohol, and a correspondingly smaller porportion drinks socially.

We can calculate the lifetime prevalence rate of abuse and/or dependence among those who are at risk for alcoholism because they have at least tried an alcoholic drink. Lifetime prevalence of alcoholism among drinkers is highest in St. Louis and lowest in New Haven (Table 5-5). Durham is near the average. This challenges a long-held theory, that is, that within environments that are relatively abstinent, those who do drink are more likely to be alcoholic.

Lifetime prevalence of alcoholism among all drinkers is 15.4%, compared to 13.8% in the total population, including abstainers. Removing abstainers from the denominator has a greater impact on female than male

Table 5-5 Lifetime Prevalence of Alcoholism Among All Drinkers and All Heavy Drinkers[a]

	Percent (SE) of All Drinkers Who Are Alcoholic			Percent (SE) of Heavy/Problem Drinkers Who Are Alcoholic		
	TOTAL (N=16,518)	MEN (N=7,821)	WOMEN (N=8,697)	TOTAL (N=5,087)	MEN (N=3,719)	WOMEN (N=1,368)
Total	15.4 (0.4)	25.1 (0.7)	5.4 (0.4)	48.5 (1.0)	53.0 (1.1)	34.7 (1.9)
New Haven	12.0 (0.6)	19.4 (0.1)	5.1 (0.6)	51.3 (2.0)	55.6 (2.4)	40.4 (3.7)
Baltimore	16.5 (0.8)	29.0 (1.4)	5.4 (0.6)	49.8 (1.8)	55.8 (2.1)	33.0 (3.3)
St. Louis	17.5 (0.9)	30.3 (1.7)	5.0 (0.8)	49.4 (2.2)	54.2 (2.4)	32.5 (4.3)
Durham	15.1 (0.9)	23.4 (1.4)	4.8 (0.8)	45.3 (2.1)	49.5 (2.4)	30.0 (4.2)
Los Angeles	16.8 (0.8)	25.6 (1.3)	7.1 (0.8)	46.7 (1.8)	50.3 (2.1)	36.2 (3.4)

[a]Total weighted to U.S. population. Site data weighted to population of the catchment areas sampled at each site.

prevalences since more women (15.4%) are abstainers than men (4.8%). Overall, the lifetime prevalence of alcoholism among female drinkers is 5.4% compared to 4.6% for all women, still far below the male rate. Thus, women's lower rate is only trivially explained by their having a disproportionate number of abstainers.

One of the theories about the male predominance among alcoholics is that many women drinkers are never exposed to enough alcohol to be at risk, either because of social custom or because women more often than men have negative physiological reactions after drinking small amounts. If this is the case, then women's advantage should disappear when only heavy drinkers are considered. Across the five sites, there were over 3,700 men who were heavy drinkers and about 1,300 women. Among heavy drinkers, the alcoholism prevalence rate for men is 53% and for women 35% (Table 5-5). The male/female prevalence ratio drops to 1.5:1, as compared to 5:1 in the total population. Thus, it is clear that women who drink heavily are much like their male counterparts in their rate of alcoholism. This would seem to support the idea that social and biological factors influencing exposure to alcohol are important contributors to the sex differential in rates.

AGE OF RISK

The ECA study defined the age of onset of disorders as the age at which the first symptom was experienced, and recency as the age of the most recent symptom. Duration is the period between these two.

Alcoholism is a disorder of youthful onset. Almost 40% of those who ever had the disorder had a symptom between 15 and 19, and the proportion of cases that have begun by age 30 is more than 80% (Figure 5-5). Furthermore, early onset has been the rule for all the generations alive in the 1980s (Figure 5-6). (For the youngest group, not yet out of their twenties, onset is, of course, entirely before 30, and mostly before 25.) However, there continues to be a small but measurable incidence of new cases of alcoholism even in the 70s.

Among men, at least half of all onsets have occurred before age 30 for all age groups; among women, this is true only for those under age 45 (Table 5-6). At all ages, women have a later age of onset than men.

Having found that alcoholism typically begins early and that the probability of having had a symptom in the current year decreases with age, we might surmise that alcoholism has a natural history of a fixed duration. Of course, we can estimate its duration only in persons no longer actively alcoholic. It is clear from clinical studies that even a full year without alcohol problems is no guarantee that remission will continue indefinitely

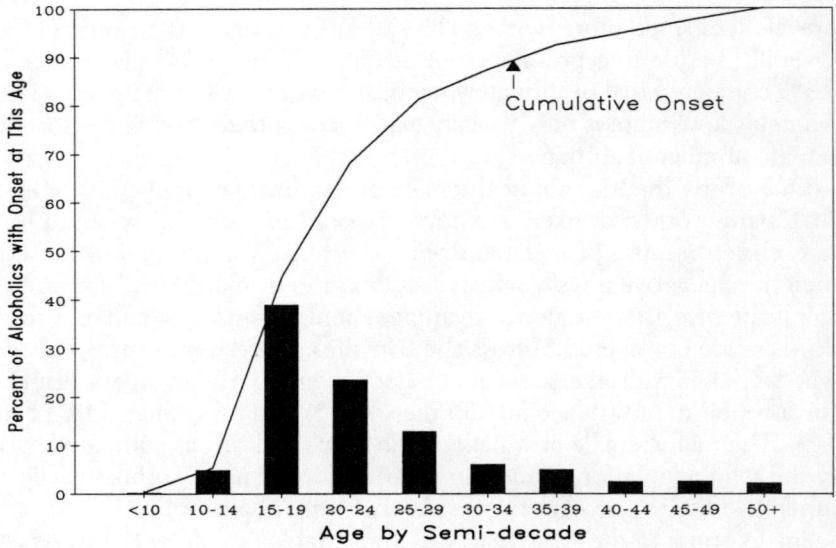

Figure 5–5 Age of Onset of First Alcoholic Symptom Among Those with Alcoholism

(Vaillant, 1983). Nonetheless, we will require only one year free of symptoms when we examine duration so as to make our definition of remission consistent with that used for the other disorders discussed in this volume; as a result, we may be including some cases who will in fact relapse later.

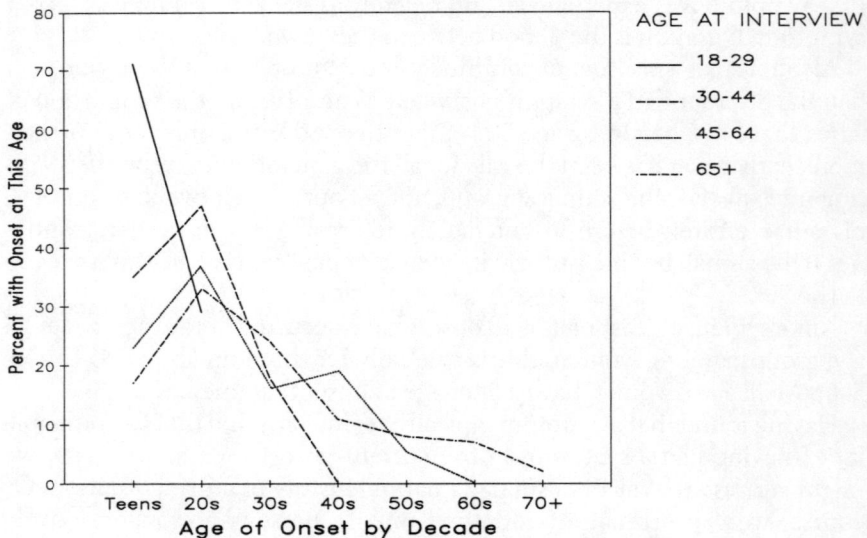

Figure 5–6 Age of Onset of Alcoholism by Age Group at Interview

Table 5-6 Age of Onset of Alcoholism by Sex and Age Groups
(Cumulative Prevalence)

	Age at Interview							
	18–29		30–44		45–64		65 +	
	Men	Women	Men	Women	Men	Women	Men	Women
18	12.2	3.0	6.4	0.7	2.8	0.1	1.0	0.1
30	26.6	6.9	23.6	3.7	13.6	1.1	6.8	0.5
45			27.9	5.5	18.5	2.2	10.8	1.0
65					21.1	3.1	13.3	1.4
Total							13.5	1.5

Most (54%) remitted cases give dates for their first and last symptoms less
than five years apart, suggesting a short duration of the disorder. In almost
three-quarters, the estimated duration is less than 11 years (Figure 5–7).
These results are very different from those seen in patients, who frequently
come to treatment for the first time only after many years of alcohol
problems. Our findings may help to explain why so few persons with

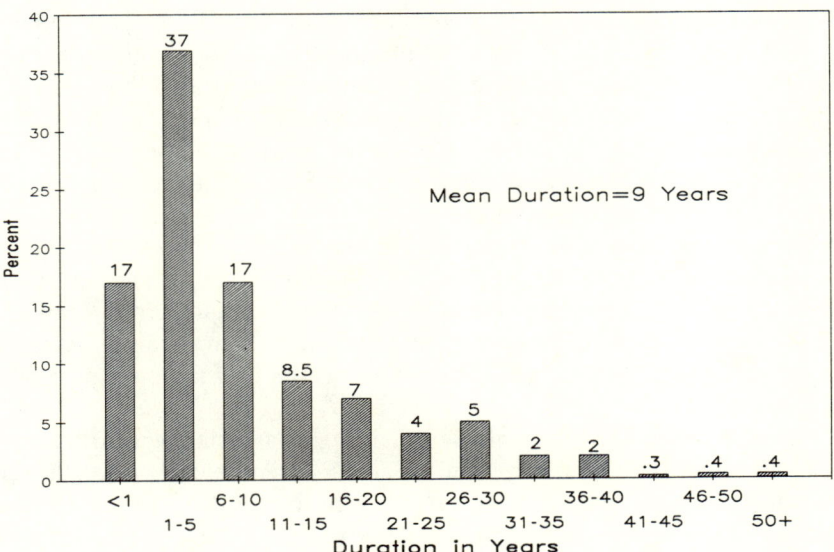

Figure 5–7 Duration of Alcoholism Among Those in Remission 12 Months
or More

alcohol problems in the general population seek care. Many appear to be able to reduce their drinking sufficiently to terminate their difficulties quite early in the course of their disorder. It is those who try and fail that appear for treatment.

ALCOHOLISM AND OTHER PSYCHIATRIC DISORDERS

There is evidence from clinical samples that alcoholism and other psychiatric disorders often occur together, but what is difficult to tell from clinical samples is whether such co-occurrence might simply be a sampling bias. It may be that alcoholics are unlikely to appear in treatment settings unless some other disorder is also present. This population sample provides us the opportunity to examine the comorbidity of alcoholism with other psychiatric disorder in the absence of such a treatment-seeking bias. One way of doing this is to examine the likelihood of a second psychiatric disorder among those with any psychiatric illness contrasted with the likelihood of a second illness among alcoholics. One-third (35%) of the total ECA sample met lifetime criteria for at least one of the psychiatric diagnoses covered in this study, and one-third (32%) of those with one diagnosis had a second. But among alcoholics, almost half (47%) had a second diagnosis. Thus, alcoholism is particularly likely to coexist with other diagnoses.

Much of this comorbidity is accounted for by drug abuse and dependence. Among those who do not meet lifetime criteria for alcohol abuse or dependence, 3.8% have a positive drug diagnosis, and for two-thirds, this is only abuse of cannabis (or tetrahydrocannabinols [THC] derived from the marijuana plant). Among those with alcohol abuse or dependence, the likelihood of a drug diagnosis is much greater (22%), and abuse is limited to cannabis for only half of those affected.

Conversely, among those using only cannabis, the lifetime prevalence rate of alcoholism is about one-third (36%) (Figure 5–8). Among users of harder drugs, the alcoholism rate is much higher, ranging from a low of 62% in users of stimulants to a dramatic high of 84% in cocaine users. In this general population sample, alcoholism occurs in a majority of those using hard drugs.

Other diagnoses with which alcoholism is highly associated are antisocial personality, mania, and schizophrenia (Table 5–7). Antisocial personality is even more strongly associated with alcoholism than is drug abuse. This is consistent for every age group, and at all five of the ECA sites. The diagnosis most often reported in the clinical literature among alcoholics is depression (Hesselbrock et al., 1985), a diagnosis only moderately elevated among alcoholics in this general population. However, our findings are not incon-

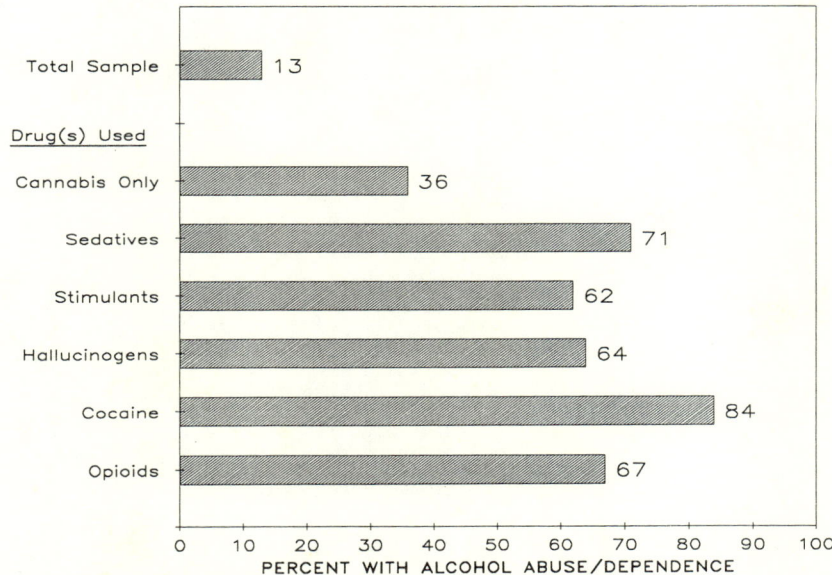

Figure 5–8 Lifetime Prevalence of Alcohol Abuse/Dependence Among Users of Specific Drugs

sistent with the clinical experience. It seems likely that the occurrence of depression motivates alcoholics to seek treatment more often than do drug abuse or antisocial personality, diagnoses with low rates of treatment. Mania and schizophrenia have high rates of treatment, but since these disorders are so infrequent compared with depression, chance alone dictates that alcoholics are more likely to show depression than either mania or schizophrenia.

Comorbidity of alcoholism with other disorders is more common in women than men. While 44% of the male alcoholics have a second diagnosis, 65% of the female alcoholics do. This higher rate is in part because women are more likely than men to have the common diagnoses of depression and phobia. But the more important reason seems to be the fact that alcoholism is so much more deviant in women than men, as indicated by a male/female prevalence ratio of over five (Table 5–3). For disorders other than cognitive impairment, obsessive compulsive, and dysthymia comorbidity ratios are higher for female than male alcoholics. Nonetheless, female and male alcoholics have highest comorbidity ratios with the same diagnoses: antisocial personality, drug abuse, mania, and schizophrenia.

Establishing Which Disorder Comes First. When two disorders are associated, the one that occurs first might be a risk factor for the other. Overall, alcoholism precedes the onset of depression in the majority of cases (78%). However, among women, depression is usually antecedent (66%). (We dropped from these analyses alcoholics with diagnoses of antisocial person-

Table 5-7 Comorbidity of Alcoholism and Other Psychiatric Disorders

Psychiatric Diagnosis	Prevalence Ratios[a]		
	Total	Men	Women
Antisocial personality	19.6	12.0	29.6
Mania	5.4	6.5	9.3
Drug abuse/dependence	5.7	4.8	8.8
Schizophrenia	3.4	4.6	5.6
Panic disorder	2.6	4.2	4.4
Obsessive compulsive	2.0	3.0	2.1
Dysthymia	1.7	2.5	2.2
Major depression	1.6	2.4	2.7
Phobic disorders	1.4	1.8	2.1
Cognitive impairment	1.1	1.2	0.7
Any diagnosis	2.0	2.4	2.2

[a]Prevalence ratios are prevalence in alcoholics divided by prevalence in nonalcoholics.

ality disorder, drug abuse/dependence, or schizophrenia since these disorders are themselves associated with depression and alcoholism, and might have explained the relationship between depression and alcoholism.) In both sexes, alcoholism is slightly less severe when depression is the antecedent diagnosis.

By definition, antisocial personality has its onset before 15. Therefore, it necessarily virtually always precedes alcoholism. However, it has the effect of lowering the age of onset of alcoholism. Consistent with findings in clinical samples that antisocial alcoholics have exceptionally early onsets, the mean age of onset for antisocial alcoholics is only 20 versus 24 in alcoholics without antisocial personality. Antisocial alcoholics also have a higher lifetime alcohol symptom count and a longer duration of alcoholism. In fact, the severity (based on symptom counts) of the two disorders is positively related, with a correlation of .37 for women and .57 for men. The association of these two disorders is stronger in older respondents than in younger ones. This suggests that in the past alcoholism was closely associated with other forms of social deviance, but that as alcoholism has become more prevalent, less antisocial portions of the population have been affected by it.

OTHER ASSOCIATED FACTORS

Education. Overall, there is a downward trend in lifetime prevalence with higher levels of education (Figure 5–9). What is more interesting is the sawtooth shape of this curve. Regardless of final level of attainment, those who finish an educational program and go no farther have lower rates of alcoholism than those who begin the next higher level but drop out. Thus, those with an eighth-grade education have lower rates of alcoholism not only than those with less education but also lower rates than those who begin but drop out of high school or college. (We include as high school dropouts those whose highest degree is the graduate equivalency [GED], available to dropouts who later pass an equivalency test.) Similarly, high school graduates who do not enter college have a lower prevalence rate of alcoholism than those who begin but do not complete college as well as a lower rate than high school dropouts have. College graduates have the lowest prevalence, but it is only slightly lower than that of eighth-grade graduates who never entered high school.

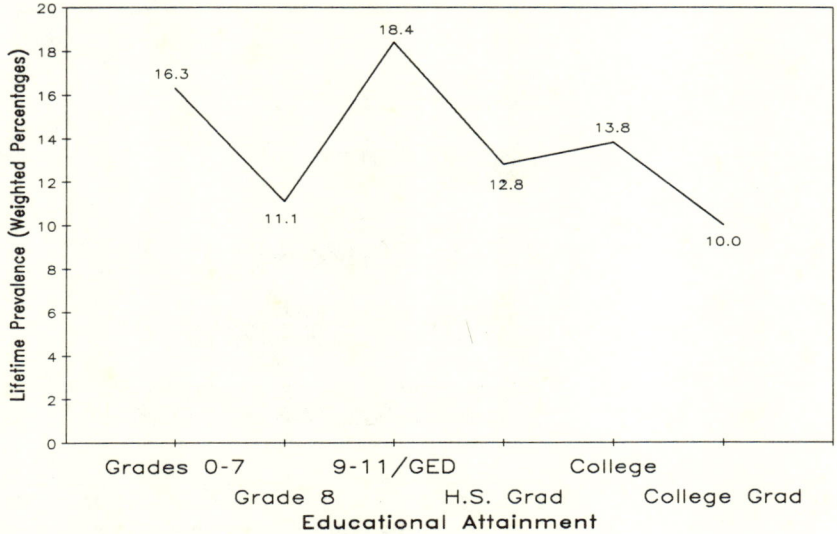

Figure 5–9 Lifetime Prevalence of Alcoholism by Educational Attainment

Age is a confounding factor, because young people have had more years of schooling than older people. For example, many of those with only an eighth-grade education are older people who went as far in school as they were expected to at the time they were growing up, and, as we have shown, older people have a low lifetime prevalence of alcoholism. Looking at specific age groups disrupts the consistency of the relationship between alcoholism and education only for the youngest age group, many of whom have not yet completed their education. The pattern shown in Figure 5–9 is quite consistent for every other age group, with one exception. For those 65 and older, prevalence of alcoholism is as low among those with some college as it is in college graduates, but relatively few in this age group have attended college, let alone graduated.

Marital Status. Marital history is distinctly related to lifetime prevalence of alcohol abuse and/or dependence (Figure 5–10). Those with a stable marriage have the lowest lifetime prevalence (9%), the never married who have not cohabited for a year or more are next, then less stable marriages, and finally highest rates (nearly 30%) occur among those who have cohabited without ever marrying.

Current marital status (as opposed to marital history) shows similar results with a one-year alcoholism prevalence among those who have never been married of 9.7%. This falls between that of the currently married (4.2%) and currently separated or divorced (9.9%), but is closer to the latter.

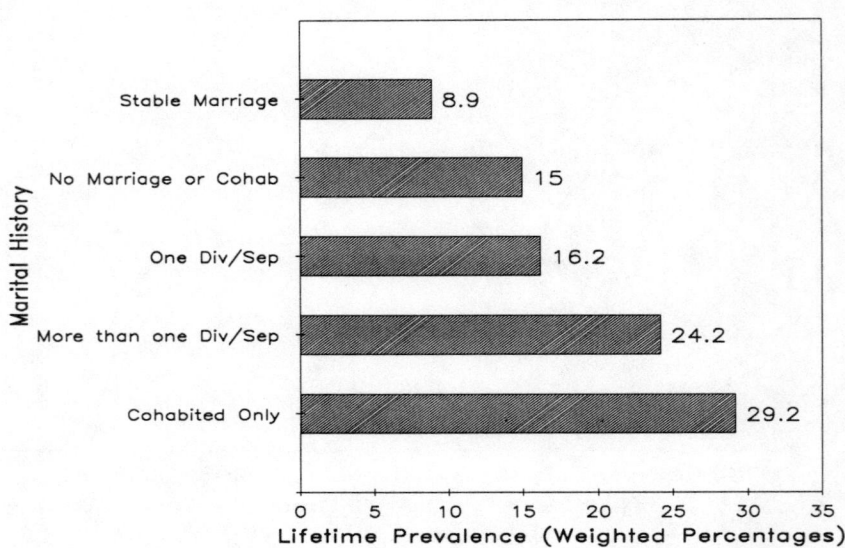

Figure 5–10 Lifetime Prevalence of Alcoholism by Marital History

Those currently widowed, a group largely made up of older women, have the lowest prevalences (2.3%).

Occupation. The lowest one-year rates of alcoholism are found among professionals and managers and highest rates among laborers (Figure 5-11). The higher rate in skilled than unskilled laborers is partly due to the fact that women are relatively uncommon among skilled workers. Alcoholism is inversely related to occupational status for men (Table 5-8). Resuts are less consistent for women, perhaps because their status depends as much on their spouse's as their own occupation.

Underemployment. We asked about employment status both as of the time of interview and over the last five years. Those currently unemployed may be either temporarily out of work or out of the work force because they are students, housewives, retired, or incapacitated. Their current status may be long-lived or brief. Because of those problems, we will use a measure we have labeled "underemployment," defined as a total of six months or more out of the five years prior to interview when expected to work— that is, excluding periods when one was not in the work force for the reasons listed above. About 13% of the total sample met this definition, with underemployment twice as common in blacks as whites (Table 5-9). The underemployed have a one-year prevalence of alcoholism of 12%

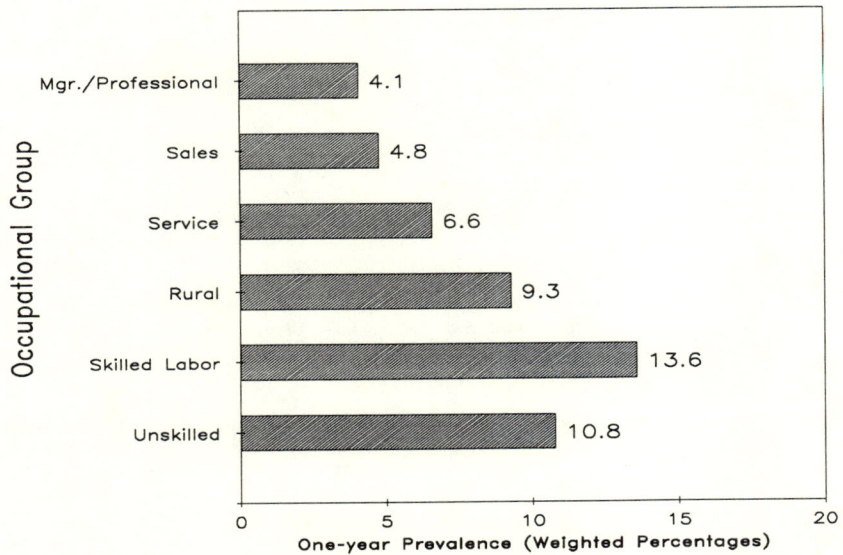

Figure 5-11 One-Year Prevalence of Alcoholism by Type of Occupation at Time of Interview

Table 5–8 Occupation and Alcoholism

Occupation at Time of Interview	Active (One-Year) Prevalence in Percent (SE)			
	Men		Women	
Unskilled labor	13.92	(1.46)	2.76	(1.12)
Skilled labor	14.79	(1.47)	0.93	(1.31)
Farm/Rural	10.57	(3.89)	0.00	—
Service occupations	10.35	(2.03)	3.35	(1.12)
Sales/Support	9.15	(1.19)	1.86	(0.46)
Management/Professional	5.97	(0.81)	1.16	(0.46)

compared to only 5% among those not underemployed. Although the rate of underemployment is highest in blacks, the difference in alcoholism prevalence between the underemployed and others is smaller for blacks than other ethnic groups, indicating that most black unemployment has other explanations.

Table 5–9 Underemployment and Prevalence of Alcoholism (Data from Three ECA Sites[a] Weighted to National Demographic Distribution)

Ethnicity	Percent Underemployed	Active (One-Year) Prevalence in Percent (SE)			
		Underemployed[b] (N=1,673)		Not Underemployed[b] (N=8,458)	
Whites	12	12.03	(1.55)	4.85	(0.38)
Blacks	23	6.71	(2.45)	4.15	(1.08)
Hispanics	18	16.80	(5.72)	5.88	(1.67)
Total	13	11.52	(1.31)	4.80	(0.35)

[a]St. Louis, Durham, Los Angeles.
[b]"Underemployed" are those unemployed six months or more in the last five years when not housewives, retired, students, or physically ill.

Financial Dependency and Income.   Because a higher proportion of black women received welfare than did other groups (Table 5–10), we looked at the relationship between financial dependency and alcoholism separately for ethnic and gender groups. For each group except Hispanic males, those receiving welfare had a somewhat higher rate of alcoholism than those who did not receive welfare, but none of the differences was statistically significant.

There was also an association between men's income and alcoholism. The higher the current income of those in full-time jobs at the time of interview, the lower the one-year prevalence of alcoholism (Table 5–11). In other words, there are fewer current alcoholics among the well paid. The pattern among women is similar but much weaker.

This negative association of alcoholism and male income holds for all age groups. It is weakest in the youngest group, where recent entry into the labor market means low incomes generally, but even among young men there is a significant negative correlation $(-.21)$. For all other age groups this correlation is a startling $-.80$ or better.

Household Size.   The modal household size was two persons, and 32% of

Table 5–10 Alcoholism and Welfare Assistance

Ethnicity	Receiving Welfare Assistance	Active (One-Year) Alcohol Prevalence in %(SE)			
		Persons on Assistance		Not on Assistance	
		Men			
	%	(N=981)		(N=6,935)	
Blacks	17	15.93	(4.40)	9.33	(1.56)
Hispanics	13	10.32	(5.57)	15.04	(2.52)
Whites	8	12.56	(1.96)	10.10	(0.53)
		Women			
	%	(N=1,726)		(N=9,072)	
Blacks	27	3.68	(1.59)	1.65	(0.66)
Hispanics	19	3.26	(2.60)	1.76	(0.93)
Whites	7	2.99	(1.00)	1.82	(0.22)

Table 5–11 Current Annual Income and Prevalence of Alcoholism Among Those Employed Full-time at Interview

Annual Income	Prevalence of Alcoholism in Percent (SE)			
	Lifetime		Active (One-Year)	
	Men	Women	Men	Women
Less than $ 5,000	23.41 (3.10)	6.82 (1.63)	15.68 (2.72)	3.76 (1.23)
$ 5,000 – $ 9,999	31.86 (2.76)	4.62 (0.90)	18.90 (2.35)	2.03 (0.63)
$10,000 – $14,999	23.89 (1.94)	6.11 (1.09)	11.59 (1.49)	2.62 (0.73)
$15,000 – $19,999	23.38 (1.90)	6.03 (1.55)	9.22 (1.32)	0.82 (0.59)
$20,000 – $24,999	19.49 (1.91)	4.86 (2.05)	6.10 (1.17)	1.10 (0.99)
$25,000 – $34,999	18.74 (1.97)	4.40 (2.17)	9.56 (1.50)	0.94 (1.03)
$35,000 – $49,999	12.77 (2.50)	3.17 (2.93)	5.28 (1.68)	0.00 —
$50,000+	14.34 (3.0)	5.08 (6.93)	1.72 (1.13)	5.08 (6.93)
Rank order correlation (income group, lowest to highest, and prevalence rate)	−.86	−.59	−.91	−.10

households fell into this category. Household size was not associated with the prevalence of alcoholism—those from small households were no more or less likely to be alcoholic than those from large ones.

Rural–Urban Residence. Of the five ECA sites, only two, St. Louis and Durham, included rural areas. In the St. Louis site, 6% of the sample was drawn from two rural counties contiguous to the metropolitan area. In the Durham site, there were four rural counties contiguous to its much smaller central city. In St. Louis, the rural counties are virtually all white, while in Durham, they are approxiately half black. Whether it is because of the discrepancy in the size of the central city, or whether rural residence has a different significance for blacks and whites, or for other reasons, the association between rural–urban residence and alcoholism differs in the two sites, and therefore will be presented separately. The one-year prevalence of alcoholism is higher in urban dwellers in St. Louis and in rural dwellers in Durham, but neither difference is statistically significant. Since there are likely to be other demographic differences between urban and rural dwellers, we examined area of residence controlling for age, race, and sex, showing the cross-site comparison for whites only in Table 5–12, and then blacks in Durham separately (Numbers in age groups are low for the St. Louis

Table 5–12 Prevalence of Alcoholism by Urban Versus Rural Residence
(White Household Dwellers Only, Weighted to Local Population)

	Active (One-Year) Prevalence by Percent (SE)			
	St. Louis		Durham	
	Rural (N=159)	Urban (N=1,597)	Rural (N=1,148)	Urban (N=1,270)
White Males				
Age:				
18–29	14.64 (7.30)	20.29 (3.17)	13.47 (4.68)	11.60 (2.71)
30–44	10.65 (9.13)	17.87 (3.20)	8.21 (3.35)	7.18 (2.25)
45–64	0.00 —	7.03 (2.03)	10.05 (3.62)	6.60 (2.23)
65+	2.14 (3.37)	3.67 (2.35)	1.45 (1.96)	1.36 (1.79)
Totals	6.76 (2.91)	13.61 (1.49)	8.90 (1.89)	7.88 (1.29)
White Females				
Age:				
18–29	0.00 —	3.75 (1.43)	2.06 (1.67)	2.80 (1.41)
30–44	4.83 (5.64)	0.49 (0.54)	0.00 —	1.30 (1.04)
45–64	0.00 —	0.44 (0.51)	0.00 —	0.20 (0.40)
65+	0.00 —	0.82 (0.85)	0.00 —	0.00 —
Totals	0.94 (1.12)	1.45 (0.48)	0.48 (0.39)	1.25 (0.52)

rural sample, ranging from 12 to 28. Standard errors are correspondingly high.)

In St. Louis, the urban predominance mentioned above for the total sample holds for both sexes and for all age groups, with the exception of 30–44 year-old women (Table 5–12). Across all age groups, this difference is significant for men but not for women.

Among white men in the Durham sample, that urban predominance is not seen; in fact, there is a slightly (nonsignificant) higher rate in rural white males. Urban white women in the Durham sample are about twice as likely to have a lifetime diagnosis of alcoholism compared to female rural dwellers; thus, their pattern is consistent with that of women in the St. Louis site. However, in neither site are the differences for women statistically significant.

For blacks in the Durham area, lifetime rates were significantly higher for male rural dwellers ($p < .01$), while for women, they were nonsignificantly higher (Table 5–13). Blazer, Crowell, and George (1987) also examined these differences and suggested a number of possible explanations including consanguinity, extreme poverty, and "reverse drift" from urban to rural areas among established black male alcoholics.

The Institutional Sample. At each of the ECA sites, representative sam-

Table 5–13 Prevalence of Alcoholism in Blacks in Durham Versus Surrounding Rural Counties (Black Household Dwellers Only, Weighted to Local Population)

	Active (One-Year) Prevalence by Percent (SE)			
	Black Males		Black Females	
	Rural (N=280)	Urban (N=196)	Rural (N=494)	Urban (N=377)
Age:				
18–29	8.11 (3.20)	1.11 (1.37)	1.21 (1.24)	1.24 (1.22)
30–44	13.47 (4.67)	8.00 (4.67)	0.30 (0.69)	0.75 (1.11)
45–64	20.37 (5.66)	6.29 (4.16)	3.94 (2.28)	0.00 —
65+	2.92 (3.62)	1.75 (2.90)	0.00 —	1.09 (1.96)
Totals	12.12 (2.32)	3.99 (1.62)**	1.57 (0.78)	0.81 (0.61)

**Urban–rural difference significant, $p < .01$.

ples of those in long term institutions were interviewed, either personally or by proxy when necessary. The institutional sample was then weighted so that it represented its true proportion in each sampled area. Up to this point, we have been presenting household and institutional data together so that the sample is representative of the whole community. As a group, institutionalized subjects have a higher one-year prevalence of alcoholism than do household residents, but there is sharp variation depending on the type of institution (Figure 5–12), with high rates among those in prison and mental hospitals but rates even lower than the household population's in nursing homes and other chronic care settings that serve the elderly.

Treatment. Alcohol problems in the past year are highly associated with recent use of mental health services, about which we have self-report information for outpatient care in the past six months and inpatient care for the past year. One-year prevalence is almost twice as high among those who have had any outpatient mental health treatment in the past six months as among those who have not (10.4% versus 5.6%). This proportion more than quadruples, to 26.8%, among those who have had any inpatient mental health treatment in the past year.

We have also examined the relationship to treatment controlling for sex, since women are more likely to receive outpatient mental health services than men. (Men and women are equally likely to have received inpatient mental health care.) The association of alcoholism with treatment is found for both men and women.

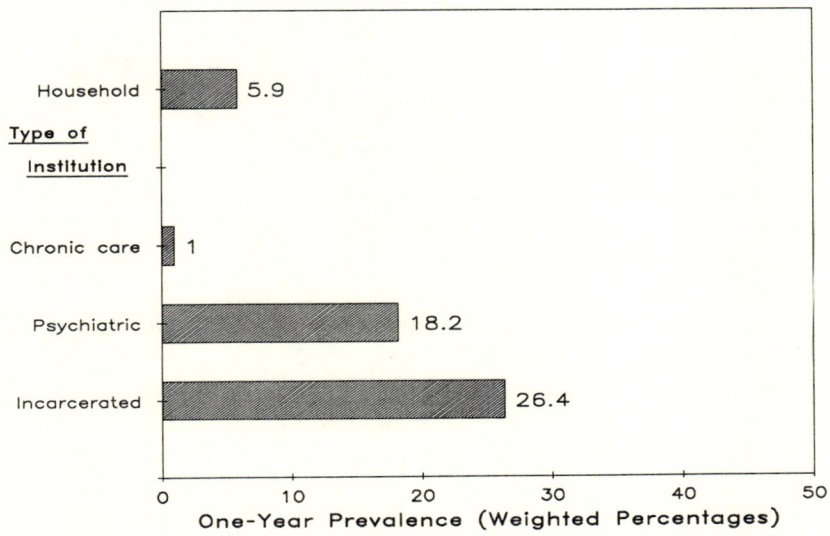

Figure 5–12 Prevalence of Alcoholism by Type of Institutional Residence

The elevated rates of alcoholism found in persons who have received mental health treatment is not found among those receiving medical (non-mental-health-related) outpatient care (5.9% for those with care versus 6.0% for those without). A different picture was seen for those who had been hospitalized. Unlike medical outpatients, the one-year prevalence of alcoholism was significantly higher among those who had had a medical hospitalization in the past year (8.1%) than in those not recently hospitalized (5.6%). This confirms the impression that alcoholism is a frequent, and perhaps frequently undetected, disorder among general medical inpatients.

Our findings of a high rate of alcoholism among those receiving mental health treatment or medical hospitalization do not necessarily suggest that these patients were being seen for their alcoholism or for medical problems it caused. We did, however, ask about specific alcohol-related contact with the health care system by asking whether the respondent had ever told a doctor about an alcohol problem. In the four sites where this question was asked, only 12% of those with alcoholism had talked to a doctor about a drinking problem. This rate was considerably higher for those with alcohol dependence (27%) than among those with abuse only (8%). Among those with neither diagnosis but at least one problem or heavy drinking, only 3% had discussed their drinking with a doctor. This low frequency among those with no diagnosis suggests that the DSM-III diagnostic threshold for alcoholism misses few cases who see themselves as requiring medical services.

CRITERIA AND SYMPTOMS
OF ALCOHOL DISORDERS

The relative frequency of specific alcohol symptoms is highly consistent across the five ECA sites. If we arrange symptoms in order of frequency of occurrence in the total sample at each site, the rank order correlations between pairs of sites range from .71 to .97. In fact, the only correlations below .90 are in New Haven, where a few of the symptoms used in all other sites were not asked about. Despite differences in the prevalence rates of alcoholism among sites, the symptomatic expression of the disorder is highly consistent.

The DSM-III diagnosis of alcohol abuse requires evidence of pathological drinking plus impairment in social or occupational function due to alcohol. Each of the specific DSM-III symptoms for pathological drinking and impairment contributes to the diagnosis of alcoholism, as shown by the fact that each is more common in those with a diagnosis than in other drinkers (Table 5-14). Among both alcoholics and other drinkers, the most common symptom of a pathological pattern was drinking a fifth or more in one day. Objections by family members is the most common of the social and occupational impairment symptoms.

A diagnosis of dependence in DSM-III requires at least one symptom of a pathological pattern or social impairment plus evidence for either tolerance or withdrawal. In the DIS, tolerance was scored positive if the person drank heavily every day for two weeks or more. Withdrawal was positive if the person drank first thing on waking—presumably to treat withdrawal symptoms—or reported any of the classic alcohol withdrawal symptoms when stopping or cutting down, including the shakes, fits, delirium tremens (DTs), or hallucinations. Tolerance was more common than withdrawal symptoms, occurring in 7% of the total population.

As we noted earlier, while it is possible to have a diagosis of either alcohol abuse or dependence with only two symptoms, persons with these diagnoses usually had many more than the minimum. Symptoms that occurred in a majority of those diagnosed as having abuse included drinking a fifth in one day, having blackouts, suffering family complaints about their drinking, and being in fights they attributed to their drinking. Symptoms that occurred in most people diagnosed as dependent included all the symptoms common among abusers, except for fighting. In addition, they were almost all tolerant to alcohol as indicated by daily heavy drinking. A very rare symptom, even among those with a positive diagnosis, was losing a job because of drinking. This was reported by 10% of the dependent and 7% of the abusers.

Alcohol symptoms generally require heavy drinking (Table 5-15). None of the alcohol symptoms occurred in as many as 10% of persons who did

Table 5–14 Lifetime Prevalence Rates of Specific Alcohol Symptoms

Abbreviated Question Covering DSM-III Criteria	Total Sample	Percent Experiencing This Symptom among Those with		
		Any Alcohol Consumption (N=16,518)	Alcohol Abuse Only (N=892)	Alcohol Dependence (with/without Abuse) (N=1,738)
A. *Pattern of Pathological Alcohol Use*				
Drank fifth (or equivalent) in one day	14	15	72	74
Blackouts	7	8	55	59
Alcohol binges or benders	4	4	12	39
Wanted to stop but couldn't	4	4	9	25
Set rules to control drinking	3	4	11	21
Drank despite serious health problem	1	2	6	19
Couldn't do daily work without alcohol	1	1	2	18
Proportion with at least one of these symptoms	17	19	100[a]	92
B. *Impairment in Social or Occupational Functioning Due to Alcohol*				
Family objects that respondent drinks too much	11	13	54	61
Physical fights while drinking	10	12	50	46
Trouble driving due to drinking	7	8	30	32
Arrested for drinking	6	7	23	32
Friends, doctor, clergyman or other professionals said drinking too much	5	6	20	32
Job or school troubles from drinking	2	3	4	20
Lost job (or expelled) due to drinking	1	1	2	10
Proportion with at least one of these symptoms	19	21	100[a]	88
C. *Symptoms of Alcohol Tolerance or Withdrawal*				
Period of daily heavy drinking	7	8	0	80
Any severe withdrawal symptoms (shakes, seizures, DTs, or hallucinations)	3	4	0	45
Drinking before breakfast	3	4	0	33
Proportion with at least one of these symptoms	9	10	0[a]	100[a]
D. *Other (Non-DSM-III) Symptoms*				
Period of weekly heavy drinking	16	18	52	90
Thought self excessive drinker	10	11	36	64
Severe health problems (liver disease, vomiting blood, paresthesias, memory loss, or pancreatitis)	3	3	10	30
Told doctor about drinking problem	3	4	8	27

[a]By definition.

111

Table 5–15 Lifetime Prevalence Rates of Alcohol Symptoms in Those Ever Drinking Heavily

Abbreviated Questions Covering DSM-III Criteria	Percent Experiencing This Symptom among:		
	Never Heavy Drinker (N=13,704)	Weekly Heavy Drinkers, Never Daily (N=1,357)	Daily Heavy Drinkers (N=1,457)
A. *Pattern of Pathological Alcohol Use*			
Drank fifth (or equivalent) in one day	7	41	72
Blackouts	2	27	53
Alcohol binges or benders	<0.5	8	37
Wanted to stop but couldn't	1	6	23
Set rules to control drinking	1	8	19
Drank despite serious health problem	<0.5	3	19
Couldn't do daily work without alcohol	<0.5	1	18
Proportion with at least one symptom	9	56	85
B. *Impairment in Social or Occupational Functioning Due to Alcohol*			
Family objects that respondent drinks too much	7	31	54
Physical fights while drinking	5	27	43
Trouble driving due to drinking	3	18	29
Arrested for drinking	2	15	29
Friends, doctor, clergyman, or other professionals said drinking too much	2	14	42
Job (or school) troubles from drinking	<0.5	4	19
Lost job (or expelled) due to drinking	<0.5	1	10
Proportion with at least one symptom	11	56	79
C. *Symptoms of Alcohol Tolerance or Withdrawal*			
Period of daily heavy drinking	0[a]	0[a]	100[a]
Any severe withdrawal symptoms (shakes,, seizures, DTs, or hallucinations)	1	8	34
Drinking before breakfast	1	4	27
Proportion with at least one symptom	1	10	100[a]
Proportions meeting DSM-III criteria for			
Abuse only	3.9	33	0
Dependence with or without abuse	1.0	9.7	91

[a]By definition.

not meet our criteria for weekly heavy drinking. And daily heavy drinking **was** virtually required to meet criteria for withdrawal or tolerance.

Those who had had a period of daily heavy drinking (seven or more drinks per day) had elevated rates of every symptom, including binge drinking. In fact, about 70% of those who had had alcoholic binges also drank heavily on a daily basis. This calls into question the claim that there are two types of alcoholics: binge drinkers, who never drink steadily, and steady drinkers.

CONCLUSION

Alcoholism is one of the most common lifetime psychiatric disorders in America. Over their lifetimes, nearly 14% of adults have met DSM-III criteria for lifetime abuse and/or dependence, and half of these had had at least one active symptom in the past year. There is variation in the prevalence by region, but even in the Durham area, it was a common disorder.

Men are about five times as likely as women to suffer from alcoholism. But the fact that the difference is least in the youngest age group suggests that women may be catching up.

Lifetime rates of alcoholism are higher in younger than in older respondents, suggesting that the illness rate has been increasing over time for both sexes, albeit more rapidly in women.

Obviously, the prevalence of a disorder depends on its definition and some would argue that the DSM-III definitions are too inclusive. A diagnosis of either alcohol abuse or dependence can be made in the presence of only two symptoms, and even these need not have been present at the same time. Most of those with four or more symptoms meet the criteria.

But one of the strengths of the DIS interview it that it ascertains a symptom profile rather than terminating an inquiry once a diagnosis can be assigned or definitely excluded. Therefore, rather than simply remarking on the very high rates of alcoholism obtained given the thresholds defined in DSM-III, we can estimate what the rates would have been had the thresholds been different.

Figure 5-2 is informative here. About 40% of those defined as alcohol abusers had the minimum of two positive lifetime symptoms. The mean number of lifetime symptoms for abusers was 3.3, more than one symptom above the minimum. Only 10% of those with a diagnosis of dependence had the minimum of two symptoms, and their mean number of lifetime symptoms was 6.4. Thus, if the symptom threshold were raised by one, rates of alcohol abuse would fall considerably, while the rate of alcohol dependence would not fall dramatically, and the ratio of those dependent to those with abuse only would increase.

We examine the threshold issue in a different way in Figure 5-13. Here we have plotted the number of positive alcohol symptoms for men and women with at least one symptom, to see if there is a plateau in symptom frequency. Such a plateau might suggest a natural threshold for the diagnosis, that is, a place to "carve nature at the joints," as Kendell has put it (1975). The minimum threshold for the diagnosis of alcoholism in DSM-III

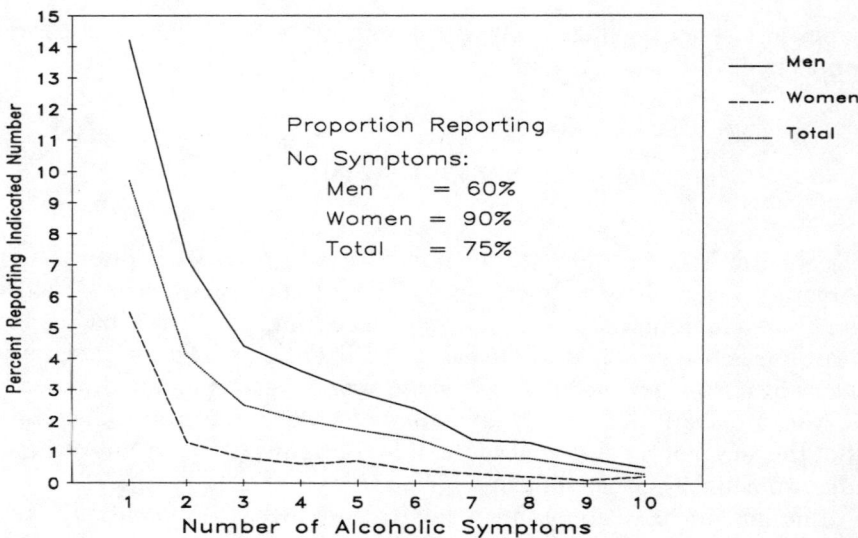

Figure 5-13 Distribution of Positive Alcoholic Symptoms Among Those with Any

is two symptoms; but the particular positive symptoms determine whether a case meets criteria and the subtype of alcoholism (abuse, dependence, or both). It is clear from the graph that for women there is a relative threshold at two symptoms; the downward slope of the curve tends to flatten at that point. For men and for the total sample there appears to be a distinct change in the slope at three symptoms. This might suggest that the minimum threshold, at least for men, should be raised or that there be a second diagnostic threshold at three symptoms. In fact, the revision of DSM-III (APA, 1987) now specifies a minimum of three symptoms for alcohol dependence, with fewer symptoms for the now residual alcohol abuse. Since DSM-III-R's criterion symptoms have been altered significantly from DSM-III's, it is difficult to judge from our data what impact the revision will have on the prevalence rates of alcoholism. But on the basis of the numbers of symptoms, there appears to be some justification for this change, at least for men. Additionally our findings suggest that a lower threshold for women might be appropriate.

Past debates about the definition of alcoholism have involved more than questions about the appropriate number of symptoms. Another issue has been the types of symptoms, that is, whether the definition should be based on the personal and social consequences of drinking, as in DSM-III, or on the quantity and frequency of alcohol intake. Since the DIS is based on DSM-III, it contains relatively few quantity/frequency questions, but it appears that groups selected on the basis of quantity and frequency would largely overlap with groups selected on the basis of personal and social consequences. We found that 80% of those who met criteria for alcohol dependence have been heavy drinkers on a daily basis (Table 5–14). Conversely, 91% of daily heavy drinkers met the DSM-III criteria for alcohol dependence (Table 5–15).

While alcoholism is approximately equally common in the three ethnic groups studied, there is an increase in the black/white ratio of lifetime prevalence with increasing age. This suggests that at least some of the fall in lifetime prevalence with age observed in the total sample is due to a true cohort effect, because if it were entirely a failure of recall in older cohorts, we would have to assume blacks have enormously better recall than whites. Second, it suggests that whites have contributed more than blacks to the increase in per capita alcohol consumption that has been seen in this country for the past two decades.

This increase in per capita consumption coupled with the finding reported here of a higher lifetime prevalence of alcoholism in younger groups is cause for considerable concern. However, other findings mitigate this concern. First, per capita consumption appears to have been tapering off since about 1980 (NIAAA, 1985). Second, we have shown that a lower proportion of the younger alcoholics are dependent (Table 5–4). Presumably this is at least partially because they have had fewer years in which to become dependent, but coupled with this is the fact that the association between alcoholism and antisocial personality disorder is not as strong in younger drinkers. Only further follow-up will tell us if alcoholism in the younger age groups is indeed less virulent, but these findings give us some hope that is the case.

Certainly, self-recognition of excessive drinking appears to be prominent. In fact, for dependent drinkers such self-recognition is slightly more prevalent than objections by family members (Table 5–14). Many alcoholics recognize that they are consuming more than they should, even if they often seem reluctant to admit it in the context of a treatment setting. Perhaps we can make increasing use of this self recognition to design ever better treatments so as to reduce what is one of the most prevalent psychiatric disorders in America.

6 Syndromes of Drug Abuse and Dependence

JAMES C. ANTHONY / JOHN E. HELZER

Alcohol, tobacco, and caffeine have been favored psychoactive drugs in American life since colonial times. Consequences of alcohol and tobacco use account for most of the nation's continuing drug problem (IOM, 1987; U.S. Department of Health and Human Services, 1988). Nevertheless, since the mid-1800s other drugs have been a continuing public concern. These other substances include derivatives of naturally occurring products such as those made from the opium poppy (laudanum, morphine, heroin), coca leaf (cocaine), and hemp (hashish, marijuana), as well as synthetic products like LSD and diazepam (Valium) (Brecher, 1972; Musto, 1973; Ray, 1983). In this chapter, we will define illicit drug use as any use of nonprescription psychoactive agents other than tobacco, alcohol, and caffeine or inappropriate use of prescription drugs (that is, taking more than was prescribed or taking drugs prescribed for someone else in order to get high, or for a novel experience).

Even with periodic strengthening and revision of drug laws, there has been a major increase in Americans' illicit use of drugs during the past 20–30 years. Good survey estimates for years before 1971 are not available, but retrospective data point toward major increases in the prevalence of illicit drug use after 1960, with continuing increases during the 1970s (Hunt, 1979; Parry, 1979). For example, in 1971 an estimated 14% of 12–17 year-old Americans had used marijuana; by 1979, the proportion had increased to 31%. Among adults, there were corresponding increases, not only for marijuana, but also for illicit use of cocaine and other controlled drugs (Fishburne, Abelson, & Cisin, 1979). All available data point toward an "epidemic" of illicit drug use in America during the most recent decades (Last, 1983).

The ECA surveys began when this recent epidemic was in full sway. Unlike prior surveys of illicit drug use, the ECA study focused on the consequent psychiatric symptoms and behavioral changes that constitute

116

the syndromes of drug abuse and dependence. This perspective stresses problems, complications, and hazards associated with drug use and is consistent with a broad consensus in international psychiatry that illicit drug use per se is not a psychiatric disorder (American Psychiatric Association, 1980, 1987; WHO, 1987).

THE DIAGNOSIS
OF DRUG ABUSE AND DEPENDENCE

The DSM-III gives case definitions and a conceptual framework that sort many psychiatric symptoms and behavioral changes due to illicit drug use into four main groups: (1) tolerance to drug effects; (2) withdrawal symptoms; (3) pathological use; and (4) impairments in social or occupational functioning due to drug use. DSM-III case definitions for drug abuse and dependence syndromes are based on the symptom groups, taken singly or combined.

Definitions are provided separately for each drug class. In general, DSM-III case definitions for abuse of a psychoactive drug require a pattern of pathological use and impaired functioning due to drug use. As a rule, DSM-III case definitions for dependence on a psychoactive drug require signs of either tolerance or withdrawal, nothing more. Cannabis (marijuana, hashish) is an exception. Like alcohol dependence (see chapter 5), cannabis dependence requires pathological use *or* impaired social functioning in addition to tolerance or withdrawal. DSM-III also requires persistence of drug-related disturbance for at least one month. Short-lived syndromes due to psychoactive drug use might qualify for diagnosis as an intoxication or some other organic mental disorder but not as drug abuse or dependence (American Psychiatric Association, 1980). Diagnoses of abuse are provided for all psychoactive drugs, and dependence for all categories except cocaine, hallucinogens, and PCP (phencyclidine and similar arylcyclohexamines). The variation in diagnostic rules for various classes of drugs has disappeared in DSM-III-R, and drug abuse is defined as a residual category. However, in DSM-III, abuse can be diagnosed separately or together with dependence.

The way in which the DIS made DSM-III case definitions operational is illustrated in Table 6-1. The table shows each symptom group that must be evaluated for the case definitions, as well as corresponding DIS questions.

Before asking the diagnostic questions in Table 6-1, interviewers first showed subjects a chart of the drug names shown in Table 6-2 and asked a series of preliminary questions. The last preliminary question, about use of drugs on more than five occasions, was used as a "gate" to exclude purely experimental users. It also addressed duration and persistence of the syn-

Table 6-1 DSM-III Drug Abuse and Dependence: Symptom Groups for the Case Definition and Corresponding Items from the NIMH Diagnostic Interview Schedule

DSM-III Criteria	Corresponding DIS Questions
Tolerance	Did you find you needed larger amounts of these drugs to get an effect—or that you could no longer get high on the amount you used to use?
Withdrawal	Have you ever had withdrawal symptoms—that is, have you felt sick because you stopped or cut down on any of these drugs?
Pattern of pathological use	Have you ever used any one of these drugs or any other illicit drug every day for two weeks or more?
	Did you have any emotional or psychological problems from using drugs—such as feeling crazy or paranoid or depressed or uninterested in things?
	Have you ever tried to cut down on any drugs, but found you couldn't do it.
	Did you have any health problems like fits, an accidental overdose, a persistent cough, or an infection as a result of using any of these drugs?
Social or occupational impairment due to drug use	Did any of these drugs cause you considerable problems with your family or friends, on the job or at school, or with police?

drome: many who use a drug more than five times might do so over a one-month span, as required by DSM-III.

Whenever a subject answered positively to one of the symptom questions in Table 6-1, the ECA interviewer asked whether the response applied to each of the drugs used on more than five occasions. At three ECA sites, the interviewer also asked when each symptom reported for each drug had last occurred (Von Korff & Anthony, 1982). For example, when subjects reported psychological problems due to marijuana use, they were asked, "When was the last time you had emotional or psychological problems from using marijuana?"

After administering the criterion-based questions, interviewers asked a series of questions about help-seeking for drug problems, global questions about age of onset of the first problem and recency of the last, and a final series of questions on problems in the year prior to interview (see Table

Table 6-2 Drugs Covered by the DIS Interview,
and Associated Global Questions

Drug Classes

Cannabis: marijuana, hashish, pot, grass

Stimulants: amphetamines uppers, speed

Sedatives: barbiturates, downers, sleeping pills, Seconal, Quaaludes, tranquilizers,
    Valium, Librium

Cocaine

Opioids: heroin, codeine, Demerol, morphine, Methadone, Darvon, opium

Hallucinogens: LSD, mescaline, peyote, psilocybin, DMT, PCP

Preliminary Questions

Have you ever used any drug on this list [see above] to get high, or without a prescription, or more than was prescribed, that is, on your own?

Have you taken any other drugs on your own either to get high or for other mental effects?

How old were you when you first used this drug (any of these drugs) on your own?

Have you ever used one of these drugs on your own more than 5 times in your life? Which ones?

Follow-up Questions for Subjects Who Reported a Drug Problem

Let's go over the problem you told me you had with drugs.
Did you tell a doctor about any of these problems with drugs?

Did you talk to any other professional about any problems with drugs?

Did you use medication more than once for any of these problems with drugs?

Did any of these problems interfere with your life or activities a lot?

When was the last time you (mention each problem)? [CODE RECENCY OF LAST PROBLEM][a]

How old were you the last time?

Which drugs have you had any of these problems with in the last year?[b]

---

[a]This was the "global" recency question asked at all five ECA sites.
[b]This was the drug-specific recency question asked at four ECA sites.

6-2). Neither DSM-III nor the DIS require that problems associated with illicit drug use co-occur within a specified time period.

A separate report describes operational definitions for each drug class covered by the DIS (Anthony, 1988b). The drug classification generally coincides with schemes used by others (for example, Ray, 1983). "Cannabis" refers to marijuana, hashish, and other cannabis products (Thai-sticks, hash oil, etc.). "Cocaine" means any form of cocaine, including crack and freebase. "Stimulants" include amphetamines and related controlled stimulants such as methylphenidate. The "sedatives" include the barbiturates, diazepam (Valium), chlordiazepoxide (Librium), methaqualone (Quaalude, Sopor), and other controlled drugs prescribed as sedatives, hypnotics (sleep promoters), or anxiolytics (anxiety relievers). "Hallucinogens" include psychedelic drugs like LSD, mescaline, peyote, and psilocybin, as well as PCP.

Heroin was asked about separately, although DSM-III combines it with other opioids, such as opium, morphine, codeine, and propoxyphene (Darvon). We use the term "heroin-like" to designate this group of opioid drugs, excluding heroin. Consistent with DSM-III, DIS diagnoses for opioid abuse and opioid dependence treat heroin and heroin-like drugs as a single group. In addition to the diagnoses of abuse and dependence on separate drug classes, we have created an overall DIS lifetime diagnosis of drug abuse/dependence to include any person with one or more of the DSM-III drug abuse or dependence diagnoses.

The 19,417 ECA participants with usable data on drug abuse and dependence provide large numbers of drug users and abusers in several categories. These large numbers are explained in part by the ECA's sampling institutional residents at a higher rate than household residents (see Chapter 2).

In all, 3,925 subjects in the ECA sample reported six or more occasions of illicit drug use. Marijuana was used by 2,977, followed by amphetamines (1,055), cocaine (975), sedatives (740), hallucinogens (647), heroin-like substances (419), and heroin itself (359).

When we compare drugs with respect to problems experienced by users, we need to keep in mind usual methods of use, sources of drugs, patterns of use, and underlying characteristics of users. If we find that heroin users experience more problems than users of other drugs, this can be seen in part as attributable to the chemical effects of the drug, but other factors may be involved as well. For example, virtually all heroin used in the United States is manufactured illicitly without the quality control that governs the licit supply of prescription drugs like barbiturates and cocaine, and sellers frequently adulterate it to increase their profits. In addition, heroin often is taken by injection; cannabis is most often smoked; cocaine is taken by nose or by mouth, sometimes by injection; amphetamines, barbiturates, and hallucinogenic drugs usually are swallowed. These factors add to heroin users' risk of harm. Another factor may be heroin's reputation as a dangerous drug, which might tend to restrict its use to the least cautious members of society. Finally, heroin is often the last drug tried after familiarity with a host of other drugs that continue to be used. Thus, heroin users are typically users of a wide variety of drug classes, making it difficult to assign adverse effects to a particular drug.

Cocaine problems also deserve special comment. The ECA data were gathered in the early 1980s, when a national epidemic of cocaine use was still escalating. They reflect illicit users' accumulation of cocaine experiences up to that point. The experience of more recent cocaine users may be different. In particular, use of cocaine in the free base form (for example, "crack") appears to have been relatively uncommon until after the survey was complete. There is some basis for expecting crack–cocaine smokers to be at higher risk of adverse consequences than earlier "snorters" (Adler et al., 1987; Washton & Gold, 1986).

ESTIMATED PREVALENCES OF ILLICIT DRUG USE

Because exposure to illicit drugs is a necessary condition to the development of abuse and dependence, it was of interest to learn how large the population exposed was. Thirty percent of the population reported illicit drug use one or more times (Table 6–3). Women were somewhat less likely to have used illicit drugs (25%) than men (36%). Not unexpectedly, estimates showed a sharp and statistically significant decline with advancing age. Overall, our estimates are statistically similar to, though somewhat lower than, corresponding estimates from the last national household survey that had drug abuse as its primary focus (NIDA, 1989). As in the national survey data, we found prevalence of illicit drug use to be lower for

Table 6–3 Lifetime History of Illicit Drug Use (Percent)

	Both Sexes	Men	Women
All persons	30.5	36.1	25.4
Age:			
18–29	60.3	65.2	55.3
30–44	35.8	43.7	28.3
45–64	7.2	9.0	5.5
65+	1.6	2.9	0.7
Race/Ethnicity:			
Hispanics	25.1	34.5	16.1
Blacks	29.9	39.0	22.4
Whites/Others	30.7	35.6	26.3
ECA sites:[a]			
New Haven	29.0	34.0	24.6
Baltimore	28.2	35.5	22.2
St. Louis	28.2	33.5	23.4
Durham	23.2	30.5	17.0
Los Angeles	37.1	44.1	30.6

[a]Weighted to population of the catchment areas sampled at each site.

Hispanic-Americans, as compared to other race/ethnicity groups, and no significant differences between blacks and the white/other category.

The sampled populations in New Haven, Baltimore, and St. Louis had essentially equivalent prevalence estimates for illicit drug use, all between 28% and 29%. Corresponding to regional differences identified in national survey data (NIDA, 1989), the estimated prevalence of illicit drug use was lower in the Durham area (23%) and higher in the Los Angeles area (37%).

Durham differed from the other sites not only in being located in the Southeast, but also in being half rural. We wondered whether its rural areas might explain its low rate of drug abuse/dependence. There was a somewhat lower rate of drug abuse or dependence in its rural than its urban men (4.18% versus 6.92%) and a markedly lower rate in rural (0.83%) than urban (5.39%) women. Thus, its large rural population is one reason that Durham's rate is low.

PREVALENCE OF SPECIFIC SUBSTANCE ABUSE DISORDERS

Cannabis abuse/dependence was the most commonly diagnosed DSM-III drug disorder, affecting an estimated 4.4% of the adult population (Table 6–4). Two-thirds of these cases had used cannabis in the prior year, one-half in the prior month. Almost two-fifths (38%) of those with a lifetime history of cannabis abuse/dependence reported active problems in the prior year.

By comparison, lifetime prevalence estimates were under 1% for DIS/DSM-III opioid abuse/dependence (0.7%), hallucinogen abuse (0.4%), and cocaine abuse (0.2%). An estimated 1.2% qualified as current or former cases of abuse or dependence involving sedative drugs, and 1.7% were stimulant abuse/dependence cases.

ESTIMATED LIFETIME PREVALENCE OF ANY DRUG ABUSE/DEPENDENCE

Combining these individual drug diagnoses into a single category of "drug abuse/dependence," we found an estimated 6.2% of the sampled populations with a history of an abuse/dependence syndrome involving controlled drugs. Thirty percent of those who had ever been cases of drug abuse or dependence reported illicit drug use in the prior year and 22% had drug-related symptoms in the prior month.

Site Differences. There were intersite differences in the estimated lifetime prevalence of drug abuse/dependence, (Table 6–5), following to some extent differences observed for illicit drug use. The prevalence estimate for drug abuse/dependence was smallest at the Durham site (3.8%), significantly lower than estimates obtained for Baltimore (5.6%), New Haven

Table 6–4 Prevalence of Specific Drug Abuse/Dependence Disorders (Percent)

	Any Drug	Cannabis	Opioids	Stimulants	Sedatives	Cocaine[b]	Hallucinogens[b]
				Abuse/Dependence Involving:			
Lifetime prevalence of abuse/dependence	6.2	4.4	0.7	1.7	1.2	0.2	0.4
Among those ever abusing/dependent:[a]	(1,316)	(837)	(364)	(314)	(289)	(101)	(97)
Used this drug in prior month	22	47	18	10	18	17	8
Used this drug in prior year	30	67	60	29	41	60	44
Problem with this drug in prior year	24	38	42	16	18	46	30

[a]The number of abuse/dependence cases for each drug is given in parentheses.
[b]Diagnosis of abuse only, in accord with DSM-III categories of disorder.

Table 6-5 Estimated Lifetime Prevalence of Drug Abuse/Dependence and Estimated Proportion of Illicit Drug Users Who Qualified as Cases, by Site

	Population Lifetime Prevalence		Lifetime Prevalence among Illicit Drug Users	
	%	(SE)	%	(SE)
ECA sites:[a]				
New Haven	5.93	(0.22)	20.46	(1.42)
Baltimore	5.82	(0.87)	20.59	(1.52)
St. Louis	5.64	(0.56)	20.00	(1.84)
Durham	3.78	(0.53)	16.22	(1.60)
Los Angeles	7.62	(0.53)	20.48	(1.33)
All sites:[b]	6.19	(0.25)	20.27	(0.75)

[a]Weighted to population of the catchment areas sampled at each site.
[b]Weighted to national distribution.

5.9%), and Los Angeles (7.6%). The Los Angeles prevalence estimate was significantly higher than the next largest estimate, 5.9%, obtained at the New Haven site. The estimate for the St. Louis site, 5.6%, was intermediate. Roughly 20% of illicit drug users qualified as current or former cases of drug abuse/dependence.

Sex and Age Differences. In parallel with illicit use, drug abuse/dependence was more common in men than women (7.7% versus 4.8%), and among younger adults (Table 6-6). We found an estimated 13.5% of 18-29 year olds to be active or former cases. By comparison, drug abuse/dependence affected 6.7% of the 30-44 year-olds, 0.8% of the 45-64 year olds, and just under 0.1% of older adults.

The higher rate of exposure to drugs among men than women largely explained men's higher rate of abuse/dependence syndromes. Among users, male and female rates of these syndromes were similar (21% versus 19%). However, even among illicit drug users, the prevalence of drug abuse/dependence declined with age, from 22% in users under 30 to 5% in users over 65. The decline with age was more dramatic in women than men. Abuse/dependence prevalence rates were similar for male and female users who were under 30 (24% versus 20%) or 30 to 44 years old (19% versus 18%). By contrast, the lifetime prevalence of abuse/dependence among all female users older than 44 was only 1%. For men these rates were 9% for those 45-64 and 4% for those 65 and older.

The intensity of exposure to illicit drug use was an important predictor of abuse, as can be seen by comparing prevalence of drug abuse/dependence among persons with and without a history of daily illicit drug use (Table

Table 6-6 Lifetime Prevalence of Illicit Drug Use and the DIS/DSM-III Drug Abuse/Dependence Syndromes, by Sex, Age, and Ethnicity, in Percent (SE)

	Both Sexes			Men			Women		
	Prevalence of Illicit Drug Use	Prevalence of Drug Abuse/Dependence in: Population	Users Only	Prevalence of Illicit Drug Use	Prevalence of Drug Abuse/Dependence in: Population	Users Only	Prevalence of Illicit Drug Use	Prevalence of Drug Abuse/Dependence in: Population	Users Only
	% (SE)	% (SE)	%	% (SE)	% (SE)	%	% (SE)	% (SE)	%
All ages combined	30.68 (0.48)	6.19 (0.25)	20	36.09 (0.72)	7.72 (0.40)	21	25.37 (0.62)	4.78 (0.31)	19
Age:									
18–29	60.29 (0.91)	13.46 (0.63)	22	65.20 (1.25)	15.96 (0.96)	24	55.30 (1.31)	10.92 (0.82)	20
30–44	35.79 (0.96)	6.68 (0.50)	19	43.72 (1.43)	8.36 (0.80)	19	28.33 (1.26)	5.09 (0.61)	18
45–64	7.18 (0.51)	0.78 (0.17)	11	9.04 (0.82)	0.77 (0.25)	9	5.50 (0.62)	0.80 (0.24)	1
65+	1.57 (0.34)	0.08 (0.08)	5	2.88 (0.71)	0.12 (0.14)	4	0.66 (0.28)	0.06 (0.09)	1
Age 18–29:									
Whites	63.10 (1.00)	14.40 (0.73)	23	66.85 (1.38)	16.84 (1.10)	25	59.25 (1.46)	11.89 (0.96)	20
Blacks	52.86 (2.68)	10.48 (1.64)	20	61.92 (3.79)	12.71 (2.60)	21	44.79 (3.67)	8.51 (2.06)	19
Hispanics	39.81 (3.41)	7.39 (1.83)	19	50.83 (4.84)	10.67 (3.00)	21	27.95 (4.51)	3.87 (1.94)	14
Age 30–44:									
Whites	37.19 (1.07)	7.02 (0.56)	19	44.31 (1.57)	8.61 (0.88)	19	30.35 (1.42)	5.49 (0.70)	18
Blacks	33.02 (2.85)	5.44 (1.38)	16	47.14 (4.47)	7.58 (2.37)	16	21.03 (3.36)	3.62 (1.54)	17
Hispanics	21.04 (3.30)	3.90 (1.57)	19	28.78 (5.32)	5.03 (2.57)	17	14.01 (3.88)	2.87 (1.87)	13

Table 6–7 Lifetime Prevalence of Sustained Daily Illicit Drug Use and DIS/DSM Drug Abuse/Dependence by Sex and Age

| | Prevalence (%) of Daily Illicit Use for Two Weeks or More | | Percent with Lifetime Diagnosis among Drug Users Who Were: | |
	Total Sample (N=19,407)	Among Drug Users[a] (N=3,925)	Daily Users (N=1,670)	Not Daily Users (N=2,255)
Total	8	27	54	31
Men:	11	31	52	36
18–29	22	34	53	36
30–44	12	28	52	24
45–64	1	13	51	14
65+	0	14	30	0
Women:	6	23	52	25
18–29	14	24	55	39
30–44	6	20	58	45
45–64	1	24	58	3
65+	0	8	—[b]	22

[a]Used any drug six times or more.
[b]Only one daily user.

6–7). Men and young persons might have higher rates of drug disorder only because more of them had been daily users. If that were the case, among those who had been daily users, men and women would have similar rates of disorder, as would young and older persons; while among those who had never used daily, similarly low rates would be found in all age/sex groups.

We found that men were almost twice as likely as women to report daily illicit drug use (11% versus 6%), and this was not entirely explained by the fact that more men than women used drugs at all. Male users were somewhat more likely than female users to engage in such heavy use (31% versus 23%). The younger the male users, the more likely they were to have used drugs daily. No age effect was seen among female drug users, except that the very small group of elderly users rarely used daily.

Among users who *never* engaged in illicit drug use on a daily basis for two weeks or more, men suffered a greater prevalence of drug abuse/dependence than did women (36% versus 25%), and young adults had a greater prevalence of disorder than did older adults (Table 6–7). Among daily illicit drug users, an estimated 54% qualified for the diagnosis of drug abuse/dependence. This high proportion was roughly similar across gender and age groups.

Race–Ethnicity. Race and ethnicity were found to be related to drug abuse/dependence as they were to illicit drug use. In Table 6–6, we have shown these relationships only for the two younger age groups, because less than 1% of older groups had drug abuse or dependence.

In both age groups, and among both men and women, blacks had a lower prevalence of drug abuse/dependence than whites, and Hispanics had a lower prevalence than blacks. However, the only statistically significant ethnic difference was found in a comparison of white with Hispanic women 18–29 years old. Not only did young Hispanic women have significantly low rates of use, those who used drugs had a significantly low rate of drug abuse/dependence compared to users of other ethnic backgrounds.

In this context, some previously reported ECA study results merit special note. Studying lifetime histories of drug abuse/dependence within the Los Angeles ECA sample of Mexican-Americans, Burnam et al. (1987) found that prevalence increased with increasing acculturation.

ESTIMATED PREVALENCE OF DRUG ABUSE VERSUS DRUG DEPENDENCE

Up to this point we have been considering drug abuse or dependence as a single disorder. This disorder can be subdivided into three components— abuse without dependence, dependence without abuse, and abuse with dependence. There is a consistent predominance of males and the young for all three of these components. In fact, in the oldest age group, drug abuse without dependence was almost nonexistent (Table 6–8).

In the revision of the *Diagnostic and Statistical Manual* (American Psychiatric Association, 1987) published since these data were collected, drug abuse is a residual category reserved for people who did not meet criteria for drug dependence. When we approximate that diagnostic scheme (Table 6–9), we find that three-fifths of our positive cases meet criteria for dependence, leaving two-fifths in the "abuse only" category. Among both men and women with a drug disorder, the proportion dependent increased with age. Among the 45–64 year olds, 82% of the male cases received a drug dependence diagnosis. The proportions dependent among cases of older women and of men 65 years or older were also high, but the number of elderly diagnosed cases was too small to merit specific attention. Among younger cases the proportions dependent ranged from 35% of black females 18–29 years up to 60% of those aged 30–44.

ASSESSING DIFFERENCES IN PREVALENCE OF ACTIVE DISORDER ACROSS SITES

So far, we have been considering lifetime prevalence of drug diagnoses. We now look at estimated prevalences for active cases. There are several options open to us for defining active cases. We will compare these with

Table 6–8 Lifetime Prevalence of Drug Abuse and Dependence by Sex, in Percent (SE)

	Men			Women		
	Abuse Only	Dependence Only	Abuse Plus Dependence	Abuse Only	Dependence Only	Abuse Plus Dependence
All ages	3.18 (0.26)	2.14 (0.22)	2.41 (0.23)	2.14 (0.21)	1.18 (0.15)	1.46 (0.17)
18–29	6.92 (0.66)	4.05 (0.52)	4.99 (0.57)	5.41 (0.60)	2.34 (0.40)	3.17 (0.46)
30–44	3.22 (0.51)	2.71 (0.47)	2.43 (0.44)	2.05 (0.40)	1.47 (0.34)	1.56 (0.35)
45–64	0.13 (0.10)	0.23 (0.14)	0.40 (0.18)	0.03 (0.05)	0.39 (0.17)	0.38 (0.17)
65+	0.00 (—)	0.10 (0.13)	0.02 (0.06)	0.01 (0.04)	0.00 (—)	0.05 (0.08)

Table 6–9 Lifetime Prevalence of Drug Dependence

	Men			Women		
	Prevalence of Drug Dependence with or without Abuse %	Proportion of All Drug Abuse/Dependence Cases Who Received a Drug Dependence Diagnosis N	%	Prevalence of Drug Dependence with or without Abuse %	Proportion of All Drug Abuse/Dependence Cases Who Received a Drug Dependence Diagnosis N	%
All ages	4.55	854	59	2.64	962	55
18–29	9.04	549	57	5.51	283	50
30–44	5.14	272	61	3.03	164	60
45–64	0.63	30	82	0.77	13	—[a]
65+	0.12	3	—[a]	0.05	2	—[a]
Age 18–29:						
Whites	9.59	292	57	6.27	178	53
Blacks	7.01	161	55	2.99	81	35
Hispanics	3.22	35	64	1.98	17	—[a]

[a]N too small to calculate percent.

respect to what they tell us about intersite differences. We begin with a definition available in all five sites: cases with a lifetime drug disorder involving any drug and at least one reported drug-related problem within one month or one year of interview. When we use this definition to look at differences across sites (Table 6–10, columns A and B), we find that Los Angeles had the highest active rate (1.7% affected in the last month; 2.9% in the last year), as it had the highest lifetime rate (Table 6–5), and its rates of active drug disorder were significantly higher than Durham's (0.6% active in the last month and 1.6% in the last year). We can now test a hypothesis about why Los Angeles had higher lifetime rates than Durham. The higher lifetime prevalence rate might be explained by the drug epidemic having begun earlier in Los Angeles, not because of a persisting high prevalence of acute drug abuse/dependence among Los Angeles area residents. If that were the sole explanation, one might expect a larger proportion of lifetime users to have become inactive in Los Angeles (for example, because they would have had more time to "mature out" of drug use). However, this was not the case—Los Angeles had the larger proportion of its lifetime cases still active in the last month (22% compared to 15% in

Table 6–10 Site Differences in Prevalence of Drug Abuse/Dependence (Weighted to Local Population)

	Prevalences in Percent (SE)									
	A		B		C		D		E	
	One-Month Based on Most Recent Problem[a]		One-Year Based on Most Recent Problem[a]		One-Year Based on Most Recent Problem[b]		One-Year Based on Most Recent Drug Use[c]		Lifetime Prevalence	
New Haven	1.1	(0.2)	2.6	(0.3)	NA[d]		NA[d]		5.9	(0.2)
Baltimore	1.4	(0.2)	2.9	(0.3)	3.3	(0.4)	4.0	(0.4)	5.8	(0.5)
St. Louis	1.5	(0.3)	2.2	(0.4)	1.8	(0.3)	NA[d]		5.6	(0.6)
Durham	0.6	(0.2)	1.6	(0.3)	1.3	(0.2)	2.2	(0.3)	3.8	(0.4)
Los Angeles	1.7	(0.3)	2.9	(0.3)	2.3	(0.3)	4.6	(0.4)	7.6	(0.5)

[a]Based on most recent problem with any drug if any drug diagnosis given (see Footnote a, Table 6–2).
[b]Based on most recent problem involving a drug for which a diagnosis was given (see Footnote b, Table 6–2).
[c]Based on most recent use of a drug for which a diagnosis was given (see text).
[d]NA = not ascertained.

Durham) and approximately an equal proportion still active in the last year (38% compared to 42% in Durham).

This first method of estimating whether a disorder is active is somewhat inexact because it relies on a question asking about the most recent problem involving any controlled substance used, not necessarily the drug for which the respondent met diagnostic criteria for abuse or dependence. In all sites but New Haven, a more exact assessment was available based on the question, Which drugs have you had any of these problems with in the last year? Using this question to restrict answers to drugs meeting diagnostic criteria (column C, Table 6-10), we again found Los Angeles's active rate higher than Durham's and equal proportions of active cases among those with lifetime disorders (33% in Durham versus 30% in Los Angeles).

A third way of estimating active problems is available in the three sites where a question was asked about the most recent use of each drug. This allowed us to estimate how many of those who ever had a substance abuse disorder continued to *use* the particular drugs accounting for the problem. This question enabled us to come close to assessing a criterion that first appeared in DSM-III-R (American Psychiatric Association, 1987): "Continued substance use despite knowledge of a persistent or recurrent social psychological or physical problem that is caused by or exacerbated by the substance" (p. 168). Counting continued use of the substance as evidence of active disorder identified 4.6% of the sampled populations in Los Angeles as active cases of drug abuse/dependence, again significantly more than the 2.2% in Durham (column D, Table 6-10), and again the rate of active use was no lower among those with a lifetime diagnosis in Los Angeles than in Durham. In both sites, approximately 60% of those who ever had a drug disorder had used that drug in the year prior to interview. This confirms the findings based on the other two methods of estimating active use. The greater lifetime prevalence in Los Angeles than Durham is not explained by early cases in Los Angeles that are now in remission. A high rate of active cases indicates that there is a continuing higher rate of drug disorders there.

Comparing the proportions recently using a drug with which they have had problems (Table 6-10, column D) with the proportion having a recent problem with one of these drugs (Table 6-10, column C) showed that about one-third of the diagnosed cases continued use without reporting recent problems.

We next compared the two younger age groups with respect to site-specific rates of active disorder. If the low rate in Durham were explained only by the fact that the drug epidemic had arrived there very recently, we would expect to find that the level of disorder in Durham was closer to levels elsewhere for the youngest group than for those over 30 (to the extent that the epidemic began everywhere among the young) and that in Durham the disorder was still active in almost all those ever affected. However, this was not the picture (Table 6-11). Drug disorders were lower in Durham

Table 6–11 Site Differences in Active Prevalence of Drug Abuse and/or Dependence, by Age (Weighted to Local Population)

	Active Prevalence in Percent (SE) of Drug Disorder				
	A	B	C	D	E
	One-Month Based on Problem[a]	One-Year Based on Problem[a]	One-Year Based on Problem[b]	One-Year Based on Drug Use[c]	Lifetime Prevalence
Age 18–29:					
New Haven	3.35 (0.64)	7.81 (0.95)	NA[d]	NA[d]	15.51 (1.28)
Baltimore	3.10 (0.61)	6.35 (0.87)	7.61 (0.94)	9.15 (1.02)	12.50 (1.17)
St. Louis	4.08 (0.87)	5.88 (1.04)	4.64 (0.93)	NA[d]	12.98 (1.48)
Durham	1.44 (0.45)	4.10 (0.74)	3.27 (0.67)	5.51 (0.85)	8.82 (1.06)
Los Angeles	3.42 (0.63)	5.71 (0.80)	4.27 (0.70)	8.58 (0.97)	12.13 (1.13)
Age 30–44:					
New Haven	0.46 (0.25)	1.27 (0.41)	NA[d]	NA[d]	5.18 (0.82)
Baltimore	1.83 (0.55)	3.62 (0.77)	3.61 (0.77)	4.44 (0.85)	7.17 (1.06)
St. Louis	0.68 (0.38)	1.30 (0.53)	1.19 (0.51)	NA[d]	5.37 (1.05)
Durham	0.50 (0.28)	1.10 (0.42)	0.87 (0.37)	1.96 (0.56)	3.83 (0.77)
Los Angeles	1.38 (0.44)	2.95 (0.64)	2.70 (0.62)	5.28 (0.85)	10.71 (1.18)

[a]Based on most recent problem with any drug if any drug diagnosis given (see Footnote a, Table 6–2).

[b]Based on most recent problem involving specific drug for which a diagnosis was given (see Footnote b, Table 6–2).

[c]Based on most recent use of a drug for which a diagnosis was given (see text).

[d]NA = not ascertained.

than elsewhere for both age groups, and the ratio of current rates to lifetime prevalence in Durham was comparable to those elsewhere.

Age. Overall, about half of the 18–29 year olds who ever met criteria for a drug disorder had a problem in the last year (Table 6–11, column B divided by column E), and for most sites the proportion dropped to about one-fourth in the 30–44 year olds. This difference might be explained by (a) greater incidence (new occurrence) of drug abuse/dependence among 18–29-year-olds; (b) longer persistence of problems among the younger adult cases, and an associated possibility of faster recovery, or remission among older adult cases; or (c) measurement errors (for example, better recall for illicit drug use than for drug problems among older cases).

Race–Ethnicity. Using the estimate of active disorder available at all sites, we found that cases active within the prior month were equally prevalent among all ethnic groups. The same was true for cases active within the prior year (Table 6–12).

Table 6–12 Prevalence of Drug Abuse/Dependence by Sex and Ethnicity

	Prevalence in Percent (SE)					
	One-Month[a]		One-Year[a]		Lifetime	
Total	1.28	(0.12)	2.67	(0.22)	6.19	(0.25)
Ethnicity:						
Whites	1.26	(0.13)	2.67	(0.24)	6.35	(0.28)
Blacks	1.39	(0.38)	2.68	(0.67)	5.46	(0.73)
Hispanics	1.40	(0.52)	1.98	(0.80)	4.36	(0.91)
Men:	1.89	(0.20)	4.09	(0.38)	7.72	(0.40)
White	1.84	(0.22)	4.15	(0.42)	7.80	(0.44)
Black	1.73	(0.62)	3.11	(1.07)	7.22	(1.24)
Hispanic	2.55	(1.00)	3.32	(1.47)	6.27	(1.54)
Women:	0.73	(0.12)	1.37	(0.21)	4.78	(0.31)
White	0.72	(0.13)	1.31	(0.23)	5.02	(0.34)
Black	1.11	(0.46)	2.33	(0.85)	4.01	(0.86)
Hispanic	0.30	(0.34)	0.69	(0.66)	2.53	(0.98)

[a]Based on most recent problem with any drug if any drug diagnosis given (see Footnote a, Table 6–2).

Gender. Active drug abuse/dependence was more common among men than women, as might be expected based on their higher lifetime prevalence. But in addition, a greater proportion of all males who had ever had a drug disorder were active cases (Table 6–12). Among men ever affected, 24% had had a problem in the last month, and 53% in the last year; for women, these prevalences were 15% and 29% respectively. Thus, a greater proportion of female cases were no longer experiencing active problems.

ONSET AND DURATION

Among current and former drug abuse/dependence cases, we found the median reported age of initiating illicit drug use to be 16 years; the mean was 17 years. For most cases of drug abuse/dependence (the 25th to the 75th percentiles), illicit use began within the four-year range of 15 to 18. Use among cases seldom began after age 20 (Figure 6–1). The first drug problem typically occurred two to three years after first use—at a median of 18 years, a mean of 20 years—and most onsets occurred between age 16 and age 21, with onset rare after age 25 (Figure 6–1).

Comparing ages of onset of use and of problems for different birth

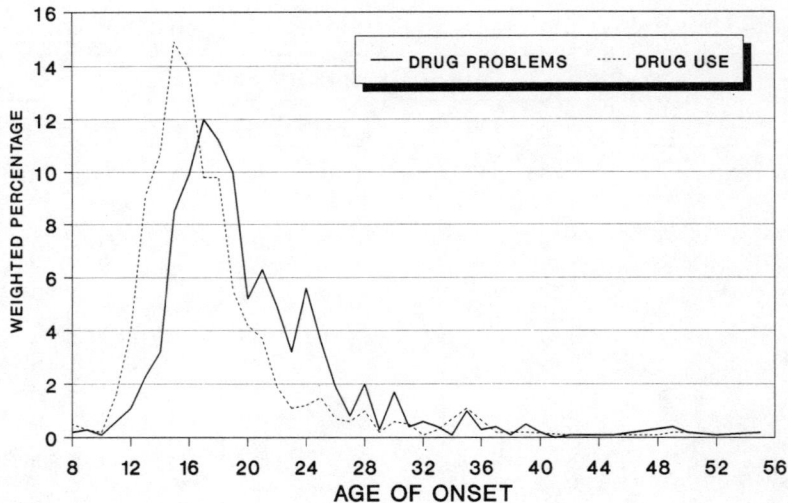

Figure 6-1 Age of Onset of Drug Use and Problems, Among Cases of Drug Abuse/Dependence

cohorts in our sample may be misleading because younger cohorts have lived through less of the risk period during which they might initiate illicit drug use, experience onset of drug problems, and develop drug abuse or dependence. Subject to these limitations, age of onset clearly is earlier in younger cohorts (Table 6–13). Thus, among male cases who were 18–29 years old at interview, 3.8% had developed an initial drug problem during the preteens, and 77% had their first drug problem by the end of their teen years. Among 30–44 year old male cases, only 22% had developed their first drug problem during the teen years. For the 45–64 year old male cases there were no onsets before 20. For female cases, onsets in each age cohort were later than for men, but women showed the same increase in age of onset in older cohorts. The late onsets in older cases can probably be explained by the fact that drugs did not become generally available until the late 1960s, when most of those over 45 at interview were already 30 or older.

A significant proportion of the 30–44 year old cases reported problem onset after 30: 13% of the male cases; 16.6% the female cases. Programs to prevent drug abuse are now focused almost exclusively on adolescents. While the adolescents are at highest risk, adults may deserve more preventive intervention than they now receive.

ESTIMATED DURATION OF DRUG ABUSE/DEPENDENCE

Since the median age of problem onset was only 18 years, it was possible for cases of drug abuse in all but the youngest respondents to have had a long duration. However, among currently active cases, the median time elapsed

Table 6–13 Age of Onset of Lifetime Drug Abuse/Dependence by Sex and Age

| Onset Before Age: | Cumulative Proportion (%) Having Experienced Onset among Those Who Ever Developed the Disorder | | | | | | | |
| | 18–20 | | 30–44 | | 45–64 | | 65+ | |
	Men	Women	Men	Women	Men	Women	Men	Women
13	3.0	2.6	0.1	0.0	0.0	0.0	0.0	0.0
20	77.1	79.8	22.0	20.6	0.0	0.0	0.0	0.0
30	100.1	100.1	87.0	83.4	77.5	15.3	0.0	0.0
40			99.7	100.0	100.0	57.3	0.0	16.9
50			100.0	100.0	100.0	81.1	15.6	16.9
60					100.0	100.0	100.0	16.9
70					100.0	100.0	100.0	16.9
Ever							100.0	100.0

from first reported problem to the present was only four to five years; the mean was 6.1 years; and most cases (75th percentile) had lasted no more than eight years. About 5% of the currently active cases had a duration of less than one year (Figure 6–2; Table 6–14).

Among cases reporting no active problems during three or more years

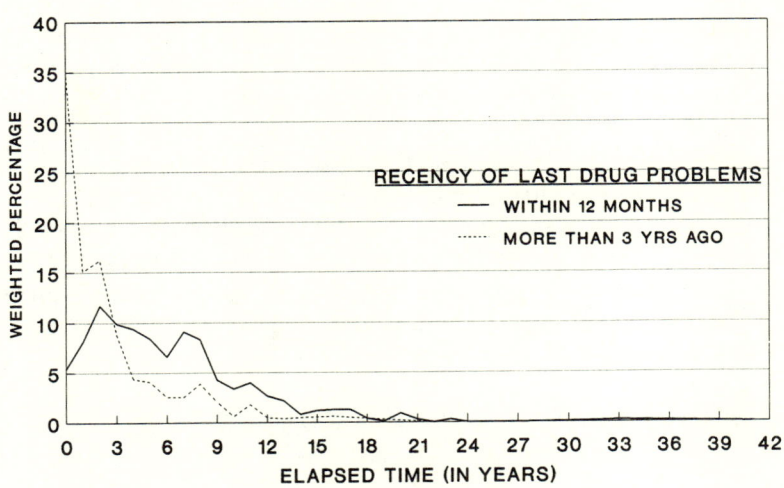

Figure 6–2 Elapsed Time Since Onset of Drug Problems for Drug Abuse/Dependence Cases

Table 6–14 Duration of Drug Abuse/Dependence in Relation to the Last Drug Problem Experienced

	Duration When:	
	Problem within Prior Year (N=598) Cumulative %	Last Problem More Than Three Years Ago (N=452)[a] Cumulative %
<1 year	5.4	35.0
<2 years	13.5	50.1
<3 years	25.1	66.3
<4 years	35.0	75.1
<5 years	44.3	83.6
<6 years	52.7	86.2
<7 years	59.3	86.2
<8 years	68.3	88.7
<9 years	76.7	92.7
<10 years	80.9	94.8
<11 years	84.3	95.4
<12 years	88.3	97.3
<13 years	91.0	97.8
<14 years	93.2	98.2
<15 years	94.0	97.8
<16 years	95.3	98.2
16 years or more	100.0	100.0
Mean (in years)	6.1	2.6
Median (in years)	4–5	1–2
Interquartile range (yrs)	7	4

[a]The exact age at last problem was not available when the last problem occurred one to three years prior to interview.

prior to time of interview, we found a median duration of only one to two years, a mean of 2.6 years, and most cases (the 75th percentile) had ended within four years. Thirty-five percent of formerly active cases had a duration of less than one year.

The distribution of duration of the disorder for those active and in remission in Figure 6–2 illustrates how surveys restricted to active cases can give biased estimates of the length a disorder typically lasts. Cases of short duration are sparsely represented in cross-sectional samples of active cases. On the other hand, the lifetime duration of active cases is underestimated because they will continue to run their course.

SUSPECTED RISK FACTORS AND CONSEQUENCES

To shed new light on suspected risk factors for drug abuse/dependence and on its consequences, we have studied variation in lifetime prevalence estimates in relation to education, marital status, and other selected character-istics of ECA participants. In some instances, it has been more appropriate to study variation in prevalence of currently active drug abuse/depen-dence.

EDUCATION

It is reasonable to suspect that a low level of schooling would be associated with a high lifetime prevalence of drug abuse/dependence syndromes. First, drug involvement might lead to dropping out of high school or col-lege, since drug problems often start before age 20 (Figure 6-1). Second, failure to achieve expected goals in education or early separation from an educational milieu may be a psychosocial risk factor for intensification of drug use and possibly for drug problems (Clayton, 1984).

The ECA estimates generally supported this expected association of drug abuse with low educational achievement. For both men and women, the proportion with a DIS lifetime diagnosis of drug abuse/dependence was highest among persons who started high school but received no di-ploma (9.3% for men; 3.9% for women), and among persons who attended college but had not earned a degree (11.2% for men; 8.7% for women). This pattern was especially apparent among men and women under 30 (Table 6-15).

Lifetime prevalence estimates were generally lower among those who did not enter high school as compared to those who attended high school, particularly in the older age groups. This might suggest that rather than being protective, getting more than an elementary school education was a risk factor, especially for adults who completed elementary schooling be-fore the drug epidemic started in the 1960s. One factor seems clear: initiat-ing but failing to complete an educational landmark is associated with relatively higher rates of drug abuse/dependence. This could mean either that drug abuse causes dropout or that failure to conform to school require-ments signals a susceptibility to substance abuse.

MARITAL STATUS AND MARITAL HISTORY

There are several reasons for expecting marital history to be associated with drug abuse/dependence. For example, the drug abuse/dependence of one partner might be disapproved of by the other, causing sufficient friction to lead to marital separation or divorce (Yamaguchi & Kandel, 1985). Drug abuse/dependence might also reduce the likelihood of first marriage; some would be reluctant to marry a person with a history of drug abuse/depen-

Table 6-15 Prevalence of Drug Abuse/Dependence by Educational Attainment, Sex, and Age

Characteristics of Subjects	Lifetime Prevalence in Percent (SE) among Persons of Age:				
	All Ages	18–29	30–44	45–64	65+
Men	7.72 (0.40)	15.96 (0.96)	8.36 (0.80)	0.77 (0.25)	0.12 (0.14)
Educational attainment:					
Completed fewer than 8 grades	2.35 (0.79)	12.33 (5.42)	5.79 (3.04)	0.53 (0.62)	0.00 (—)
Completed Grade 8, but no high school	2.35 (0.92)	14.50 (6.07)	4.95 (4.67)	0.47 (0.69)	0.00 (—)
Attended high school, but no diploma	9.31 (1.03)	22.45 (2.53)	6.76 (1.88)	0.42 (0.41)	0.00 (—)
Received diploma, but no college	7.54 (0.79)	14.44 (1.65)	6.29 (1.50)	0.74 (0.48)	0.09 (0.30)
Attended college, but earned no degree	11.17 (1.03)	16.76 (1.89)	12.24 (1.88)	1.19 (0.79)	0.11 (0.36)
Received college degree	6.79 (0.83)	11.36 (1.96)	8.01 (1.39)	1.12 (0.69)	0.00 (—)
Women	4.78 (0.31)	10.92 (0.82)	5.09 (0.61)	0.80 (0.24)	0.06 (0.09)
Educational attainment:					
Completed fewer than 8 grades	0.17 (0.21)	0.36 (1.10)	1.01 (1.31)	0.00 (—)	0.00 (—)
Completed Grade 8, but no high school	1.32 (0.60)	8.77 (6.57)	3.09 (2.97)	1.54 (1.08)	0.05 (0.16)
Attended high school, but no diploma	4.51 (0.70)	11.15 (1.98)	4.40 (1.43)	0.90 (0.58)	0.26 (0.40)
Received diploma, but no college	3.92 (0.50)	9.46 (1.34)	2.33 (0.73)	0.87 (0.44)	0.00 (—)
Attended college, but earned no degree	8.68 (0.89)	13.99 (1.69)	9.42 (1.77)	0.85 (0.61)	0.00 (—)
Received college degree	5.68 (0.87)	9.27 (1.91)	6.46 (1.45)	0.31 (0.47)	0.00 (—)

dence and its attendant social and health risks (Kandel, 1978; Newcomb & Bentler, 1985).

We found that an exceptionally low proportion of married men and women with no prior separations or divorces qualified for a lifetime diagnosis of drug abuse/dependence, only 3.6% of the men and 1.8% of the women (Table 6–16). By comparison, for unmarried adults who had cohabited for a year or more, the lifetime prevalence was exceptionally large (30.2% of men; 19.9% of women), a finding that is consistent with prior research (O'Donnell et al., 1976; Newcomb & Bentler, 1985). Those who had neither married nor cohabited and those with a history of separation or divorce were at intermediate levels. There was some tendency for a history of drug abuse/dependence to be more common when there had been repeated separations or divorce than when there had been only one.

OCCUPATION AND FINANCIAL STATUS

Drug abuse is thought to be a cause of poor job performance, and some employers have introduced drug counselors at the work site. We would expect, therefore, to find unemployment associated with drug disorders. However, we found no more active drug abuse/dependence in men and women not currently employed than in those currently working (Table 6–17, column 5 versus column 6). In fact, there was a tendency, not statistically significant, for more employed than unemployed 18–29 year olds who ever had the disorder to be using drugs currently. A similar trend has been observed among high school students, where increased drug use was found among those with after-school jobs (O'Malley, Johnston, & Bachman, 1985). Drug use may be promoted by a relative abundance of disposable income.

However, the picture with respect to income among currently employed men suggests that chances of being an active case of drug abuse or dependence, as well as an active drug user if ever dependent, *decreased* as income rose (Table 6–18, columns 3 & 5). Also, lifetime prevalence was highest (over 16%) among men earning less than $10,000 (Table 6–18, column 1). This rate fell to 4.0% among those earning $50,000 or more. A similar pattern was observed in the estimates of current prevalence based on any *use* of the illicit drug in the prior year.

These findings at first seem inconsistent with our previous findings that employment was unrelated to drug abuse, given that low wages often result from having to reenter employment at an entry level wage after losing a job. However, these observed associations between annual income and drug abuse/dependence might be confounded by age. Younger workers earn

Table 6–16 Prevalence of Drug Abuse/Dependence by Marital History, Sex, and Age

Characteristics of Subjects	Lifetime Prevalence in Percent (SE) among Persons of Age:				
	All Ages	18–29	30–44	45–64	65 +
Men	7.72 (0.40)	15.96 (0.96)	8.36 (0.80)	0.77 (0.25)	0.12 (0.14)
Marital history:					
Married					
Never separated or divorced	3.59 (0.40)	13.98 (1.90)	4.25 (0.80)	0.27 (0.19)	0.14 (0.19)
Separated/divorced only once	6.31 (0.96)	20.35 (4.12)	8.83 (1.89)	0.42 (0.43)	0.00 (—)
Separated/divorced more than once	12.04 (1.53)	28.15 (5.53)	16.61 (2.76)	3.46 (1.48)	0.00 (—)
Never married,					
Never lived as if married	11.57 (0.98)	13.07 (1.15)	9.87 (2.77)	0.00 (—)	0.41 (1.31)
Lived as if married	30.24 (3.59)	34.28 (4.64)	26.08 (6.36)	12.89 (11.40)	0.00 (—)
Women	4.78 (0.31)	10.92 (0.82)	5.09 (0.61)	0.80 (0.24)	0.06 (0.09)
Marital history:					
Married,					
Never separated or divorced	1.75 (0.26)	6.14 (1.16)	2.17 (0.59)	0.37 (0.21)	0.00 (—)
Separated/divorced only once	5.06 (0.78)	12.83 (2.71)	6.76 (1.54)	0.92 (0.59)	0.00 (—)
Separated/divorced more than once	6.66 (0.99)	14.65 (3.30)	7.53 (1.65)	2.75 (1.19)	0.73 (1.03)
Never married,					
Never lived as if married	9.14 (1.00)	11.22 (1.27)	6.30 (2.36)	0.00 (—)	0.00 (—)
Lived as if married	19.91 (3.15)	21.02 (3.81)	22.12 (6.87)	0.00 (—)	0.00[a] (—)

[a]Too few cases to produce a usable estimate.

140

Table 6–17 Employment Status and Prevalence of Drug Abuse/Dependence

Age	Lifetime Prevalence Among				Active (1-Year) Prevalence Based on Most Recent Use (3 Sites Only)				Active (1-Year) Prevalence Based on Most Recent Problem (4 Sites Only)			
	Persons Not Working for Pay %	(SE)	Persons Working for Pay %	(SE)	Persons Not Working for Pay %	(SE)	Persons Working for Pay %	(SE)	Persons Not Working for Pay %	(SE)	Persons Working for Pay %	(SE)
18–29:												
Men	13.32	(1.95)	16.67	(1.20)	9.88	(2.85)	12.46	(1.38)	7.82	(1.99)	7.04	(1.00)
Women	11.14	(1.34)	11.37	(1.21)	4.91	(1.50)	5.23	(1.08)	2.91	(0.91)	2.87	(0.78)
30–44:												
Men	9.64	(3.10)	7.56	(0.81)	10.39	(5.13)	4.60	(0.84)	1.61	(1.60)	1.89	(0.51)
Women	3.10	(0.83)	5.77	(0.89)	1.28	(0.99)	3.48	(0.85)	1.05	(0.64)	1.57	(0.56)
45–64:												
Men	1.00	(0.76)	0.56	(0.24)	1.04	(1.15)	0.36	(0.26)	0.00	(—)	0.23	(0.19)
Women	0.53	(0.32)	1.06	(0.43)	0.00	(—)	0.00	(—)	0.00	(—)	0.00	(—)
65+:												
Men	0.00	(—)	0.18	(0.58)	0.00	(—)	0.00	(—)	0.00	(—)	0.00	(—)
Women	0.10	(0.14)	0.00	(—)	0.00	(—)	0.00	(—)	0.12	(0.19)	0.00	(—)

Table 6–18 Annual Income and Prevalence of Drug Abuse/Dependence Among Those Fully Employed at Time of Interview

Current Annual Income	Lifetime Prevalence				Active (1-Year) Prevalence Based on Most Recent Use				Active (1-Year) Prevalence Based on Most Recent Problem			
	Men		Women		Men		Women		Men		Women	
	%	(SE)	%	(SE)	%	(SE)	%	(SE)	%	(SE)	%	(SE)
All ages:												
Less than $ 5,000	16.48	(2.72)	9.95	(1.94)	13.15	(3.29)	4.44	(1.80)	6.02	(2.71)	2.00	(1.44)
$ 5,000 – $ 9,999	16.32	(2.19)	6.32	(1.09)	13.27	(2.43)	2.82	(0.96)	8.95	(2.37)	1.40	(0.80)
$10,000 – $14,999	9.34	(1.32)	8.17	(1.25)	5.81	(1.37)	3.30	(0.96)	3.39	(1.23)	1.92	(0.87)
$15,000 – $19,999	7.23	(1.16)	6.48	(1.60)	4.69	(1.23)	4.18	(1.51)	2.91	(1.15)	2.44	(1.38)
$20,000 – $24,999	5.83	(1.13)	4.08	(1.89)	4.32	(1.27)	1.04	(1.02)	2.55	(1.17)	0.00	(—)
$25,000 – $34,999	6.89	(1.28)	7.32	(2.76)	4.46	(1.25)	2.91	(1.78)	2.11	(1.04)	3.48	(2.33)
$35,000 – $49,999	3.12	(1.30)	13.22	(5.66)	2.11	(1.31)	1.50	(2.06)	0.78	(0.96)	0.00	(—)
$50,000 +	4.05	(1.68)	8.56	(8.83)	3.16	(1.73)	6.54	(8.15)	2.79	(1.95)	0.00	(—)
Age 18–29:												
Less than $ 5,000	17.63	(3.13)	15.26	(3.16)	13.31	(2.48)	6.30	(2.87)	6.98	(3.37)	2.58	(2.21)
$ 5,000 – $ 9,999	22.29	(3.08)	11.11	(2.20)	19.48	(3.56)	5.39	(2.06)	13.43	(3.56)	1.87	(1.45)
$10,000 – $14,999	14.60	(2.42)	15.41	(2.78)	9.44	(2.57)	5.11	(1.98)	5.42	(2.32)	3.31	(1.92)
$15,000 – $19,999	13.52	(2.92)	14.82	(4.56)	9.33	(3.16)	7.70	(4.13)	6.63	(3.18)	7.47	(4.83)
$20,000 – $24,999	16.50	(4.27)	4.26	(3.92)	12.29	(4.20)	0.00	(—)	6.12	(3.60)	0.00	(—)
$25,000 – $34,999	18.79	(4.73)	9.00	(7.27)	15.02	(4.82)	6.39	(6.04)	8.16	(4.36)	0.00	(—)
$35,000 – $49,999	0.00	(—)	a		0.00	(—)	a		0.00	(—)	a	
$50,000 +	0.00	(—)	a		0.00	(—)	a		0.00	(—)	a	

[a]Too few sampled subjects to produce usable estimate.

142

less than older workers, and as we have seen, older workers have little drug abuse/dependence. Indeed, among the youngest age group, there was no clear relationship between income and disorder. Young men earning $5,000–$10,000 per year had slightly higher lifetime and current rates than those earning more, but this difference was not statistically significant (Table 6–18, lower panel). No clear pattern emerged for women either. Therefore, we still find no evidence that drug disorders either lead to low earnings or that they require higher levels of disposable income.

There is a long history of speculation about social class differences in the occurrence of drug abuse/dependence. DeQuincey (*Confessions of an English Opium Eater*, 1821) and other upper-class cases were well-known in the 19th century, and iatrogenic morphine dependence was common among middle-class housewives early in the 20th century. Thereafter, drug abuse/dependence became relatively more common among the lower working classes, as doctors became more cautious in their dispensing practices, and perhaps as drug abuse/dependence limited upward advancement to more prestigious occupations (Terry & Pellens, 1928).

There also has been speculation about occupation as a modifier of risk of drug use. Performers of popular music, movie actors, as well as hospital personnel with easy access to scheduled substances, are believed to have increased risks.

As with income levels, ECA data on occupational level do not suggest occupational differences in frequency of drug abuse/dependence syndromes. Among men, there is an overall tendency for active prevalence to be lowest in top level occupations (Table 6–19). However, the observed difference could be explained by chance alone. The absence of relationship with occupational level, however, does not mean that certain specific occupations may not have a high risk.

Because like age and income, age and occupation are confounded, we again looked for associations between occupation and drug disorders in a single age cohort, the 18–29 year olds. In young men we found manual workers to have a higher prevalence than white-collar workers. Again, however, none of these differences was statistically significant. Among women, as well, differences were not large enough to be statistically significant.

Whereas we found no significant association between drug abuse/dependence and unemployment, physical disabilities resulting from illicit drug use might qualify an unemployed person for disability payments, or more chronic unemployment might lead them to require welfare support. For these reasons, we asked whether drug abuse/dependence was associated with current receipt of disability or welfare payments.

Because being either a former case or a current case might affect beneficiary status, we looked at persons who *ever* qualified as drug abusing or dependent. We found no evidence of an association (Table 6–20). When

Table 6-19 Male Occupational Status and Drug Abuse/Dependence

Occupation at Time of Interview	Lifetime Prevalence %	(SE)	Active (One-Year) Prevalence Based on Most Recent Drug Use[a] %	(SE)	Active (One-Year) Prevalence Based on Most Recent Drug Problem[b] %	(SE)
All ages:						
Unskilled labor	9.26	(1.19)	6.71	(1.42)	4.37	(1.02)
Skilled labor	11.63	(1.29)	8.78	(1.42)	5.40	(1.09)
Farm/Rural	6.87	(3.14)	7.94	(3.65)	5.11	(2.90)
Service occupations	8.09	(1.78)	4.14	(1.81)	3.89	(1.54)
Sales/Support	6.83	(1.03)	4.15	(1.00)	1.47	(0.59)
Management/Professional	6.27	(0.82)	4.24	(0.93)	0.93	(0.42)
Age 18-29:						
Unskilled labor	16.54	(2.48)	12.92	(3.24)	8.09	(2.26)
Skilled labor	23.87	(2.89)	21.88	(3.60)	13.01	(2.76)
Farm/Rural	16.72	(7.21)	19.65	(8.43)	12.25	(6.70)
Service occupations	13.69	(3.69)	8.01	(3.93)	8.65	(3.63)
Sales/Support	13.37	(2.31)	7.40	(2.15)	3.50	(1.48)
Management/Professional	14.29	(2.58)	8.28	(2.64)	1.15	(1.00)

[a]Based on most recent use of a drug for which a diagnosis was given (based on data from three sites).
[b]Based on most recent problem involving a drug for which a diagnosis was given (see Footnote b, Table 6-2).

age was controlled, men and women with a lifetime history of drug disorder had a nonsignificantly greater chance of financial dependence.

The same lack of statistically significant differences in beneficiary status were found when we looked at active disorder (Table 6-21), although in the youngest age group, there was some over-representation of active abusers in both men and women of all ethnic groups.

RESIDENCE IN INSTITUTIONAL AND NONINSTITUTIONAL GROUP QUARTERS

The extent to which institutions and group quarters promote or prevent drug abuse/dependence syndromes has not been studied, but there is a clear basis for expecting that drug abuse/dependence might lead to institutionalization. Unauthorized possession of drugs like marijuana and heroin is a crime punishable by imprisonment. Moreover, users of these drugs—es-

Table 6–20 Receipt of Disability or Welfare Assistance by Persons With and Without a Lifetime History of Drug Abuse/Dependence

| | Proportion Receiving Assistance among: | | | |
| | Persons with Lifetime Abuse/Dependence | | Persons with No Lifetime Abuse/Dependence | |
	%	(SE)	%	(SE)
Men:				
All ages	7.75	(1.45)	9.28	(0.46)
18–29	6.97	(1.68)	5.73	(0.67)
30–44	7.42	(2.62)	7.08	(0.77)
45–64	30.66	(15.05)	13.18	(0.98)
65+		a	12.98	(0.44)
Women:				
All ages	13.24	(2.23)	9.90	(0.44)
18–29	11.26	(2.54)	10.90	(0.88)
30–44	17.66	(4.71)	9.06	(0.83)
45–64	15.59	(11.08)	8.71	(0.78)
65+		a	11.58	(1.13)

[a]Too few subjects to produce a usable estimate.

Table 6–21 Prevalence of Active Abuse/Dependence in Relation to Receipt of Disability-Unemployment-Welfare Assistance, by Sex and Race-Ethnicity, for All Ages and for 18–29 Year Olds

	Active Prevalence[a]							
	All Ages				Age 18–29			
	Receiving Assistance		Not Receiving Assistance		Receiving Assistance		Not Receiving Assistance	
	%	(SE)	%	(SE)	%	(SE)	%	(SE)
Males:								
All males	3.51	(0.92)	3.62	(0.30)	13.17	(3.66)	8.32	(0.75)
White males	3.67	(1.09)	3.51	(0.32)	14.58	(4.56)	8.41	(0.84)
Black males	2.89	(1.99)	4.11	(1.05)	9.88	(7.29)	7.81	(2.23)
Hispanic males	4.18	(3.69)	3.46	(1.26)	12.33	(12.44)	5.96	(2.42)
Females:								
All females	2.12	(0.65)	1.47	(0.18)	4.60	(1.68)	4.08	(0.56)
White females	1.96	(0.81)	1.50	(0.20)	4.40	(2.28)	4.33	(0.63)
Black females	2.96	(1.43)	1.78	(0.68)	5.48	(2.97)	4.09	(1.78)
Hispanic females	0.75	(1.27)	0.63	(0.56)	2.25	(3.79)	1.28	(1.25)

[a]Based on most recent problem with any drug if any drug diagnosis given (see Footnote a, Table 6–2).

pecially heroin—have been found to commit other crimes for income needed to buy drugs (Goldstein, forthcoming). Second, patients in psychiatric hospitals and other residential treatment programs have been reported to have high rates of illicit drug use, and many of these facilities have special programs for the treatment of drug abuse and dependence. Further, drug use may cause other types of psychopathology. For these reasons, one might expect residents of prisons, mental hospitals, and other residential treatment programs to receive a DIS lifetime diagnosis for drug abuse/dependence more frequently than household residents. One type of institution—nursing homes—should be an exception because its residents are mostly elderly.

For men and women (all ages combined), for men age 18–64, and for women age 18–29, we found that prisoners and patients in residential treatment programs for alcohol and drug problems were most likely to have a history of drug abuse/dependence syndromes (Table 6–22). Mental hospital residents had intermediate lifetime prevalences; household residents had the lowest values. Generally, as expected, nursing home rates were low, but there were few residents under 64 for comparison.

Unlike household residents, among whom men had more drug abuse than women, there was no preponderance of male drug abuse among residents of institutions. Except in nursing homes, women's rates were comparable to men's. And rates for both men and women were extraordinarily high in prisons. More than half the prison residents of either sex had a history of substance abuse disorder.

Notwithstanding the restrictive environments of institutions, residents in prisons and jails, mental hospitals, and residential alcohol-drug treatment programs were more likely to qualify as active cases of drug abuse/dependence than were household residents. Because of the small numbers in institutions, many of the apparent differences were not statistically significant, but the general tendencies followed those seen in the lifetime prevalence data.

In the prison and mental hospital samples, men aged 30–44 were as likely as those aged 18–29 to qualify for a lifetime or active diagnosis of drug abuse/dependence. (There were too few women over 30 in prison to do a similar comparison by age.) This was in sharp contrast to the age relationship observed for men in the household sample, where the rates for 30–44 year olds were about one-half those estimated for younger adults. There are a number of plausible explanations for this difference in age relationships across the types of residence, but a likely one is that the few persons who enter prison at older ages have not yet given up their illicit drug use, as most of their contemporaries have. Another plausible explanation is that older drug users who come to police attention are especially likely to be incarcerated because their legal difficulties are unlikely to be first offenses.

Table 6-22 Prevalence of Drug Abuse/Dependence by Type of Residence, Sex, and Age

Place of Residence	All Ages	18–29	30–44	45–64	65 +
			A. Lifetime Prevalence		
Men	7.72 (0.40)	15.96 (0.96)	8.36 (0.80)	0.77 (0.25)	0.12 (0.14)
Households	7.58 (0.40)	15.65 (0.96)	8.23 (0.79)	0.75 (0.25)	0.12 (0.15)
Prison	55.50 (13.93)	59.08 (16.16)	55.23 (29.93)	10.73 (37.60)	a
Mental hospital	21.74 (26.11)	27.78 (40.43)	24.67 (50.12)	4.96 (35.09)	a
Treatment program[b]	54.39 (49.15)	63.95 (70.54)	66.92 (83.62)	a	a
Nursing home[b]	2.27 (4.60)	a	0.00 (—)	3.24 (12.18)	0.00 (—)
Women	4.78 (0.31)	10.92 (0.82)	5.09 (0.61)	0.80 (0.24)	0.06 (0.09)
Households	4.79 (0.31)	10.89 (0.82)	5.07 (0.61)	0.80 (0.24)	0.06 (0.09)
Prison	70.31 (55.99)	73.44 (65.14)	a	a	a
Mental hospital	21.62 (40.00)	a	34.20 (78.44)	0.00 (—)	a
Treatment program[b]	47.21 (68.50)	49.58 (91.63)	a	a	a
Nursing home[b]	0.00 (—)	a	a	0.00 (—)	0.00 (—)
			B. Active Cases		
Men	2.98 (0.31)	6.91 (0.80)	2.41 (0.54)	0.17 (0.14)	0.00 (—)
Households	2.94 (0.31)	6.81 (0.80)	2.38 (0.54)	0.17 (0.14)	0.00 (—)
Prison	19.45 (13.94)	22.89 (17.45)	11.88 (24.01)	6.32 (37.05)	a
Mental hospital	5.88 (19.07)	8.30 (31.09)	5.45 (34.18)	0.00 (—)	a
Treatment program[b]	22.12 (44.35)	34.74 (73.46)	18.33 (78.73)	a	a
Nursing home[b]	0.52 (2.65)	a	0.00 (—)	0.00 (—)	0.00 (—)
Women	1.22 (0.19)	2.77 (0.53)	1.44 (0.40)	0.05 (0.07)	0.00 (—)
Households	1.22 (0.19)	2.75 (0.52)	1.43 (0.40)	0.05 (0.07)	0.00 (—)
Prison	44.94 (75.93)	44.95 (98.58)	a	a	a
Mental hospital	1.31 (11.38)	a	4.07 (34.88)	0.00 (—)	a
Treatment program[a]	17.42 (54.54)	25.81 (84.44)	7.07 (55.77)	a	a
Nursing home[a]	0.00 (—)	a	a	0.00 (—)	0.00 (—)

[a]Indicates too few cases to provide for a usable estimate.

[b]"Nursing home" includes chronic hospitals. "Treatment program" refers to residential treatment, including halfway houses.

DRUG ABUSE/DEPENDENCE
AND OTHER PSYCHIATRIC DISORDERS

When illicit drug use or drug problems coexist with other diagnoses, it is difficult to know whether the drug use has exacerbated already existing symptoms and provoked the development of new psychiatric symptoms, or whether the other disorders have promoted illicit drug use and drug abuse or dependence, perhaps as an effort at self-medication to relieve these symptoms.

The DIS offers only reported ages of onset as a way of deciding the order in which disorders appeared, and therefore their likely causal relationships. A longitudinal research design would be preferred. However, we can estimate how frequently cases of DIS-diagnosed drug abuse/dependence also qualified as cases of other mental disorders and their apparent sequence.

We present ratios of lifetime prevalence estimates: the estimated lifetime prevalence of each disorder among active and former cases of drug abuse/dependence, divided by the estimated lifetime prevalence of the disorder among all others. A prevalence ratio of 1.0 indicates no association. We found that former and active cases of drug abuse/dependence frequently qualified for other DIS-diagnosed mental disorders (Table 6–23). The lifetime prevalence ratio for drug abuse/dependence versus every other mental disorder except cognitive impairment was greater than 3.0.

Among men, drug abuse/dependence had especially strong associations with antisocial personality disorder, mania, and schizophrenia, as indicated by a ratio of lifetime prevalence estimates of 6.0 or greater. Among women, associations involving antisocial personality, mania, alcohol abuse/dependence, and schizophrenia were of comparable strength. These findings are generally consistent with prior research on psychiatric comorbidity among cases of drug abuse/dependence.

There was considerable comorbidity between drug and alcohol disorders. Among persons with both disorders, we found that the age of initial alcohol intoxication was lower than the age of first illicit drug use in 64.2% of cases (Table 6–24). An additional 22.1% reported the same age for initiating illicit drug use and initial alcohol intoxication. For only 13.7%, was an illicit drug used before the initial alcohol intoxication.

When we looked at the age of first problems with controlled drugs and alcohol, we found that in 43.3% of the doubly diagnosed cases the age of first alcohol problem was lower than the age of first drug problem; in 36.1% the age of first drug problem was lower than the age of first alcohol problem. For 20.6% of these cases, the reported ages of onset for alcohol problems and drug problems were identical (Table 6–24).

In short, whether we use age of first use or age of first problem as our starting point, usually the alcohol preceded the illicit drugs, but the earlier

Table 6–23 Comorbidity of Drug Abuse/Dependence and Other Psychiatric Disorders

Psychiatric Diagnosis	Lifetime Prevalence (%) of Other Disorders among Cases of Drug Abuse/Dependence			Prevalence Ratios[a]		
	Both Sexes	Men	Women	Both Sexes	Men	Women
Antisocial personality	17.2	22.2	9.8	10.6	7.3	26.6
Mania	5.5	4.6	6.7	10.7	11.3	11.1
Alcohol abuse/dependence	47.7	59.8	29.7	4.1	2.9	9.0
Schizophrenia	6.0	4.6	8.0	5.9	6.2	6.4
Panic disorder	4.2	3.2	5.6	3.0	4.1	2.9
Obsessive compulsive	7.4	6.1	9.4	3.3	3.6	3.5
Dysthymia	10.0	8.8	11.8	3.5	5.1	3.1
Major depression	19.6	14.2	27.5	3.6	4.9	3.6
Phobic disorders	22.9	19.2	28.5	1.9	2.4	1.9
Cognitive impairment	0.0	0.0	0.0	0.0	0.0	0.0
Any diagnosis	71.2	75.6	64.7	2.5	2.5	2.5

Note. A comparison of the ratios estimated for both sexes with those estimated for males and females separately shows Simpson's paradox.
[a]Prevalence ratios are prevalence of the diagnosis in those with drug abuse/dependence divided by its prevalence in those with neither drug abuse nor dependence.

Table 6-24　Order of Appearance of Alcohol and Drug Use and Problems Among Persons with Both Alcohol and Drug Abuse/Dependence

	Prevalence (%) among Those with Both Alcohol and Drug Abuse/Dependence
Use	(N = 634)
Alcohol intoxication before illicit drug use	64.2
Same year	22.1
Illicit drug use before alcohol intoxication	13.7
	100.0
Problems	(N = 607)[a]
Alcohol problem before illicit drug problem	43.3
Same year	20.6
Illicit drug problem before alcohol problem	36.1
	100.0

[a]Age of onset data missing for 27 subjects.

onset of alcohol was clearer for first drug use than first alcohol problem, indicating a more rapid induction of drug than alcohol problems.

TREATMENT

Only a minority of drug abuse/dependence cases bring their drug problems to the attention of doctors or other treatment professionals. At four ECA sites, it was possible to investigate how frequently they seek help (Table 6-25). Among the illicit drug users who reported daily use or at least one drug problem, only 22.8% said they had talked to a doctor or another professional about their drug use. Among those meeting criteria for drug abuse/dependence, a slightly higher proportion (30.4%) reported talking to a doctor or other professional about their problems. Females in all use categories were somewhat more likely than males to have told professionals about drug problems.

Those with a drug diagnosis, especially cases with at least one problem active in the prior year, were more likely than others to have used mental health services (Table 6-26). But, it is not known whether they received services for drug problems per se, associated mental disorders, or for other problems.

Table 6–25 Help Seeking for Drug Problems

	Proportion (%) Who Told a Doctor about a Drug Problem[a]	Proportion (%) Who Told a Doctor or Another Professional about a Drug Problem[a]
Persons with at least one drug problem	17.96	22.78
Males	15.74	19.86
Females	21.88	27.71
Current and former cases of drug abuse/dependence	23.03	30.35
Males	19.86	26.39
Females	28.30	36.92

Note. Data from all sites except New Haven weighted to national distributions.
[a]Problems include daily use.

Drug cases also received more outpatient medical care than others, and as much general medical in-patient care. This is particularly striking given the fact that older adults, who have little drug abuse, receive more general medical services than those younger. The medical needs of drug abusers apparently were sufficient to make up for their youth.

A noteworthy finding was that 60% to 70% of currently active cases had received health services during the prior six months. Yet, many of these had never spoken with a doctor or other professional about their drug problems. This finding directs attention toward a need for health service providers to take a more active role in the identification, prevention, and control of drug abuse/dependence.

CONCLUSION

Using general population samples and epidemiologic survey methods to study syndromes of drug abuse and drug dependence, we have found that the estimated prevalence of current and past drug abuse/dependence in the population exceeded 6%. Still higher rates were found among men, among younger adults, among those who had dropped out of high school or college, and among cohabitating or formerly married adults. The prevalence estimates did not vary greatly with race–ethnicity, current employ-

Table 6–26 Recent Mental Health Care and Other Medical Care for Those with Drug Abuse/Dependence

	Percent with at Least One Recent Visit or Admission for:			
Drug Abuse/Dependence Status	Outpatient Mental Health Services[d]	Inpatient Mental Health Services[d]	Outpatient General Medical Services	Inpatient General Medical Services
Cases active in prior year:				
Based on recent drug use[a]	15.77	1.04	62.58	11.02
Based on specific drug problem[b]	14.96	3.24	65.97	12.74
Based on any drug problem[c]	16.19	3.59	68.86	15.39
Inactive cases	7.37	0.72	57.15	12.51

[a]Based on most recent use of a drug for which a diagnosis was given.
[b]Based on most recent problem involving specific drug for which a diagnosis was given (see Footnote b, Table 6–2).
[c]Based on most recent problem with any drug if any drug diagnosis was given (see Footnote a, Table 6–2).
[d]Includes specialized drug and alcohol services.

152

ment status, current annual income, occupational status, or receipt of disability, unemployment, or welfare benefits. However, there was a tendency for Hispanic women to have lower rates and those financially dependent to have higher rates as compared to their counterparts in the rest of the population.

There was an important degree of comorbidity between drug abuse/dependence and other psychiatric disorders. In the association between alcoholism and drug abuse/dependence, the age of onset data suggested that the alcoholism most often came first. More definitive research on this association and on associations involving other psychiatric disorders is under way.

Persons with drug abuse/dependence get more health care than average, but many do not broach the topic of their drug problems in that context, and doctors do not routinely ask about drug use. Many missed cases could be found if health care providers pursued the drug issue. Beginning with gentle inquiry and dialogue, the professional can open the door for interventions to shorten or lessen ongoing symptoms connected with illicit drug use, as well as for services to prevent a worsening of these problems and the development of new problems.

THE PREVALENCE OF SUBSTANCE ABUSE: COMBINING ALCOHOL AND DRUG DISORDERS

This chapter has reported on drug-related disorders; chapter 5 discussed alcohol-related disorders. In DSM-III, both appear in the section entitled "Substance Use Disorders." DSM-III provides slightly different criteria for each class of drugs, and none is identical with the criteria for alcohol; in DSM-III-R (American Psychiatric Association, 1987), all drugs and alcohol have identical criteria.

If we lump alcohol- and drug-related disorders as "substance abuse," we find an estimated 17% of the population qualify as active or former cases. Consistent with patterns observed for alcohol and controlled drugs looked at separately, the lowest rate was obtained for the Durham site (12.8%), the highest for the Los Angeles site (18.8%) (Table 6–27), and there was a strikingly higher lifetime prevalence for men (26.9%) than for women (7.9%), and for adults 18–29 (23.8%) than for those over 65 (6.4%).

Among 18–29 year olds, substance abuse/dependence was about twice as common among men as women. Gender differences increased with age, reaching male estimates more than nine times the female estimates in the oldest group.

Although these disorders are extremely common, affecting one-third of young males, they are rarely treated. The strong association of the disorders

Table 6–27 Lifetime History of Substance Abuse/Dependence (Alcohol and/or Illicit Drugs): Prevalence Estimates in Relation to Sex, Site, and Age

| | Both Sexes | | Males | | Females | |
	%	(SE)	%	(SE)	%	(SE)
All sites	17.00	(0.30)	26.94	(0.60)	7.94	(0.30)
ECA sites:[a]						
New Haven	15.00	(0.67)	22.41	(1.16)	8.56	(0.72)
Baltimore	18.59	(0.78)	30.66	(1.37)	8.55	(0.76)
St. Louis	18.31	(0.94)	31.24	(1.66)	6.95	(0.85)
Durham	12.83	(0.70)	22.51	(1.29)	4.64	(0.60)
Los Angeles	18.78	(0.79)	28.84	(1.31)	9.32	(0.82)
Age groups:						
18–29	23.85	(0.70)	33.06	(0.12)	14.50	(0.90)
30–44	20.02	(0.80)	31.41	(0.13)	9.31	(0.80)
45–64	11.96	(0.60)	21.30	(1.10)	3.49	(0.50)
65+	6.43	(0.60)	13.58	(1.40)	1.50	(0.43)

[a]Site data weighted to population of catchment areas sampled at each site. Other data were weighted to national population distributions.

with curtailed education, disrupted marriages, and crime show that they have profound effects on our society as a whole as well as on those directly affected by them. Their variation by site and age group show them to be strongly influenced by the social environment, making them promising targets for prevention and intervention.

7 Panic and Phobia

WILLIAM W. EATON / AMY DRYMAN /
MYRNA M. WEISSMAN

THE DIAGNOSIS OF PANIC DISORDER
AND PHOBIC DISORDER

Panic disorder and phobic disorder are the two major anxiety disorders included in all sites of the ECA program. Some researchers feel that panic disorder should not be considered an entity distinct from agoraphobia because of the seemingly spontaneous nature of the precipitation of episodes of fear, in both panic and phobia. It is also true that panic attacks occur during the episodes of fear associated with all the variety of phobias. Therefore panic and phobia are brought together here in a single chapter. An underlying theme of this chapter, on which all the results can be focused, is the value of the distinction between panic and phobia and, especially, between panic disorder and agoraphobia.

A panic attack is a sudden feeling of apprehension or fear during which symptoms occur that are related to the nervous system (for example, feeling dizzy or faint); to the cardiovascular system (palpitations and shortness of breath); or to psychosensory functioning (the fear one is going crazy). The DIS opens the inquiry about panic attacks with the question, "Have you ever had a spell or attack when all of a sudden you felt frightened, anxious, or very uneasy in a situation when most people wouldn't be afraid?" Panic attacks can be caused by being in a very dangerous situation, but these types of attack are excluded from consideration here because most people would be afraid then. Panic attacks can result from ingestion of substances (for example, cocaine, marijuana, psychedelic drugs, or prescribed medications) or from physical illness or injury. Therefore, the interviewer must be sure that the attack cannot be explained by ingestion of substances or physical illness. The DSM-III diagnosis of panic disorder requires that panic attacks occur with 4 out of 12 concomitant psychophysiological symptoms, that the attacks are severe enough and happen often enough to be disruptive or distressing to the individual, and that at least one attack was spontaneous, that is, occurred in the absence of a phobic stimulus.

A phobia is an unreasonable fear of a particular situation. There are no credible causes of phobias due to medication, drugs, alcohol, physical ill- ness, or injury. The diagnosis of phobic disorder requires that the phobia be severe. Phobias seldom meet severity criteria by causing help seeking or taking medication, and when respondents are asked, Does your fear of [heights, for example] interfere with your life or activities a lot? They often answer something like, It doesn't interfere with my life because I don't go near [heights]. Interviewers were trained, at each ECA site, to respond to that answer with the further probe, Does having to avoid [heights] interfere with your life or activities a lot? To meet criteria of severity, therefore, the fear must either itself cause help-seeking, medication, or severe interfer- ence with activities or having to avoid the phobic stimulus is disruptive.

There are so many types of situations that are potentially fearful, and so many explanations for the fearfulness, that it is difficult to classify the phobias, and there is research underway currently to attempt to arrange the phobias into more meaningful classes than those provided by DSM-III. Following DSM-III, the DIS computer algorithm sorts phobias into three types: simple phobia, social phobia, and agoraphobia. In simple phobia, the fearful situation is an easily identified object or setting, such as animals, heights, bugs, closed places, or water. Social phobia includes fears of situa- tions involving meeting new people, eating in front of people, or speaking in public. Agoraphobia is more difficult to describe. It is a fear of entering a situation from which escape is impossible or difficult, and where help would not be available if something disabling occurred. One possibility for the "something disabling that might occur" is a panic attack. The DIS asks about the settings listed in DSM-III: tunnels, bridges, crowds, and public transportation, going out of the house alone, and being alone. Agoraphobia is regarded as the most severe form of phobia because agoraphobics often severely limit their travel and activities. Later publications from the ECA program will present more details on the specific phobias. For reasons of space we concentrate here, for the most part, on the broad category of phobic disorders.

There has been considerable clinical and theoretical research on panic and phobias, most of it conducted under the rubric of more encompassing nosologic categories such as neurosis (Marks, 1987). This research is un- usual in the field of psychopathology because it runs the gamut from biochemical to behavioral to use of animal models. Many disparate disci- plines contribute important information, theories, and perspectives to this varied research, which has produced an array of therapies, especially for the phobias. But since the delineation of panic and phobia into major, discrete diagnostic categories is relatively new with the DSM-III, the epidemiologic data are sparse. For this reason data from the ECA program may make an especially important contribution.

Table 7–1 (adapted from Marks, 1987, Table 9–5) compares selected

Table 7-1 Prevalence in Percent of Panic and Phobic Disorders: Community Surveys

Place of Study	Citations	Type of Rate	Sample Size	Panic Disorder	Agoraphobia	Other Phobia	Any Phobia	Phobic Symptoms
						Rate for:		
Vermont	Agras, S., et al., 1969	Point	325		0.6		2.2	7.7
Florida	Schwab, J., et al., 1979		1,645		0.2			16.0
London	Bebbington, P., et al., 1981	1 mo	800					17.4
New Haven	Weissman, M.M., et al., 1978	Point	511	0.4			1.4	
U.S.	Uhlenhuth, E.G., et al., 1983	1 yr	3,161		1.2	2.3		
Switzerland	Angst, J., & Dobler-Mikola, A., 1983	1 yr	600		1.8	1.2		
Munich	Wittchen, H.-U., 1987	6 mo	1,504		3.6	4.1		
U.S.	This chapter	1 yr	15,490	0.9	4.2	8.6	9.7	9.7

community studies published in English with the current study, which forms the bottom row of the table. If one expects a prevalence rate of 10% for these disorders, then a sample of 250 would provide 25 cases, which is the minimum for credible analysis: therefore, only studies with a sample size greater than 250 have been included. Only one study (Weissman et al., 1978) presents a prevalence rate for panic disorder—0.4%—, and this rate is based on only two cases found in a sample of 511 respondents. The ECA prevalence rate is 0.9%, twice as large but based on an interval of one year instead of a point prevalence. The published rates of agoraphobia are considerably lower than the ECA rate, except for the Munich study, which also used the DIS (version II). The rates for "other phobia" and "any phobia" are also much lower in earlier surveys than in the ECA data. However, the rate of phobic symptoms reported in this chapter is lower than the "phobic symptoms" rates reported in Florida (16%) and London (17.4%).

Phobic disorders are more common than any other specific disorder in the ECA program. This could be due, in part, to the fact that the DSM-III lists fewer criteria for the diagnosis of phobia than for other disorders. Two "yes" answers to DIS questions can satisfy the diagnostic criteria: a positive response to the initial specific phobia (for example, Have you ever had an unreasonable fear of heights?); and a positive response to the first probe question (for example, Did you tell a doctor about your fear of heights?). A second aspect of the DIS implementation of DSM-III phobic disorder is that there are 14 questions on specific phobias and one general question (Anything else you were unreasonably afraid of?); each of these 15 questions provides an opportunity to satisfy the diagnostic criteria in the simple two-question manner described above. Because DSM-III requires only a single phobic object, random measurement error may create a bias toward high rates of this disorder.

Data from New Haven have been omitted from analyses of phobias in the current chapter because version II of the DIS was used at the New Haven site and version III used at later sites. Version III inquires about eight additional phobias. The omission of these phobias in New Haven results in an undercount of phobic disorders there compared to the other four sites. The sample size for analyses of panic disorder is 19,498, representing those with complete responses for the panic disorder section at five ECA sites. The population estimates for panic disorder are obtained by weighting to the national U.S. population using the combined distribution on age, race/ethnicity, and sex for the five sites. For phobic disorder the sample size is 14,263, representing those with complete responses for the phobic disorder section at four sites (Baltimore, St. Louis, Durham, and Los Angeles). The population estimates for phobic disorder are obtained by weighting the combined four-site sample to the U.S. population with respect to age, race/ethnicity, and sex.

There have been several publications about panic and phobic disorders from the ECA program. Weissman and colleagues have provided several earlier reviews of anxiety disorders in general (1985, 1988); collaborators at Johns Hopkins have conducted analytic studies of panic disorder (Keyl and Eaton, 1989; Von Korff, Eaton & Keyl, 1985) and taxonomic studies of anxiety and depression (Eaton & Ritter, 1988; Eaton & Bohrnstedt, 1989).

PREVALENCE OF PANIC AND PHOBIC DISORDERS

Panic disorder is not very prevalent in the population, with less than 1% meeting criteria for diagnosis in the year prior to the interview, and less than 2% over their lifetime (Table 7–2a). The one-month rate is about half the size of the rate for one year, and about one-third the size of the lifetime rates. These ratios of one-half and one-third are found across the various subgroups (Table 7–2a) except for the minority group males, where the rates differ less by time periods, suggesting longer durations of the disorder for black and Hispanic than for white males.

Table 7–2a Prevalence of Panic Disorder by Sex and Ethnicity

| | | Prevalence in Percent (SE) | | | | | |
	Sample Size	One-Month		One-Year		Lifetime	
Total	19,498[a]	0.53	(.07)	0.91	(.10)	1.57	(.13)
Both Sexes							
White	12,968	0.50	(.08)	0.90	(.11)	1.62	(.14)
Black	4,668	0.64	(.26)	1.00	(.32)	1.31	(.37)
Hispanic	1,604	0.51	(.32)	0.66	(.36)	0.87	(.41)
Men							
All groups	8,375	0.35	(.09)	0.58	(.11)	0.99	(.15)
White	5,573	0.33	(.09)	0.58	(.12)	1.02	(.16)
Black	1,855	0.27	(.25)	0.57	(.36)	0.57	(.36)
Hispanic	818	0.31	(.36)	0.32	(.36)	0.41	(.41)
Women							
All groups	11,123	0.69	(.12)	1.22	(.16)	2.10	(.21)
White	7,395	0.65	(.13)	1.20	(.17)	2.17	(.23)
Black	2,813	0.94	(.42)	1.37	(.51)	1.93	(.60)
Hispanic	786	0.69	(.52)	1.00	(.62)	1.31	(.71)

[a]For lifetime prevalence, the total sample size is 19,501. These three additional cases are also included when calculating lifetime prevalence for the subgroups.

Females have about twice the rate of panic disorder as males throughout all the groups. This large difference is consistent with the literature.

There are no consistent differences in rates of panic disorder between race/ethnic groups, although blacks and Hispanics have lower lifetime prevalence rates than whites.

Phobic disorder is more prevalent than panic disorder, with a one-month rate of 6.7% and a lifetime rate of 14.2% (Table 7–2b). The lifetime prevalence figures are about 50% higher than the one-month figures for whites but two to three times higher for blacks and Hispanics. These results suggest briefer durations for the disorder in the two minority groups, contrary to the pattern for panic disorder.

Rates of phobic disorder are about twice as high for females as males. These differences are statistically significant ($p < .05$) for all race/ethnic groups combined and at the margin of significance for each of the three race/ethnic subgroups. The strongest and most consistent gender difference is found among the Hispanics, where the female rate is more than twice the male rate for one-month, one-year, and lifetime prevalence.

Table 7–2b Prevalence of Phobic Disorder by Sex and Ethnicity

		Prevalence[a] in Percent (SE)		
	Sample Size	One-Month	One-Year	Lifetime
Total	14,263[b]	6.67 (0.31)	9.72 (0.37)	14.25 (0.44)
Both Sexes				
White	8,409	6.17 (0.33)	9.06 (0.40)	9.68 (3.22)
Black	4,116	11.30 (1.24)	16.19 (1.45)	23.41 (0.47)
Hispanic	1,517	6.16 (1.30)	8.14 (1.48)	12.21 (1.62)
Men				
All groups	6,159	4.21 (0.37)	6.26 (0.44)	10.42 (0.56)
White	3,666	3.82 (0.38)	5.73 (0.46)	9.89 (0.59)
Black	1,610	7.88 (1.57)	11.54 (1.86)	16.52 (2.15)
Hispanic	768	3.77 (1.47)	4.70 (1.64)	8.23 (2.12)
Women				
All groups	8,104	8.92 (0.50)	12.88 (0.58)	17.74 (0.66)
White	4,743	8.34 (0.53)	12.13 (0.63)	16.65 (0.71)
Black	2,506	14.17 (1.86)	20.08 (2.13)	26.94 (2.34)
Hispanic	749	8.45 (2.11)	11.44 (2.41)	17.46 (2.87)

[a]Four sites' combined respondents (Baltimore, St. Louis, Durham, Los Angeles) weighted to the U.S. by age, sex, and ethnicity.

[b]For lifetime prevalence, the total sample size is 14,409, due to fewer missing data.

Blacks have higher rates of phobic disorders than whites or Hispanics (Table 7–2b). The difference is apparent for one-month, one-year, and lifetime prevalence and occurs in both gender groups. This difference is significant ($p < .05$) for both sexes combined and on the margin of significance for all the subgroups. Combining the effects of race/ethnicity and gender produces a considerable range in rates. Rates of lifetime prevalence among subgroups range from 8% (Hispanic males) to 27% (black females).

Simple phobia is the most common of the three subtypes, as shown in Table 7–2c. The figures given are for lifetime prevalence only: data on subtypes are available only for lifetime prevalence, since a single recency question grouped all the phobias experienced. About 11% of the population met criteria for simple phobia during their lifetime, compared with 5.6% for agoraphobia and 2.7% for social phobia. The relationships of gender and ethnicity to these phobia subtypes are generally similar to the relationships for phobic disorder as a whole; that is, rates are higher among women and among blacks, although there is less variation across groups for social phobia. Almost one-quarter of black women (24.4%) met criteria for simple phobia over their lifetime.

Table 7–2c Lifetime Prevalence[a] of Phobia Subtypes by Sex and Ethnicity, in Percent (SE)

		Lifetime Prevalence of		
	Sample Size[b]	Agoraphobia	Simple Phobia	Social Phobia[b]
Total	14,436	5.63 (0.29)	11.25 (0.40)	2.73 (0.20)
Both Sexes				
White	8,501	5.21 (0.31)	10.35 (0.42)	2.68 (0.22)
Black	4,185	9.19 (1.13)	19.70 (1.55)	3.39 (0.71)
Hispanic	1,526	5.37 (1.22)	9.63 (1.59)	2.46 (0.84)
Men				
All groups	6,212	3.18 (0.32)	7.75 (0.49)	2.53 (0.29)
White	3,694	2.85 (0.33)	7.12 (0.51)	2.71 (0.32)
Black	1,630	5.81 (1.35)	14.06 (2.01)	1.87 (0.78)
Hispanic	733	2.90 (1.29)	6.33 (1.88)	1.66 (0.99)
Women				
All groups	8,224	7.86 (0.47)	14.45 (0.61)	2.91 (0.29)
White	4,807	7.38 (0.50)	13.30 (0.65)	2.65 (0.31)
Black	2,555	12.00 (1.71)	24.38 (2.27)	4.66 (1.11)
Hispanic	753	7.74 (2.02)	12.79 (2.52)	3.21 (1.33)

[a]Four sites' combined respondents (Baltimore, St. Louis, Durham, Los Angeles) weighted to the U.S. by age, sex, and ethnicity.

[b]Sample sizes given are for agoraphobia. For simple phobia, the total sample is 14,429 and for social phobia, the total is 14,400.

SITE DIFFERENCES

For panic disorder the variation across sites is not very large (Table 7–3); the lifetime prevalence rates of panic disorder vary only from a low of 1.5% to a high of 1.6%. None of the differences between sites is statistically significant. (The figures in the "total" row at the top of Table 7–3 are slightly different from those in Table 7–2 because here the sample is weighted to the population in these sites, not to the total U.S population).

In contrast to panic disorder, there is considerable variation in rates for phobic disorders across sites (Table 7–3), ranging from 4.1% one-month prevalence at St. Louis to 11.2% at both Baltimore and Durham. As noted above, data from New Haven are not included because the structure of the questionnaires differed. The Baltimore and Durham sites have significantly higher rates than St. Louis or Los Angeles. It is not obvious why rates of sites should vary. To produce such a large difference between sites, a

Table 7–3 Prevalence of Panic and Phobic Disorders by Site

| | Sample Size | Prevalence[a] in Percent (SE) | | |
		One-Month	One-Year	Lifetime
Total				
Panic	19,498[b]	0.55 (0.09)	0.91 (0.10)	1.51 (0.11)
Phobic	14,263[c]	8.21 (0.29)	11.78 (0.34)	17.02 (0.40)
New Haven				
Panic	5,105	0.37 (0.11)	0.81 (0.17)	1.47 (0.23)
Baltimore				
Panic	3,567	0.68 (0.16)	1.08 (0.21)	1.47 (0.24)
Phobic	3,523	11.23 (0.63)	16.30 (0.74)	23.66 (0.85)
St. Louis				
Panic	3,210	0.60 (0.19)	1.09 (0.25)	1.54 (0.30)
Phobic	3,192	4.08 (0.48)	6.36 (0.60)	9.47 (0.71)
Durham				
Panic	4,122	0.53 (0.15)	0.77 (0.18)	1.64 (0.26)
Phobic	4,073	11.23 (0.66)	15.72 (0.76)	21.12 (0.85)
Los Angeles				
Panic	3,494	0.62 (0.16)	0.87 (0.19)	1.64 (0.26)
Phobic	3,475	5.18 (0.45)	7.25 (0.52)	11.56 (0.64)

[a]Each site's respondents weighted to population of its sample catchment areas by age, sex, and ethnicity.
[b]For lifetime prevalence, the sample size is 19,501.
[c]For lifetime prevalence, the sample size is 14,409.

characteristic would have to be strongly related to the occurrence of phobia and have a very different distribution at the two "high" versus the two "low" sites. There are variables with moderate associations with phobia discussed below, but none with very strong associations. Furthermore, the site differences in such variables tend to be small. There may be cultural differences related to living along the East Coast, but this hypothesis is difficult to test with the data at hand. This issue of intersite differences in phobic disorders is the subject of continuing exploration in the ECA program.

AGE

Older persons have low rates of panic disorder (Table 7–4a); adults aged 30–44 have the highest rates. This relationship to age occurs among whites

Table 7–4a Prevalence of Panic Disorder by Age, Sex, and Ethnicity

| | Prevalence in Percent (SE) | | | |
| | Men | | Women | |
Ethnicity	One-Year	Lifetime	One-Year	Lifetime
All Groups				
18–29	0.57 (0.20)	0.64 (0.21)	1.11 (0.28)	1.39 (0.31)
30–44	0.73 (0.24)	1.76 (0.38)	1.94 (0.38)	3.67 (0.52)
45–64	0.68 (0.24)	1.04 (0.29)	1.13 (0.29)	2.23 (0.40)
65+	0.04 (0.08)	0.08 (0.12)	0.41 (0.22)	0.67 (0.29)
Whites				
18–29	0.58 (0.22)	0.67 (0.24)	1.10 (0.31)	1.45 (0.35)
30–44	0.72 (0.27)	1.80 (0.42)	2.08 (0.44)	4.04 (0.61)
45–64	0.68 (0.25)	1.10 (0.32)	1.04 (0.30)	2.17 (0.43)
65+	0.04 (0.09)	0.09 (0.13)	0.33 (0.21)	0.59 (0.29)
Blacks				
18–29	0.59 (0.59)	0.60 (0.60)	1.49 (0.89)	1.49 (0.89)
30–44	0.87 (0.83)	0.87 (0.83)	2.17 (1.20)	3.07 (1.42)
45–64	0.41 (0.62)	0.41 (0.62)	0.96 (0.86)	2.04 (1.24)
65+	0.00 (—)[a]	0.00 (—)[a]	0.00 (—)[a]	0.36 (0.75)
Hispanics				
18–29	0.55 (0.71)	0.55 (0.71)	0.18 (0.42)	0.18 (0.42)
30–44	0.01 (0.10)	0.34 (0.68)	0.00 (—)[a]	0.41 (0.72)
45–64	0.36 (0.83)	0.36 (0.83)	2.92 (2.25)	3.73 (2.52)
65+	0.00 (—)[a]	0.00 (—)[a]	3.41 (3.83)	3.41 (3.83)

[a]No standard error computed for rate of zero.

and blacks and in both sexes. Only the group over 65 years of age is significantly different from the other age groups.

The lower level of lifetime prevalence for older persons is curious, because older persons have had a longer period in which to develop an occurrence of the disorder. One explanation could be that individuals with panic disorder are less likely to reach old age—perhaps the leading speculation consistent with this hypothesis would be that they have concomitant cardiovascular disturbances that raise mortality. Another explanation might be that individuals born earlier constitute a cohort that is somehow protected against panic disorder; or conversely, that younger individuals are in a cohort that has a heightened risk of panic disorder. The most probable explanation for the higher lifetime rate of panic disorder is that older people fail to recall episodes of panic because they have not experienced them recently, or because they are more likely than younger individuals to find them shameful.

The relationship of age to panic disorder is distinctly different for Hispanics. The group aged 30–44 years has a lower one-year rate than those younger (18–29 years) and also lower than the middle-aged group, those 45–64 years. This pattern is found for both men and women. In the group aged 65 years and older, there are strong sex differences. The rate for men in this age group drops to zero, while for Hispanic women, the rate is large. The overall pattern for Hispanic women suggests a linear increase in the prevalence of panic disorder with increasing age. The differences shown in Table 7–4a are in general not statistically significant, but the patterns are strong and clear.

Age differences in rates of phobic disorder are not as strong as for panic disorder (Table 7–4b). The group aged 65 and older tend to have the lowest rate, but since the differences are not very large, the overall conclusion is that there is no consistent pattern relating age to phobic disorder.

SYMPTOMS AND DISORDERS

This section focuses on the symptoms of panic and phobia, the way the symptoms are combined to form disorders, and the relationship of the two disorders to each other. Table 7–5a presents the lifetime prevalence of the various symptoms of phobia and panic. It includes a single question from the DIS—Have you ever considered yourself a nervous person?—which is not used for any DSM-III disorder but is relevant to this general area.

Table 7–5a shows symptoms aggregated into diagnostic categories. The table also shows use of services by persons with each symptom to aid in judging its importance. The figures presented are unweighted; that is, they are percentages of respondents, not population estimates. The left column,

Table 7-4b Prevalence of Phobic Disorder by Age, Sex, and Ethnicity

| Ethnicity | Sample Size | Prevalence[a] in Percent (SE) | | | |
| | | Men | | Women | |
		One-Year	Lifetime	One-Year	Lifetime
All Groups					
18-9	3,945	6.50 (0.78)	11.13 (0.99)	13.38 (1.09)	16.26 (1.18)
30-44	3,721	6.12 (0.84)	10.46 (1.07)	16.13 (1.25)	22.58 (1.41)
45-64	3,319	6.73 (0.87)	10.73 (1.07)	11.64 (1.07)	17.09 (1.25)
65+	3,271	4.90 (1.11)	7.78 (1.37)	8.84 (1.22)	13.74 (1.47)
Whites					
18-29	2,020	5.84 (0.83)	10.65 (1.09)	12.24 (1.18)	14.84 (1.28)
30-44	1,997	5.82 (0.90)	10.27 (1.17)	16.35 (1.40)	22.33 (1.56)
45-64	2,146	6.23 (0.91)	9.93 (1.12)	10.49 (1.11)	15.56 (1.30)
65+	2,244	4.20 (1.10)	7.18 (1.41)	8.45 (1.27)	13.01 (1.53)
Blacks					
18-29	1,285	11.46 (3.00)	16.18 (3.46)	22.99 (3.81)	27.23 (4.00)
30-44	1,156	10.48 (3.35)	14.29 (3.81)	18.04 (3.83)	24.60 (4.26)
45-64	851	12.71 (4.01)	20.26 (4.78)	21.03 (4.40)	30.63 (4.90)
65+	822	12.04 (5.96)	15.30 (6.58)	14.80 (5.37)	24.17 (6.42)
Hispanics					
18-29	564	7.12 (3.05)	10.55 (3.63)	9.58 (3.60)	13.50 (4.16)
30-44	509	2.68 (2.29)	6.84 (3.59)	12.12 (4.43)	22.19 (5.63)
45-64	280	2.62 (2.67)	6.44 (4.10)	15.77 (5.91)	20.54 (6.56)
65+	161	4.97 (6.70)	4.97 (6.70)	6.43 (6.28)	10.36 (7.80)

[a]Four sites' combined respondents (Baltimore, St. Louis, Durham, Los Angeles) weighted to the U.S. by age, sex, and ethnicity.

headed "severe," shows the percentage reporting the symptom on the initial DIS question (for example, Have you ever had an unreasonable fear of heights?) who met criteria of severity (that is, the symptom was mentioned to a doctor or other health professional, medication was taken for it more than once, or it interfered with life or activities a lot). For phobias, this column is equivalent to the DSM-III diagnosis for the specific phobia named. It also gives lifetime prevalences for "any simple phobia," "any social phobia," "any agoraphobia," and "any phobia." The second column, headed "non-severe," is the percentage of persons who reported the symptom on the initial question but did not answer positively to any of the questions assessing its severity. These two columns are mutually exclusive and can be added to yield the total percentage reporting each symptom or *any* symptom of a disorder.

Unreasonable fears of heights and bugs or other small animals are the

Table 7–5a Unweighted Lifetime Prevalence of Anxiety Symptoms by Severity, with Use of Services

Symptoms	Prevalence of Symptom (%)		Mental Health Services in Prior Six Months for Persons with This Symptom (%)	
	Severe[a]	Non-Severe	Specialty Settings	Other Medical Settings
Nervous Person	—[b]	26.7	8.7	8.0
Simple Phobias				
Heights	4.7	13.5	7.0	6.5
Closed places	2.4	5.6	12.0	8.2
Storms[c]	2.8	6.5	4.6	6.8
Water[c]	3.3	9.2	5.0	7.9
Bugs, mice,, snakes, bats	6.1	16.3	6.7	7.5
Animals	1.1	2.8	9.1	12.3
Other fears	2.1	4.2	12.2	7.9
Any simple phobia[c]	15.1	35.1	6.6	6.8
Social Phobias				
Eating in public[c]	0.9	1.8	10.2	8.6
Speaking in public[c]	1.8	4.7	9.3	8.5
Speaking to new acquaintances	1.4	3.3	14.2	7.4
Any social phobia	3.2	8.5	9.9	8.4
Agoraphobia				
Being alone	1.4	2.4	21.4	8.7
Tunnels or bridges[c]	2.1	4.9	6.0	6.7
Crowds	2.6	4.2	13.4	10.0
Public transport[c]	3.2	7.3	6.6	7.3
Going out by oneself	1.4	1.9	13.5	10.6
Any agoraphobia[c]	7.6	15.7	9.4	8.2
Any Phobia[c]	18.5	41.7	7.5	7.0
Panic[c]				
Any attack	5.5	4.2	20.6	10.4
Any Anxiety Symptom[c]	21.0	54.8	9.1	7.4

[a]Severe symptoms are those meeting one of three criteria: a professional was told about it, medication was taken for it more than once, or it interfered with life or activities a lot. In addition, for panic attacks to be severe, at least one attack was not explained by alcohol, drugs, physical illness, exertion, or a situation that would be expected to be frightening.

[b]This symptom was not rated as to severity.

[c]Because not all questions were asked in New Haven, that site was dropped for this item, reducing sample size to 14,263.

most common fears reported—over 18% responded positively to each of these questions, and about 5% met criteria of severity. Two other symptoms—unreasonable fears of water and of public transport—were reported by over 10% of the sample, with over 3% meeting criteria of severity.

A comparison of the relative magnitude of the first two columns suggests that many symptoms of phobia usually occur in trivial or innocuous form, instead of being an experience quite different from the normal. While more than half of those reporting the occurrence of a panic attack (5.5%/9.7%) said it met severity criteria and was not explained by medication, drugs, alcohol, physical illness, or injury, an "unreasonable fear of bugs or small animals" met severity criteria for less than one-third of those responding positively (6.1%/22.4%). Indeed, all anxiety symptoms except three met severity criteria less than one-third of the time; the exceptions were panic attacks and two symptoms of agoraphobia, an unreasonable fear of being alone and of going out by oneself. These three symptoms appear to represent less of a continuum with normal experience than other anxiety symptoms.

The symptoms of anxiety are widely distributed in the population. Half reported a simple phobia, ignoring whether or not it met severity criteria; 12% a social phobia; and 23% a symptom of agoraphobia, a total of 60% reporting one or more phobic symptoms after overlaps are removed. More than three-quarters (75.8%) of the population responded positively to one or more of these symptom questions. This high frequency is reminiscent of the Midtown Manhattan study in the 1950s (Srole et al., 1962), and underscores the importance of the DIS's follow-ups of positive responses to separate trivial fears and responses to the stresses and strains of everyday life from psychiatric disorders.

Table 7-5b concerns the relationship of panic attacks to agoraphobia. Here the reader can follow the DSM-III algorithm explicitly, examining prevalences at each step. DSM-III requires a panic attack to have four or more concomitant physiological symptoms. These "intense" attacks occurred in 5.9% of the sample. Intense attacks usually are severe and not explained by drugs, medication, alcohol, physical illness, or injury ("intense and severe," 3.8%). In only 1.7% of the population, or less than half of those with intense and severe attacks, have the attacks occurred at least three times in three weeks, that is, often enough to meet the DSM-III criteria of recurrence. Persons with intense, recurrent attacks are diagnosed as having panic disorder if the attacks have occurred at least once with no obvious phobic stimulus. It is rare for severe, intense, and recurrent panic attacks to have occurred solely in the presence of a phobic stimulus: 0.1% occurred only when confronted by a social or simple phobic situation and 0.2% in an agoraphobic situation (and perhaps in other phobic situations as well) but not spontaneously. Thus 17% of all persons experiencing severe recurrent panic attacks had them only in phobic situations (.3%/1.7%).

Table 7–5b Overlap Between Panic Attacks and Phobia and Use of Services (Unweighted)

Type of Panic Attack	Prevalence of This Type of Attack (%)		Mental Health Services in Prior Six Months for Persons with This Type of Attack (%)	
	Severe[a]	Non-Severe	Specialty Settings	Other Medical Settings
Intense	3.8	2.1	21.3	11.8
Intense, recurrent	1.7	0.5	26.8	12.8
Solely in phobic situations:				
Social/Simple only	0.1	0.0	—[c]	—[c]
Agoraphobic	0.2	0.0	33.3	7.4
In phobic situation and spontaneous:				
Social/Simple only	0.2	0.0	32.1	14.3
Agoraphobic	0.5	0.0	27.5	12.5
No phobia	0.7	0.2	23.5	15.6
Panic Disorder[b]	1.4	0.3	26.0	14.3

[a]Severe symptoms are those meeting one of three criteria: a professional was told about it, medication was taken for it more than once, or it interfered with life or activities a lot. In addition, for panic attacks to be severe, at least one attack was not explained by alcohol, drugs, physical illness, exertion, or a situation that would be expected to be frightening.

[b]Because not all questions were asked in New Haven, that site was dropped for this item, reducing sample size to 14,263.

[c]Sample size for this cell below 25; percentage not estimated.

The remainder (1.4%) had severe, intense, recurrent panic attacks at least once in the absence of a phobic stimulus (rows headed "Phobic Situation and Spontaneous" plus "No Phobia"), and thus met DSM-III criteria for panic disorder. Almost two-thirds (64%) of the cases of panic disorder [(.2% + .7%)/1.4%] were panic disorder without agoraphobia, while the remainder could be termed panic disorder with agoraphobia. Thus, DIS/DSM-III panic disorder is not inevitably tied to DIS/DSM-III agoraphobia. Of those with agoraphobia (7.6% of the sample), only a few have panic disorder (.5%/7.6%, or about 7% of those with agoraphobia).

The third and fourth columns of Tables 7–5a and b show the degree to which the occurrence of a severe anxiety symptom or disorder over the individual's lifetime was associated with use of medical services for emotional problems during the six months prior to the interview. The fourth column shows the percentage with the severe symptom who visited a nonpsychiatric medical setting because of an emotional problem. The third column shows the percentage visiting a psychiatric setting. These columns suggest which symptoms produce demand for mental health-related services in both psychiatric and nonpsychiatric settings. Over 20% of those reporting ever having had a severe panic attack or a severe unreasonable fear of being alone had visited a psychiatric setting during the six months prior to the interview. Persons with recurrent panic attacks were the ones most likely to visit the mental health sector (over 25% did). Persons with an unreasonable fear of going out alone—the third symptom suggested above as being severe—also had a relatively high rate of services use, with about 14% reporting a recent psychiatric visit. Unreasonable fears of tunnels, bridges, and public transport, although defined as part of agoraphobia, are associated with the low rates of treatment typical of simple phobias, while an unreasonable fear of closed places, defined as a simple phobia, has the higher rate associated with other agoraphobia symptoms and panic attacks.

Figure 7–1 provides additional insight into the overlaps between panic, agoraphobia, and other phobias for men and women. About 5% of both males and females with one or more of these disorders have panic disorder only, and about 10% of both males and females meet criteria for agoraphobia only. For men and women with one of these disorders, the most common pattern is "other phobia" alone (64% of affected males; 51% of affected females). The next most common pattern is agoraphobia plus another type of phobia (16% of men; 28% of women). The combination of agoraphobia and panic accounts for 3% of affected men and 4% of affected women. This overlap between panic and agoraphobia accounts for 11% of

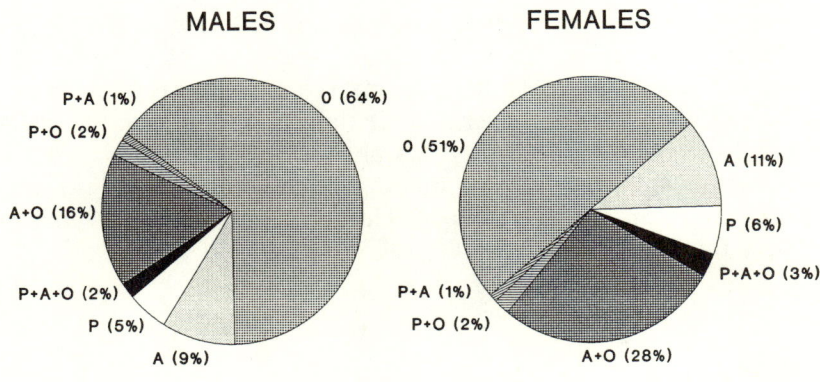

P = PANIC
A = AGORAPHOBIA
O = SIMPLE OR SOCIAL PHOBIA

Figure 7–1 Overlap of Panic and Phobic Disorders in Males and Females with Either

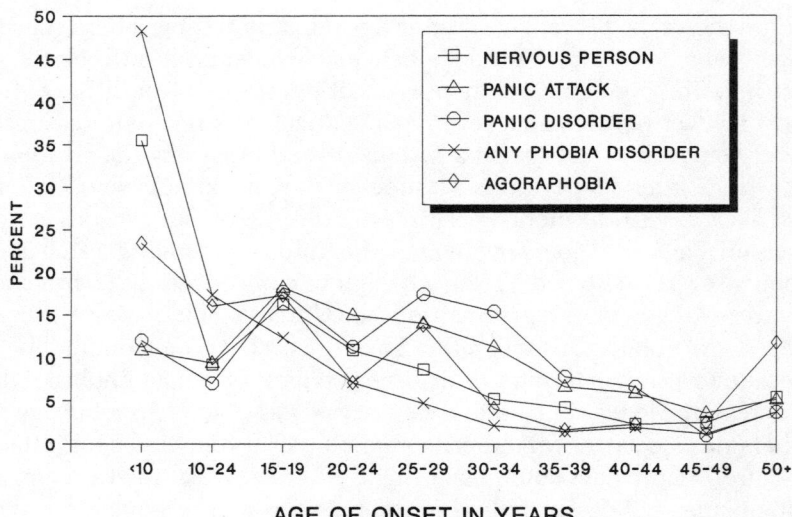

Figure 7-2 Age of Onset for Anxiety

men with agoraphobia (3%/28%), 30% of men with panic disorder (3%/10%), 9% of women with agoraphobia (4%/43%) and 33% of women with panic disorder (4%/12%). Therefore, a minority of affected men and women with either disorder has the other, but agoraphobia is more typical of people with panic than panic is of people with agoraphobia, because panic disorder is less common than agoraphobia.

Another aspect of the distinction between panic and phobia is the possible difference in age of onset. Figure 7-2 shows age of onset for those reporting a panic attack over their lifetime, those meeting criteria for panic disorder or phobic disorder over their lifetime, and those meeting lifetime criteria for agoraphobia but no other phobia. Phobic disorders generally begin early in life, whereas panic attacks and panic disorder typically occur for the first time in young adulthood. The age of onset of agoraphobia falls between that of other phobias and panic disorder.

POTENTIAL RISK FACTORS

In this section we consider potential risk factors for panic disorder and phobic disorder that derive from the socioeconomic placement of individuals in society. In the next section we consider potential risk factors deriving from individuals' immediate social networks—that is, their marital status and the situation of their household or residence.

Because these data are cross-sectional in nature, the interpretation of an association between a given status and an elevated rate of disorder is subject to two competing explanations. One explanation for the association is that the sociodemographic status causes the disorder in some way; the second general type of explanation is that individuals with specific mental disorders are selected into certain sociodemographic statuses. Both panic and phobia are symptoms connected to fear, which is a natural response to certain situations. Fear is likely to be heightened in situations where the individual is not in control of the environment. Inability to control the environment—especially the social environment—provides one general framework for understanding how sociodemographic statuses might be causally related to the prevalence of panic and phobia. Low socioeconomic status, for example, might lead to less control over the environment with regard to where one lives, with whom one associates, how one copes with unexpected crises, and so forth. On the other hand, low socioeconomic status could be an indication that the disorder has caused disability, perhaps in work performance. With cross-sectional data it is impossible to establish the truth of the competing causation versus selection interpretations. Hence we use "potential risk factor" to describe the variables under study.

SOCIOECONOMIC VARIABLES

Educational status is one indicator of socioeconomic status (SES). Lower educational attainment means less knowledge and earnings, which may be related to a general feeling of lack of control over the environment, thus relating to the causation interpretation; it also reflects a lower level of achievement, which relates to the selection interpretation. Either way, respondents with lower educational attainment are expected to have higher rates of panic and phobia. Table 7–6 shows that there is not much relation between women's education level and either panic or phobia. For men, there is no regular relationship for panic, but there is a tendency for men with lower education to have higher rates of phobia. Since average educational attainment has increased in recent decades, we examined these relationships within distinct age groups. Age-specific data are not reported because the patterns within age groups did not differ from those seen for the total sample in Table 7–6.

Average educational attainment also varies by race/ethnic status. Lower educational achievement may constitute a special stress for members of disadvantaged minority groups. Therefore, Table 7–7 presents prevalence rates by education and race/ethnic group for panic and phobia. For panic disorder, there is no discernible relationship of educational attainment to prevalence for any of the three race/ethnic groups. For phobia, there is no

Table 7-6 One-Year Prevalence of Panic and Phobic Disorders by Sex and Education, in Percent (SE)

Years of Education	Panic Disorder		Phobic Disorder[a]	
	Male	Female	Male	Female
0-7	1.82 (0.69)	1.12 (0.53)	10.81 (1.86)	12.60 (1.94)
8	0.17 (0.25)	1.80 (0.70)	7.77 (1.93)	15.02 (2.24)
9-11	0.78 (0.31)	1.15 (0.36)	8.16 (1.16)	16.74 (1.48)
12	0.24 (0.15)	1.08 (0.27)	5.59 (0.84)	12.24 (1.01)
13-15	0.64 (0.26)	1.48 (0.38)	4.11 (0.78)	11.46 (1.30)
16+	0.38 (0.20)	0.95 (0.36)	5.05 (0.92)	10.01 (1.42)

[a]Four sites' combined respondents (Baltimore, St. Louis, Durham, Los Angeles) weighted to the U.S. by age, sex, and ethnicity.

clear relationship of educational attainment to prevalence for the two minority groups, but there is a barely significant linear trend evident for whites, with lower educational attainment associated with a higher rate of phobic disorder.

When we examine differences between ethnic groups with equal levels of educational attainment, no difference is found with respect to panic disorder, but minority groups have higher levels of phobia at every level of educational attainment.

Another measure of socioeconomic status is the relative standing of the occupation. The index created by Nam and Powers (1965) measures this standing in percentiles, and Table 7-8 presents rates of panic and phobia by the Nam scores grouped into quintiles. The causation and selection interpretations both lead to the prediction that those in the lower quintiles will have higher rates of disorder. Table 7-8 shows that there is not much difference in rates of phobic disorder according to socioeconomic standing of the occupation. For panic disorder, the pattern of findings differs by sex, in that lower SES males have higher rates of disorder, as expected; but lower SES females have lower rates of disorder, contrary to the expectation. This pattern, however intriguing, is not statistically significant.

Another measure of SES is whether the individual is financially dependent on the government, as indicated by receiving payments such as welfare or disability benefits. Being financially dependent is stressful and clearly reduces the ability to control the environment; therefore, one expects a higher rate of disorder among the financially dependent. It is also probably true that persons prone to various types of mental disorders,

Table 7-7 One-Year Prevalence of Panic and Phobic Disorders by Race/Ethnic Group and Education, in Percent (SE)

Years of Education	Panic Disorder			Phobic Disorder[a]		
	White	Black	Hispanic	White	Black	Hispanic
0–7	1.74 (0.62)	1.33 (1.01)	0.91 (0.70)	11.95 (1.74)	19.95 (4.23)	5.63 (2.04)
8	1.09 (0.44)	1.77 (1.77)	0.00 (—)[b]	11.05 (1.58)	23.14 (7.20)	10.29 (7.44)
9–11	0.87 (0.26)	1.28 (0.66)	0.95 (0.93)	11.80 (1.06)	17.63 (2.74)	11.61 (3.81)
12	0.75 (0.18)	0.45 (0.42)	0.33 (0.61)	9.03 (0.73)	13.59 (2.64)	8.10 (3.50)
13–15	1.14 (0.26)	0.94 (0.77)	0.04 (0.24)	7.13 (0.78)	13.30 (3.37)	8.57 (3.99)
16+	0.58 (0.20)	0.89 (1.11)	1.28 (2.28)	6.78 (0.83)	14.67 (5.01)	10.49 (7.95)

[a]Four sites' combined respondents (Baltimore, St. Louis, Durham, Los Angeles) weighted to the U.S. by age, sex, and ethnicity.
[b]Standard error not computed for rate of zero.

Table 7-8 One-Year Prevalence of Panic and Phobic Disorders by Sex and Occupational Status

| Quintile of Occupational Status | One Year Prevalence in Percent (SE) | | | |
| | Panic Disorder | | Phobic Disorder[a] | |
	Males	Females	Males	Females
0–20 (Low)	0.56 (0.47)	0.49 (0.43)	6.68 (1.83)	14.94 (2.54)
21–40	0.38 (0.25)	0.99 (0.46)	5.07 (1.08)	11.51 (1.75)
41–60	0.32 (0.22)	0.65 (0.36)	6.54 (1.15)	12.04 (1.73)
61–80	0.19 (0.14)	1.42 (0.52)	3.70 (0.75)	11.44 (1.73)
81–100 (High)	0.14 (0.17)	1.23 (0.80)	5.68 (1.36)	11.58 (2.87)

[a]Four sites' combined respondents (Baltimore, St. Louis, Durham, Los Angeles) weighted to the U.S. by age, sex, and ethnicity.

including panic and phobia, are more likely to become financially dependent. Table 7-9 shows that, as expected, financially dependent individuals, whether males or females, have higher rates of both disorders.

THE FAMILY AND HOUSEHOLD

The immediate social environment of the individual can be described in terms of his marital status, the number of individuals living in the household, and his residential setting. It might be expected that the sharing of

Table 7-9 One-Year Prevalence of Panic and Phobic Disorders by Sex and Financial Dependence in Percent (SE)

| Financial Dependency | Panic Disorder | | Phobic Disorder[a] | |
	Males	Females	Males	Females
No	0.44 (0.11)	0.97 (0.15)	5.59 (0.44)	12.09 (0.61)
Yes	1.94 (0.68)	3.23 (0.80)	12.98 (2.04)	19.63 (2.17)

[a]Four sites' combined respondents (Baltimore, St. Louis, Durham, Los Angeles) weighted to the U.S. by age, sex, and ethnicity.

resources that takes place between spouses would remove certain sources of stress and provide help to meet unexpected crises. This line of reasoning, within the framework of the causation interpretation, leads to the prediction that the nonmarried (never married or separated, widowed, or divorced) have higher rates of disorder than the married, although some have argued that marriage is beneficial only to men, not to women. The selection view argues that psychopathology decreases chances of marrying and increases the likelihood of becoming separated or divorced if one marries. Both lines of reasoning lead to the prediction that the never married and the separated and divorced will have higher rates of psychopathology than the married, but the two arguments diverge in their prediction for the widowed category. Under the causation interpretation, the widowed suffer the same stresses as other nonmarried groups and should have higher rates; under the selection interpretation the widowed have not participated in a selection process involving their own psychological attributes, and, therefore, their rates should be equal to those of the married (see Eaton, 1986). Since marital status varies with age, it will be necessary to control for age in examining these hypotheses.

The data support the causation argument for males, because the widowed have a rate similar to that for other nonmarried categories while those married have the lowest rates of panic and phobia (Table 7–10). For women, the data do not support either argument, because the never mar-

Table 7–10 One-Year Prevalence of Panic and Phobic Disorders by Sex, Age, and Current Marital Status in Percent (SE)

	Panic Disorder		Phobic Disorder[a]	
	Males	Females	Males	Females
18–44:				
Never Married	0.66 (0.24)	1.06 (0.35)	6.50 (0.89)	11.50 (1.34)
Married	0.48 (0.19)	1.34 (0.30)	5.58 (0.77)	15.04 (1.13)
Separated/Divorced	1.56 (0.83)	3.15 (0.91)	9.89 (0.24)	20.23 (2.51)
Widowed	[b]	2.19 (3.25)	[b]	17.48 (10.08)
45 +:				
Never Married	1.37 (1.14)	0.71 (0.77)	7.21 (2.98)	11.06 (3.54)
Married	0.25 (0.13)	1.14 (0.31)	5.71 (0.77)	9.91 (1.06)
Separated/Divorced	1.02 (0.17)	0.75 (0.56)	7.96 (2.45)	16.18 (2.83)
Widowed	1.55 (1.09)	0.38 (0.25)	7.34 (2.72)	9.47 (1.45)

[a]Four sites' combined respondents (Baltimore, St. Louis, Durham, Los Angeles) weighted to the U.S. by age, sex, and ethnicity.

[b]Less than 25 respondents in this cell; rate not computed.

ried have low rates of panic and phobia in both age groups, and among those over the age of 45 years the widowed have lower rates of both panic and phobia than do the currently married. There is some support for the view that marriage is more beneficial for men than women: married men have the lowest rate for both disorders and for both age groups, but for married women the differences are either not strong or in the wrong direction.

Additional data on the living situation are presented in Table 7–11, which shows the relationship of number of individuals living in the household to prevalence of panic disorder and phobic disorder by sex. There are two predictions here. The first prediction is that living alone probably elevates the risk for disorder. This prediction is supported by the pattern of the data for panic disorder in that males living alone have the highest rate and females living alone the second highest rate, but the same pattern is not evident for phobic disorder. The second prediction is that there is increased stress with an increase in the number of individuals—beyond two—living in the household. Larger households are generally those with children, although our data do not distinguish households with children from others. Since women are more likely to stay home with the children, the effects of increased numbers should be more evident for them. This is, indeed, what the data suggest for both panic disorder and phobic disorder, although the differences are not statistically significant.

The residential setting of the individual is important to consider, and the ECA program involved samples from the major types of setting—the

Table 7–11 One-Year Prevalence of Panic and Phobic Disorders by Sex and Number in the Household

Number in Household	Household Residents in Percent (SE)			
	Panic Disorder		Phobic Disorder[a]	
	Males	Females	Males	Females
One (living alone)	0.94 (0.44)	1.23 (0.42)	6.83 (1.34)	11.65 (1.46)
Two	0.50 (0.19)	0.97 (0.26)	5.33 (0.72)	11.62 (1.01)
Three	0.27 (0.18)	1.57 (0.39)	7.22 (1.09)	12.74 (1.27)
Four	0.71 (0.28)	1.12 (0.36)	6.41 (1.03)	13.51 (1.48)
Five or more	0.62 (0.27)	1.23 (0.37)	6.16 (1.04)	15.78 (1.53)

[a]Four sites' combined respondents (Baltimore, St. Louis, Durham, Los Angeles) weighted to the U.S. by age, sex, and ethnicity.

Table 7-12 One-Year Prevalence of Panic and Phobic Disorders by Sex and Residential Setting, in Percent (SE)

Residential Setting	Panic Disorder		Phobic Disorder[a]	
	Males	Females	Males	Females
Household	0.57 (0.11)	1.22 (0.16)	6.21 (0.44)	12.89 (0.59)
Chronic care	1.16 (3.25)	0.04 (0.46)	11.38 (11.59)	9.10 (7.59)
Correctional	2.77 (4.42)	6.06 (21.81)	15.21 (11.99)	23.50 (45.83)
Psychiatric	5.67 (14.33)	19.95 (38.99)	24.15 (34.07)	34.72 (48.57)

[a]Four sites' combined respondents (Baltimore, St. Louis, Durham, Los Angeles) weighted to the U.S. by age, sex, and ethnicity.

household and three institutional settings: chronic care, correctional, and psychiatric (Table 7-12). The household setting holds the generally healthiest portion of the population, and rates are expected to be lower there—a prediction that is confirmed in these data. Since chronic care settings contain many older persons, the expectation is that rates of panic and phobic disorder will be lower there also, and this prediction is confirmed. The rates of panic and phobic disorder are expected to be high in the psychiatric setting, and this expectation is confirmed, too. What is a little surprising is the relatively high rates of these disorders in correctional institutions.

USE OF SERVICES

About half (58%) of persons without either panic or phobia visited a doctor for physical health reasons in the six months prior to interview (Table 7-13). Those with panic disorder had used services much more; 86% had an outpatient visit for physical health reasons. Those with phobic disorders had an intermediate rate of use (68%). Those with panic disorder also made more use of the mental health sector; 51% of those with an attack in the last year reported an outpatient visit to the mental health sector during the prior six months. This compares with only 17% of those with phobic disorder, and only 8% of individuals without one of these two disorders. Thus, the odds of obtaining help for emotional problems is about seven times as great if the individual has panic disorder, and a little over twice as great if there is phobic disorder than if these disorders are absent.

Table 7-13 Use of Health Services by Household Residents With and Without
Panic and Phobic Disorders

| | Percent Using Health Services among Active (One-Year) Cases of: | | | |
| | Panic Disorder | | Phobic Disorder[a] | |
Use of Services	Yes	No	Yes	No
Physical health				
Outpatient within 6 months	86.2	58.1	68.4	55.4
Inpatient within 1 year	34.7	16.1	21.0	15.8
Mental health				
Outpatient within 6 months	51.0	8.1	17.3	7.6
Inpatient within 1 year	17.1	1.7	4.1	1.5

[a]Includes four sites (New Haven omitted).

CONCLUSION

Panic disorder and phobic disorder are closely related in terms of symptomatology and, probably, etiology. Females have higher prevalence than males
for both disorders, and the elderly have lower prevalence rates than other
age groups for both disorders. Findings regarding the relationship to measures of socioeconomic status, including education, occupational standing,
and financial dependence are not different for the two disorders. Likewise,
patterns of association with household factors, such as marital status, number in the household, and residential setting, do not markedly distinguish
the two disorders.

But there are important differences between the two disorders. Panic
disorder is much rarer. Panic disorder appears to be more distressing to the
individual than phobic disorder, as indicated by a much higher rate of
services use. The prevalence of panic disorder is also much more similar
across sites of the ECA program than is the prevalence of phobic disorder.
Phobic disorder begins younger than does panic disorder. The pattern for
minority groups is complementary instead of parallel: blacks and Hispanics
have a *lower* lifetime prevalence of panic disorder than whites, but a *higher*
rate of phobic disorders.

These patterns of similarities and differences may be explained by agoraphobia, which has similarities to both panic and the other two phobic
disorders, simple and social phobia. It is rarer than simple phobia, and

similar to panic disorder in prevalence. Certain of its subtypes (fear of being alone, going out alone, and crowds) are associated with almost as great use of psychiatric services as is panic disorder. Its age of onset is somewhere between the pattern for phobic disorder and that for panic disorder. Thus, it may be that the epidemiologic similarities of panic and phobic disorders are explained by a common etiology for panic disorder and agoraphobia, and their epidemiologic differences may be explained by separate etiologies for panic disorder and simple phobia. The patterns of similarities and differences reinforce the value of studying these disorders separately but in parallel.

8 Generalized Anxiety Disorder

DAN G. BLAZER / DANA HUGHES /
LINDA K. GEORGE / MARVIN SWARTZ /
RICHARD BOYER

THE DIAGNOSIS
OF GENERALIZED ANXIETY DISORDER

Twentieth-century views of both laymen and psychiatrists in confronting modern psychopathology have utilized no construct more than anxiety neurosis. The incorporation of anxiety into the social consciousness is exhibited in W. H. Auden's "The Age of Anxiety" (Auden, 1946). Though some have suggested that in the late 20th century we have moved into the age of melancholy, for much of the 20th century, anxiety and "nerves" were synonomous with psychopathology. Anxiety neurosis according to Freud (1979) was distinct from neurasthenia and was manifested by symptoms of general irritability, anxious expectation, and anxiety attacks that could either be based on anxious feelings alone or could be linked to one or more other bodily functions such as respiration, heart action, motor function, or glandular activity (Merikangas & Weissman, 1987).

Even Freud, however, recognized the overlap of anxiety neurosis with other symptom complexes, such as agoraphobia and simple and social phobias. In recent years, the overlap of anxiety and depression has dominated the clinical and epidemiologic literature (Racagni & Smeraldi, 1987). The overlap is not a new but a reemerging construct. Kraepelin distinguished a "gloomy, hopeless" depression from an anxious depression (Clayton, 1987; Kraepelin, 1921). Breslau (1985) reported that a widely used screening instrument for depression, the Center for Epidemiologic Studies Depression Scale (CES-D), was as useful in detecting generalized anxiety as it was in detecting major depression in a study of mothers of handicapped children. She concluded that the inability of the CES-D to discriminate

180

between generalized anxiety and major depression in these women may result from their having a more severe variety of depression that included anxiety symptoms, whereas either depression or anxiety alone may predominate in a milder version of the same disorder.

Despite the central role of generalized anxiety in psychopathology, other anxiety disorders such as panic disorder, agoraphobia, and obsessive compulsive disorder have been predominant in recent clinical research. The fact that these disorders are better defined and more discrete than generalized anxiety has contributed to this shift in emphasis. In fact, the Washington University Department of Psychiatry did not include generalized anxiety among the "Feighner" criteria, but diagnosed as "anxiety neurosis" a close approximation to what is called panic disorder in DSM-III—unlike generalized anxiety, a diagnosis requiring that persons experience discrete panic episodes (Feighner et al., 1972). In the Research Diagnostic Criteria (RDC) (Spitzer, Endicott, & Robins, 1978), generalized anxiety disorder appears as a residual disorder for "non-psychotic episodes of illness in which the most prominent disturbance is generalized anxiety without panic attacks" (p. 778).

The authors of DSM-III continued the role of generalized anxiety disorder as primarily a residual category. The diagnosis is not made if symptoms of phobias, panic disorder, or obsessive-compulsive disorder are present. In addition, the diagnosis cannot be made if the disturbance is due to another physical or mental disorder, such as hyperthyroidism, schizophrenic disorder, or major depression (American Psychiatric Association, 1980).

Even after these exclusions, a relatively large number of subjects in community and clinical surveys meet criteria for a DSM-III diagnosis of generalized anxiety disorder. Breslau and Davis (1985) felt the criteria were excessively weak and suggested that six months' duration and six symptoms be required instead of DSM-III's requirements of only one month of continuous anxious mood along with a symptom in each of three out of four categories—motor tension, autonomic hyperactivity, apprehensive expectations, and vigilance and scanning. Giving the Diagnostic Interview Schedule (DIS) to a probability sample of 357 mothers of medically ill children, they found that DSM-III criteria produced a lifetime prevalence of generalized anxiety of 45%, a six-month prevalence of 11.5%, and a current rate of 2.5%. By using the more stringent criteria, the lifetime prevalence was reduced to 9.1%, the six-month rate to 2.4%, and the current rate to 1.2%. The reduction in prevalence by the utilization of the new criteria was due chiefly to requiring the longer duration. It should be noted, however, that in this sample the lifetime prevalence would be expected to be considerably higher than in the general population, because these were mothers of chronically ill children.

Based on the work of Breslau, Davis, and other investigators, the authors of DSM-III-R (1987) changed the criteria for generalized anxiety. In contrast to the essential feature of DSM-III (1980), that is, the "persistence of anxiety of at least one month's duration," the essential feature for DSM-III-R generalized anxiety is "unrealistic or excessive anxiety and worry (apprehensive expectation) about two or more life circumstances, e.g. worry about possible misfortune to one's child (who is not in danger) and worry about finances (for no reason) for six months or longer" (p. 252).

Questions to evaluate DSM-III criteria for generalized anxiety disorder were not added to the DIS until after the ECA study had already begun, and the diagnosis was not one of the "core" diagnoses assessed at all ECA sites. In this chapter, generalized anxiety disorder is reported from the Wave 2 interviews carried out in three ECA sites, Durham, St. Louis, and Los Angeles, one year after the interview providing data on the other disorders in this volume.

Although most chapters in this book have used only positive criteria—ignoring hierarchies—for generalized anxiety, major depression and panic are allowed to preempt the disorder in most of our analyses, because of the recognized overlap between generalized anxiety and these diagnoses.

During the first 70 years of this century, generalized anxiety in epidemiologic surveys was usually subsumed under psychoneurotic or "nonpsychotic" disorders. In the Stirling County study (Leighton et al., 1963) however, the psychoneurotic disorders were disaggregated. In that study a sample of approximately 1,000 subjects from eastern Canada were evaluated by psychiatrists on the basis of the Health Opinion Survey (HOS) plus information from physicians and others. They were diagnosed according to DSM-I criteria. The overall prevalence of anxiety, with no distinction made between anxiety and panic disorder, was 2.9%. Anxiety was more prevalent in females than males and especially high in females over the age of 45. In contrast, among men, those under the age of 45 had a higher prevalence of anxiety than those older.

Warheit and colleagues (1986) surveyed the mental health problems of urban and rural household residents of northern Florida in the late 1960s. They used an anxiety scale containing 12 items and found that 14.6% of the sample had significant symptoms of anxiety. Blacks, females, the elderly, those in the lowest socioeconomic levels, and the separated, widowed, and divorced had the highest scores. The larger the number of these associated factors, the greater the likelihood of high scores on the anxiety scale.

Uhlenhuth and colleagues (1983) used a symptom checklist format as part of a study assessing the use of psychotherapeutic medications by 3,161 dwelling in the community. Among the disorders evaluated, generalized anxiety disorder was the most common, with a one-year prevalence of 6.4%. All anxiety disorders were more common in women than men (8% versus 4.3%).

In the late 1970s, epidemiological studies assessed diagnoses according to Research Diagnostic Criteria (RDC) through the Schedule for Affective Disorders and Schizophrenia—Lifetime Version (SADS-L) interview. In a New Haven study, the prevalence of generalized anxiety was 2.5% (Weissman et al., 1978). Over 80% of the persons who met positive criteria for generalized anxiety disorder in that study would have been excluded had DSM-III criteria been used because they also met criteria for phobic disorder, panic disorder, or obsessive-compulsive disorder. Generalized anxiety was slightly more common in middle-aged and younger women, nonwhites, persons not currently married, and those in lower socioeconomic classes than in others. In a similar study, Angst and colleagues (1985) evaluated 6,193 subjects in Zurich, Switzerland. The four-week prevalence of generalized anxiety was 1.5% and the one-year prevalence 5.2%. Generalized anxiety with panic attacks occurred in 0.6% within the last four weeks and in 1.5% within the last year.

Despite the varying definitions of generalized anxiety used in these studies, the range of prevalence estimates of generalized anxiety is no greater than the range reported for disorders such as major depression, and in each study the same collection of associated factors emerges. Specifically, generalized anxiety appears to be more common in younger persons (except for the Stirling county study), in blacks, in persons from lower socioeconomic classes, and in women. The ECA data provided an excellent opportunity to replicate these findings and pursue the correlates of generalized anxiety in more detail.

METHODS FOR THE DIAGNOSIS
OF GENERALIZED ANXIETY DISORDER

The DSM-III criteria for generalized anxiety were operationalized by the DIS as shown in Table 8-1. Specific questions are not presented because the questions used to assess these symptoms varied slightly across the Durham, St. Louis, and Los Angeles sites. However, all criteria were covered, allowing common diagnostic algorithms to be applied, and prevalences in the three sites to be compared. Immediately after asking about panic attacks, in each of these sites at Wave 2, an almost identical gate question was asked: Now I want to ask you about longer periods of feeling anxious or afraid. Have you ever had a period of a month or more when most of the time you felt worried or anxious (perhaps afraid that something bad was going to happen either to you yourself or to someone you cared about)? The Los Angeles site's gate question replaced "a month or more"

Table 8–1 Coverage of DSM-III Criteria by DIS Questions for Generalized Anxiety Disorder

DSM-III Criteria		DIS Items
A. *Symptoms in Three of These Four Categories*		
1. Motor tension:		
Shakiness	Inability to relax	Eyelids twitched
Jitteriness	Eyelid twitch	Jittery or fidgety
Trembling	Furrowed brow	Body trembled
Fatigability	Strained face	Tired very easily
Restlessness	Fidgeting	Restless
Tension	Easy startle	Tense or jumpy
Jumpiness		Easily startled
Muscle aches		Trouble relaxing
2. Autonomic hyperactivity:		
Sweating	Light-headedness	Sweating a lot
Heart pounding	Hot or cold spells	Heart pounding
Dizziness	Lump in the throat	Dizziness or light-headedness
Paresthesias	Pallor	Tingling in hands/feet
Stomach discomfort	Cold, clammy hands	Upset stomach
Diarrhea		Diarrhea
Frequent urination		Frequent urination
Flushing		Face flushing or turning pale
Dry mouth		Mouth dry
High resting pulse		Breathing too fast
and respiration rate		Hands cold or clammy
3. Vigilance and scanning:		
Hyperattentiveness		Trouble sleeping
Difficulty in		Trouble concentrating
concentrating		Irritable/impatient/on edge
Insomnia		
Impatience		
Feeling on edge		
4. Apprehensive expectation:		
Anxiety		Anxious, afraid, worried
Rumination		
Fear		
Worry		
Anticipation of		
misfortune		
B. *Anxious Mood Continuous for at Least One Month*		Period of a month or more
C. *Not Due to Another Disorder*		
D. *Age at Least 18 Years*		

with "two weeks or more," but the question was otherwise the same. A negative answer ended the investigation of generalized anxiety. A positive answer met one of the criteria for the diagnosis—the symptom of apprehensive expectation.

Subjects who answered "yes" to this gate question were then asked about 22 symptoms grouped into 3 categories: motor tension, autonomic hyperactivity, and vigilance and scanning (see Table 8-1). To meet diagnostic criteria, at least one symptom in each category must be reported.

In St. Louis, once a subject met one of these criteria by responding positively to one of the questions relevant to it, the interviewer skipped over the remaining questions relevant to that criterion, and began asking questions relevant to the next criterion. Therefore, the number of symptoms positive in each category can be reported only for Durham and Los Angeles. The frequency distribution of symptoms for these three categories is presented for those 98 subjects in the Durham ECA study and 51 subjects in the UCLA sample who met criteria for generalized anxiety disorder by having at least one symptom in each category and not being excluded from the diagnosis because of a preceding major depression and/or panic disorder. On average, positive cases reported about half the available symptoms of motor tension and vigilance but only one-fourth of the available autonomic symptoms (Table 8-2).

Because the prevalence of generalized anxiety was derived from the second wave of the ECA survey at all three sites, some explanation is in order concerning how the second wave sample differed from the sample that provided data for all other diagnoses. Attrition of the Wave 1 sample varied from 16% to 21% across sites. Respondents' responses were weighted as for assessing other diagnoses, to correct for varying probability of selection due to household size and the oversampling of the elderly and blacks, and to represent the demographic profile (age, sex, race) of the site as of 1980. An additional weight corrected for attrition between Waves 1 and 2.

We report the prevalence of generalized anxiety disorder according to three definitions: subjects who met positive DSM-III criteria regardless of other DSM-III diagnoses; subjects who met positive criteria and who suffered no other DSM-III diagnoses; and subjects who met positive criteria and who did not suffer current major depressive episodes or panic disorder. While we present prevalence results for all three methods, we selected the last of these options for looking at most correlates of the disorder.

The prevalence data presented and the association of that prevalence with various demographic, socioeconomic, educational, and other factors not only raise all of the issues of interpretation discussed in chapter 2, but additional cautions must be exercised because data for this chapter come from an interview conducted a year later and in only three sites.

Table 8–2 Number of Symptoms During the Past Year (%) When at Least One Symptom in the Group Was Present (Durham and Los Angeles Regions Only) (Weighted to the Site's Demographic Distribution)

Number of Symtoms Reported	Symptoms of Motor Tension[a]		Symptoms of Automatic Hyperactivity[b]		Symptoms of Vigilance and Scanning[c]	
	Durham	Los Angeles	Durham	Los Angeles	Durham	Los Angeles
1	3.7	1.1	33.2	8.9	19.7	53.3
2	19.8	4.8	29.0	6.5	30.2	29.0
3	15.4	12.5	7.5	18.3	50.1	17.7
4	12.5	21.6	11.3	21.4		
5	17.8	25.6	6.1	14.8		
6	14.0	24.4	8.1	8.3		
7	12.8	8.3	1.9	10.7		
8	4.1	1.8	1.1	5.1		
9			0.6	6.0		
10			0.0	0.0		
11			1.0	0.0		
	100.0	100.0	100.0	100.0	100.0	100.0
Median Number	4	4	2	4	2	1

[a]Eight possible symptoms in group.
[b]Eleven possible symptoms in group.
[c]Three possible symptoms in group.

PREVALENCE BY AGE, SEX, AND RACE

A NATIONAL ESTIMATE

One-year prevalence estimates weighted to reproduce demographic distributions in the nation as a whole are presented in Table 8–3. The three approaches to the operationalization of generalized anxiety are presented by age, sex, and race. As noted, these estimates are more tenuous than for other diagnoses because data are derived from only three sites, from second wave data, and from assessment procedures that differ somewhat across

Table 8–3 One-Year Prevalence Rates (%) of Generalized Anxiety (Different Exclusionary Criteria) by Sex, Race, and Age Groups for Three Sites Combined[a] (Weighted to National Demographic Distribution)

		Generalized Anxiety No Exclusions[b]	Generalized Anxiety No Panic or Major Depression[c]	Generalized Anxiety No DIS/ DSM-III Disorder[b]
Total		3.76	2.66	1.72
Sex:	Males	2.40***	1.86***	0.94***
	Females	4.95	3.37	2.41
Race:	Whites	3.47	2.48*	1.64
	Blacks	6.09	4.71	2.74
	Hispanic	3.66	1.39	0.86
Age:	<30 years	4.83*	3.51	2.35
	30–44 years	3.58	2.12	1.46
	45–64 years	3.74	2.81	1.75
	65 + years	2.22	1.90	1.05
Male white:		2.07	1.59	0.73
Age:	<30	3.10	2.88	1.59
	30–44	2.06	1.11	0.23
	45–64	1.35	0.91	0.38
	65 +	1.50	0.83	0.82
Male black:		5.45	4.81	2.90
Age:	<30	8.80	7.38	4.24
	30–44	2.28	1.68	0.73
	45–64	6.76	6.71	5.16
	65 +	0.90	1.02	0.00
Male Hispanic:		1.84	0.47	0.47
Age:	<30	1.98	0.01	0.00
	30–44	1.85	0.75	0.75
	45–64	2.13	0.90	0.90
	65 +	0.00	0.00	0.00

Table 8-3 continues

Table 8–3 continued

	Generalized Anxiety No Exclusions[b]	Generalized Anxiety No Panic or Major Depression[c]	Generalized Anxiety No DIS/ DSM-III Disorder[b]
Female white:	4.72	3.27	2.45
Age: <30	5.42	3.14	2.70
30–44	4.69	3.03	2.67
45–64	5.35	4.24	2.72
65+	2.82	2.28	1.35
Female black:	6.62	4.63	2.61
Age: <30	10.55	8.24	4.77
30–44	6.89	3.97	2.80
45–64	3.44	1.68	0.61
65+	2.76	2.71	0.83
Female Hispanic:	5.25	2.21	1.21
Age: <30	1.84	1.84	0.52
30–44	6.47	1.87	0.73
45–64	10.35	4.22	3.45
65+	0.85	0.00	0.00

[a]Analysis restricted to respondents (Rs) with complete data on sex, age, race, and the specified generalized anxiety variable. Age missing for 13 Rs, sex missing for 1 R, and race missing for 138 Rs.

[b]Data missing on generalized anxiety variable for 388 Rs.

[c]Data missing on generalized anxiety variable for 733 Rs.

*$p < .05$

**$p < .01$

***$p < .001$

sites. But our best estimate is that the one-year prevalence without exclusions is 3.8%; excluding depression and panic, 2.7%; and excluding all disorders, 1.7%. Generalized anxiety is clearly a common disorder. The combined data, with or without exclusions, reveal that the disorder is significantly more prevalent in females, in blacks, and in persons under age 30, but differences are significant for age only without exclusions and for race only when panic and depression are excluded.

PREVALENCE IN THREE SITES

Because the questions asked varied somewhat by site, in the remainder of this chapter we will present results for the three sites in parallel rather than combined. The three approaches to the operationalization of generalized anxiety disorder are presented by age, sex, and race for each of the three sites separately in Table 8-4. The overall one-year weighted prevalence

Table 8-4 One-Year Prevalence Rates (%) of Generalized Anxiety (Different Exclusionary Criteria) by Sex, Race, and Age Group for Three Sites[a] (Weighted to the Site's Demographic Distribution)

	Generalized Anxiety No Exclusions			Generalized Anxiety No Panic or Major Depression			Generalized Anxiety No DIS/DSM-III Disorder		
	Durham	St. Louis	Los Angeles	Durham	St. Louis	Los Angeles	Durham	St. Louis	Los Angeles
Total	4.94	3.84	3.42	3.55	2.86	1.99	2.23	1.80	1.30
Males	3.37	2.98	1.63	3.06	2.34	0.73	1.82	1.05	0.52
Females	6.25**	4.57	5.01*	3.96	3.31	3.12***	2.58	2.43*	1.99**
Whites	3.29	3.60	3.39	2.17	2.63	2.46	1.34	1.82	1.58
Blacks	7.72***	4.84	2.12	5.92***	3.82	1.60	3.74**	1.71	1.60
Hispanics	—	—	3.59	—	—	1.38	—	—	0.86
Age: <30	7.95**	5.71	2.37	5.81*	4.46	1.44	3.46	2.86	1.03
30–44	4.28	3.78	3.39	2.71	2.23	1.65	1.95	1.50	1.05
45–64	4.35	2.67	5.46*	3.11	2.23	3.41	2.15	1.51	1.97
65+	2.24	2.40	1.56	1.92	2.18	1.12	0.90	0.86	1.11

Table 8-4 continues

189

Table 8–4 continued

	Generalized Anxiety No Exclusions			Generalized Anxiety No Panic or Major Depression			Generalized Anxiety No DIS/DSM-III Disorder		
	Durham	St. Louis	Los Angeles	Durham	St. Louis	Los Angeles	Durham	St. Louis	Los Angeles
Male white:	1.99	2.40	1.59	1.68	1.89	0.96	0.71	0.83	0.59
Age: <30	4.18	3.59	1.49	3.87	3.59	0.87	1.53	2.23	0.58
30–44	1.28	2.63	1.74	0.99	1.10	1.18	0.70	0.00	0.24
45–64	1.40	0.82	2.24	1.06	0.68	1.23	0.00	0.08	1.23
65 +	1.03	2.68	0.00	0.68	2.68	0.00	0.72	1.41	0.00
Male black/Hisp.[b]	5.82	5.59	1.85	5.58	4.26	0.48	3.79	2.04	0.47
Age: <30	9.28	9.65	2.01	7.87	7.88	0.01	6.33	2.32	0.00
30–44	2.30	2.60	1.86	2.35	1.40	0.74	0.77	0.79	0.74
45–64	7.95*	5.98*	2.17	8.53	5.10	0.97	5.66	5.10	0.97
65 +	0.27	2.36	0.00	0.33	2.36	0.00	0.00	0.00	0.00
Female white:	4.42	4.65	5.07	2.60	3.28	3.86	1.88	2.68	2.51
Age: <30	3.38	7.02	3.67	1.16	4.30	2.30	0.71	3.66	2.24
30–44	4.69	5.01	4.13	2.74	3.34	2.88	1.93	3.20	2.45
45–64	5.92	3.54	7.90	3.74	3.15	6.54	3.05	2.60	2.55
65 +	2.92	2.37	3.67	2.26	1.97	2.96	1.34	0.61	2.94

Table 8-4 continues

190

Table 8–4 continued

	Generalized Anxiety No Exclusions			Generalized Anxiety No Panic or Major Depression			Generalized Anxiety No DIS/DSM-III Disorder		
	Durham	St. Louis	Los Angeles	Durham	St. Louis	Los Angeles	Durham	St. Louis	Los Angeles
Female black/Hisp.[b]	9.21	4.27	5.11	6.18	3.40	2.17	3.70	1.45	1.20
Age:									
<30	16.07	4.80	1.87	11.38	4.84	1.87	6.18	2.63	1.87
30–44	10.57	4.48	6.39	6.08	2.99	1.81	5.16	1.36	0.70
45–64	3.15	4.50	10.06	1.16	2.68	4.13	1.11	0.00	3.35
65+	3.70	1.49	0.86	3.74	1.49	0.00	0.89	0.86	0.00

Note. Sample sizes on which the prevalence rates are calculated can be found in Appendix Table A-4. — indicates that number was less than 25 and so no rate was computed.

[a]Analysis restricted to respondents (Rs) with complete data on sex, age, race, and the specified generalized anxiety variable.

[b]Because of small samples of blacks in Los Angeles and of Hispanics in Durham and St. Louis, rates are reported for blacks only in Durham and St. Louis, for Hispanics only in Los Angeles.

*p < .05

**p < .01

***p < .001

191

varies from 4.9% to 2.2% across these three operationalized definitions for Durham and varies similarly for the other two ECA sites. By each of the three definitions, the prevalence of generalized anxiety is lower in St. Louis than Durham and still lower in Los Angeles. According to all three definitions, and in all sites, women have more generalized anxiety than men. The disorder is more common in blacks than non-blacks in Durham. In two of the three definitions in Durham the disorder is most common in the youngest adults, and the same trend appears in St. Louis. The low prevalence in Los Angeles compared to the other two sites is accounted for by a much lower prevalence in the youngest and oldest men.

Because patterns of demographic correlates are consistent whether or not exclusions are used, in the remainder of the chapter we will present data for generalized anxiety excluding only those cases in which its first appearance was preceded by panic attacks or a depressive episode.

LIFETIME PREVALENCES AND REMISSION

Approximately 6.6% of the population in Durham and St. Louis had ever experienced a generalized anxiety disorder. In Los Angeles, the lifetime prevalence was only 4.1%. As we had noted for one-year prevalence, rates were higher in women than men, and in Durham only, in blacks and the youngest age group (Table 8–5). Remission is defined as meeting criteria for a lifetime diagnosis but not suffering from the disorder during the year prior to the interview. Approximately 50% of the subjects who reported a lifetime prevalence of the disorder reported no disorder within the last year. Remission is lowest in the youngest group, as one might expect, since the disorder had begun only recently, and somewhat more common in whites than blacks.

CORRELATES OF GENERALIZED ANXIETY

Correlates of generalized anxiety might be expected to be indicators of social stress. Living in a large city, economic hardship, and marital maladjustment could be the subjects of the anxiety and worry that are essential to the diagnosis. On the other hand, the disorder might also occur in persons with few objective reasons for worry.

RURAL–URBAN RESIDENCE

There is little difference in prevalence across urban–rural boundaries for one-year prevalence, but a trend exists toward higher lifetime prevalence in urban areas (Table 8–6).

Table 8–5 Prevalence Rates (%) of Generalized Anxiety (No Panic or Major Depression) for One Month, One Year, Lifetime, and Remission (%) by Sex, Race, and Age Group for Three Sites (Weighted to the Site's Demographic Distribution)

	One Month			One Year			Lifetime			Remission (%)[b]		
	Durham	St. Louis	Los Angeles	Durham	St. Louis	Los Angeles	Durham	St. Louis	Los Angeles	Durham	St. Louis	Los Angeles
Total[a]	1.23	1.28	1.40	3.55	2.86	1.99	6.58	6.59	4.14	48.56	58.33	58.56
Males	1.06	1.42	0.45	3.06	2.34	0.73	5.73	5.20	2.62	50.17	54.97	75.34*
Females	1.36	1.16	2.25***	3.96	3.31	3.12***	7.29	7.78*	5.50*	47.51	60.29	51.37
Whites	0.68	1.15	1.62	2.17	2.63	2.46	5.15	6.73	4.73	69.90*	63.13	56.41
Blacks	2.16**	1.83	0.14	5.92**	3.82	1.60	9.05*	5.98	3.85	37.48	36.17	—
Hispanics	—	—	1.24	—	—	1.38	—	—	3.33	—	—	62.94
Age: <30	1.61	1.96	0.62	5.81*	4.46	1.44	8.35	6.97	2.50	37.02	33.38	68.84
30–44	0.69	1.08	1.12	2.71	2.23	1.65	5.81	6.75	4.91	53.34	72.95**	53.64
45–64	1.49	0.80	2.70	3.11	2.23	3.41	6.77	7.31	5.75*	54.81	70.88	—
65+	1.06	1.23	1.12	1.92	2.18	1.12	4.57	4.25	2.58	57.96	[48.76]	—

Note: — indicates the number of respondents was less than 25, and so no rate was computed. [ ] indicates the number was 25 to 29, and rates may be unstable.

[a] Analysis restricted to respondents (Rs) with complete data on sex, race, age, and generalized anxiety.

[b] Remission = Lifetime minus one-year divided by lifetime: (Lt − 1Yr)/Lt.

*p < .05

**p < .01

***p < .001

193

Table 8-6 Prevalence Rates (%) of Generalized Anxiety (No Panic or Major Depression) and Remission (%) by Residence for the Durham and St. Louis Sites (Weighted to the Site's Demographic Distribution)

	One Year		Lifetime		Remission	
	Durham	St. Louis	Durham	St. Louis	Durham	St. Louis
Total	3.55 (2,958)	2.84 (2,460)	6.56	6.56	48.46 (175)	58.53 (157)
Rural	2.71 (1,571)	1.24	5.57	2.47 (125)	51.88 (79)	— (<25)
Urban	4.30 (1,387)	2.99 (2,335)	7.45	6.95*	46.17 (96)	58.82 (152)

Note. Parentheses contain the unweighted numbers of respondents on whom prevalence rates are based. Under "Remission," the parenthetical numbers are the unweighted number of lifetime cases of generalized anxiety. — indicates the number of respondents was less than 25, and so no rate was computed.

SOCIOECONOMIC STATUS

Workers in the service sector and persons in technical, sales, and support occupations had somewhat more generalized anxiety disorder during the year prior to interview than did other workers (Table 8–7). The relationship becomes clearer when occupations are ranked by the Nam quintiles (Nam & Powers, 1965), which reflect education and earnings. One-year prevalence decreases as occupational status increases (Table 8–7).

Since the Nam ranking takes typical earnings into account in ranking occupations, we would expect to find low income also associated with a higher prevalence of generalized anxiety disorder. This indeed is the case. Those in households with incomes of less than $10,000 per year suffer the highest one-year prevalence (Table 8–8). The inference that a precarious financial situation is associated with generalized anxiety disorder is further strengthened by the finding that individuals dependent upon unemploy-

Table 8–7 One-Year Prevalence Rate of Generalized Anxiety (No Panic or Major Depression) by Type and Level of Occupation for the Durham and Los Angeles Sites (Weighted to the Site's Demographic Distribution)

	Durham		Los Angeles	
	N	%	N	%
Total[a]	(1,367)	4.40	(1,568)	1.83
Type of occupation:				
Management/Professional	(323)	2.24	(518)	1.82
Technical/Sales support	(365)	4.86	(490)	1.98
Service	(178)	7.43	(174)	3.68
Farm/Forest/Fish	(46)	0.00	(187)	0.00
Skilled labor	(181)	5.08	(140)	0.00
Laborers	(274)	4.81	(228)	1.41
Occupational level:[b]				
0–20 (Low)	(221)	8.47	(185)	3.47
21–40	(268)	5.05	(328)	1.20
40–60	(343)	3.42	(354)	1.97
61–80	(358)	3.86	(452)	1.90
81–100 (High)	(177)	1.55	(249)	0.99

[a]Analysis in Durham restricted to Rs in community currently employed full-time. Data were missing for 10 Rs. Analysis for Los Angeles restricted to community Rs currently employed full-time or part-time. Data missing on 1,010 Rs in Los Angeles.
[b]Based on Nam & Powers (1965).

Table 8–8 One-Year Prevalence Rate of Generalized Anxiety (No Panic or Major Depression) by Income for the Durham and Los Angeles Sites (Weighted to the Site's Demographic Distribution)

	Durham N[a]	%	Los Angeles N[a]	%
Total	(1,286)	4.69	(1,450)	1.99
< $5,000	(111)	7.54	(126)	4.03
$5,000–$9,999	(262)	9.16*	(199)	3.24
$10,000–$14,999	(357)	4.51	(248)	1.67
$15,000–$19,999	(199)	4.08	(203)	2.24
$20,000–$24,999	(151)	1.67	(199)	0.63
$25,000–$34,999	(110)	0.29	(244)	1.08
$35,000–$49,999	(46)	1.48	(142)	0.63
$50,000+	(50)	0.00	(89)	2.98

[a]The unweighted number of employed persons (Los Angeles) or full-time employed (Durham) for whom income was known.
*$p < .05$, controlled for sex.

ment compensation, disability payments, social security, the Veterans Administration, or welfare experience a higher prevalence of generalized anxiety than others. Overall, the one-month prevalence for persons receiving some type of supplemental income is 3.8% compared to 1% for those who do not receive such support in Durham and 4.6% versus 1% in Los Angeles.

Popular opinion suggests both that persons with higher education who hold "pressure filled" jobs and those whose low educational level limits them to poorly paid work would experience significant symptoms of anxiety. Data from the ECA study do not substantiate these opinions (Table 8–9). Indeed, no clear association of either lifetime or one-year prevalence of generalized anxiety with education is found.

MARITAL STATUS

Marital problems could be expected to be another source of anxiety. In Durham those never married and in Los Angeles those multiply divorced had the highest one-year prevalence (Table 8–10). In both sites, those who married and remained married experienced the lowest prevalence. No signficant differences by marital status were found in St. Louis.

Table 8–9 Prevalence Rates (%) of Generalized Anxiety (No Panic or Major Depression) by Education for Three Sites[a] (Weighted to the Site's Demographic Distribution)

	Number[b]			One-Year			Lifetime		
	Durham	St. Louis	Los Angeles	Durham	St. Louis	Los Angeles	Durham	St. Louis	Los Angeles
Total	(3,061)	(2,607)	(2,537)	3.54	2.88	1.88	6.61	6.64	4.11
0–7 grades	(615)	(236)	(400)	4.22	2.38	1.82	6.78	5.48	3.26
8th grade (no high school)	(178)	(274)	(77)	1.28	3.01	0.00	4.91	3.73	2.01
High school, no diploma	(602)	(584)	(419)	5.39	2.17	2.41	9.15	6.53	3.17
High school graduate, no college	(761)	(716)	(551)	3.55	4.29	1.67	7.24	8.20	3.36
Some college, no diploma	(435)	(509)	(552)	3.29	1.57	1.34	5.40	5.14	4.39
College graduate	(470)	(288)	(538)	1.74	2.70	2.71	4.14	7.76	6.36

[a]Education categories for St. Louis based on Wave-1 data. Education categories for Durham and Los Angeles based on Wave-1 and Wave-2 data. Missing data for 334 respondents (Rs) in Durham, 273 Rs in St. Louis, and 25 Rs in Los Angeles explain differences in totals from Table 8.4

[b]Unweighted numbers of respondents for whom education data available.

197

Table 8–10 Prevalence Rates (%) of Generalized Anxiety (No Panic or Major Depression) by Marital History for Three Sites (Weighted to the Site's Demographic Distribution)

	One-Year Prevalence		
	Durham	St. Louis	Los Angeles
Total[a]	3.55	2.86	2.03
	(3,114)	(2,655)	(2,560)
No divorce/separation	2.30	2.43	1.01
	(1,762)	(1,101)	(944)
Never married	7.95***	3.37	1.22
	(396)	(490)	(516)
Divorced/separated once	2.98	1.12	3.63
	(492)	(437)	(406)
Divorced/separated more than once	3.27	5.88	4.38**
	(397)	(498)	(421)
Cohabit only	4.41	1.85	2.82
	(67)	(129)	(243)

Note: Parentheses contain the unweighted numbers of respondents (Rs) for whom marital history was known. Data on marital history missing for 4 Rs in Durham, 15 Rs in St. Louis, and 2 Rs in Los Angeles.
**$p < .01$; sex was controlled in testing for significant group differences.
***$p < .001$

AGE OF ONSET AND DURATION

The onset of generalized anxiety disorder can occur across the life cycle (Table 8–11). There were no significant differences in age of onset by sex.

A duration of only one month is required to meet criteria, but among remitted cases, half had lasted more than one year (see Table 8–12). About 40% of the still active cases have suffered symptoms of generalized anxiety disorder over more than 5 years and more than 10% over more than 20 years, though not necessarily continuously. No significant difference by sex was found in duration of symptoms.

COMORBIDITY

People with generalized anxiety often suffer from at least one other DIS/DSM-III disorder. Those who have ever had generalized anxiety have

Table 8-11 Age of Onset of Generalized Anxiety (No Panic or Major Depression) (Weighted to the Site's Demographic Distribution)

Age at First Symptom	Among Persons with the Disorder (%)		
	Durham	St. Louis	Los Angeles
18, 19	20.6	17.0	11.1
20–24	19.5	27.4	20.6
25–29	16.4	15.4	18.8
30–44	23.0	21.9	36.4
45–64	17.5	14.2	10.3
65 +	3.0	4.1	2.8
	100.0	100.0	100.0
Number of cases	180	180	120
Mean age at interview	31.36	31.05	32.74
(Standard deviation)	(14.04)	(14.08)	(12.58)

also had at least one other DIS/DSM-III disorder in between 58% to 65% of cases (depending on the site). If an individual suffered from generalized anxiety, he/she was especially likely to suffer from a panic disorder or major depression.

TREATMENT EXPERIENCE

Generalized anxiety disorder is associated with the increased use of mental health services (see Table 8-13). Those suffering from generalized anxiety disorder during the past year were significantly more likely to have received outpatient mental health services in the past six months in all three sites. Use of inpatient mental health services was more common for persons with this disorder in Durham but not in other sites. Use of general health services was not significantly affected by this disorder. The slightly higher rate of outpatient general medical use by those *without* the disorder merely reflects the youth of those with generalized anxiety.

CONCLUSION

Generalized anxiety disorder is a common condition, even among people not suffering from any other disorder. Its association with a number of social risk factors makes us wonder whether it is a disorder in the ordinary sense of the word. Could it be a residual of symptoms reflecting poor life satisfaction or generalized stress?

Table 8-12 Percentage of Respondents Reporting Generalized Anxiety (No Panic or Major Depression) by Duration of Symptoms for Current and Remitted Cases at Three Sites (Weighted to the Site's Demographic Distribution)

	Active Cases (%)			Remitted Cases (%)		
	Durham	St. Louis	Los Angeles	Durham	St. Louis	Los Angeles
Duration:[a]						
<1 year	24.3	27.3	11.2	58.7	35.7	53.0
1–5 years	42.0	31.5	39.3	22.8	33.3	27.1
6–10 years	13.9	15.1	8.1	4.6	10.6	5.8
11–20 years	9.7	13.9	25.4	4.1	12.6	11.0
21+ years	10.1	12.2	16.0	9.8	7.8	3.1
	100.0	100.0	100.0	100.0	100.0	100.0
Number of cases	87	90	44	93	86	75
Mean years duration	6.45	8.79	10.38	4.26	5.82	3.33
(Standard deviation)	(9.97)	(13.37)	(11.35)	(8.68)	(7.92)	(6.45)

[a]Data missing on duration for 356 Rs in Durham, 349 Rs in St. Louis, and 28 Rs in Los Angeles.

Table 8-13 Utilization of Health Services by Persons with Generalized Anxiety, and No Panic or Major Depression (%), for Three Sites, Weighted to the Site's Demographic Distribution

	Outpatient Mental Health			Inpatient Mental Health			Outpatient Physical Health			Inpatient Physical Health		
	Durham	St. Louis	Los Angeles	Durham	St. Louis	Los Angeles	Durham	St. Louis	Los Angeles	Durham	St. Louis	Los Angeles
Total	8.06	4.00	9.92	0.83	0.36	0.12	47.46	56.86	44.17	6.89	9.97	5.01
Active cases (one-year)												
No	7.70 (3,016)	3.69 (2,562)	9.12 (2,507)	0.63 (3,016)	0.37 (2,562)	0.13 (2,455)	47.93* (3,016)	56.83 (2,562)	44.56* (2,507)	6.86 (3,016)	9.91 (2,562)	4.97 (2,457)
Yes	17.95** (98)	14.71*** (93)	48.46**** (51)	6.15*** (98)	0.00 (93)	0.00 (50)	34.76 (98)	57.78 (93)	25.10 (51)	7.76 (98)	11.77 (93)	6.78 (50)

Note: Based on respondents (Rs) for whom health service utilization was ascertained.
*p < .05
**p < .01
****p < .001

201

The propensity of individuals suffering from the symptoms of generalized anxiety to seek mental health services is reminiscent of the group said to be suffering from "demoralization" (Dohrenwend et al., 1980). Demoralization is a psychological (and psychosocial) construct that cuts across specific psychiatric disorders, sharing some features of major depression, somatization disorder, and anxiety, and, according to Dohrenwend, that predicts the use of mental health services. The symptoms of generalized anxiety disorder, however, do not clearly overlap with those of demoralization. Such cardinal symptoms of demoralization as poor self-esteem and sadness are not usually encountered in subjects with generalized anxiety disorder, though the dread and anxiety seen in demoralization are present. Dohrenwend estimates that demoralization affects one-quarter of the population, whereas generalized anxiety, as operationalized in DSM-III, affects no more than seven to eight percent of the population, even when exclusionary criteria are used. Thus, if generalized anxiety disorder is merely a measure of nonspecific psychological and psychosomatic stress, it is a more restrictive measure than is "demoralization."

A barrier to accepting generalized anxiety disorder as a specific psychiatric illness is the frequent overlap of its symptoms with those of other disorders, especially major depression. However, as exhibited in this report, generalized anxiety disorder cases remain even when other DIS/DSM-III diagnoses are excluded. This ability to "stand alone," however, does not imply that when persons with major depression also have symptoms of generalized anxiety disorder, they have two separate psychopathological disorders. Rather, as noted by Clayton (1987), major depression can express itself in at least two ways—as melancholic depression and as anxious depression. In the latter, symptoms found in generalized anxiety may occur but have an etiology different from that of the "stand-alone" form of generalized anxiety disorder.

Generalized anxiety disorder without depression and/or panic has an identifiable risk factor profile and leads to increased utilization of mental health services. With increased emphasis placed upon the psychobiological etiology of psychiatric disorders, the potential of chronic stress to induce a psychiatric disorder has been neglected. Some clinicians consider it axiomatic that internal unresolved psychological conflicts and external chronic stress play a role in inducing symptoms of anxiety. Yet our current conceptions of psychopathology have tended to ignore generalized anxiety. Rather, psychiatrists have concentrated upon the sometimes more severe but rarer "anxiety attack" or "panic attack." As pharmacotherapy has tended to supplant psychotherapy, and as the economics of mental health care have rendered ongoing psychotherapy by psychiatrists in an outpatient setting less feasible, psychiatrists have become less interested in generalized anxiety. With the more restrictive criteria for the disorder that have appeared in DSM-III-R, its prevalence according to official criteria will decline, but making the criteria more restrictive will not change the common presentation of enduring anxiety symptoms in the general population nor reduce the need of those experiencing them for therapeutic intervention.

The high utilization of mental health services by individuals suffering from DIS/DSM-III generalized anxiety disorder is noteworthy. Most of these mental health services are provided by primary care physicians rather than mental health specialists. Anxious individuals are often treated with benzodiazepines, which are among the most frequently prescribed medications (Balter, Levine, & Manheimer, 1974). Most benzodiazepines are prescribed by primary care physicians (Hasday & Karch, 1981).

Given the high frequency of the disorder and the large demand for treatment it accounts for, more attention should be devoted to the epidemiology, phenomenology, psychobiology, and treatment of individuals suffering from generalized anxiety disorder.

9 Obsessive Compulsive Disorder

MARVIN KARNO /
JACQUELINE M. GOLDING

The intrusion into consciousness of intense, repetitive, disgusting, frightening, absurd, or otherwise alien thoughts is a dramatic and remarkable experience. That is the nature of obsessions. The compelling necessity to carry out repeatedly small and private or elaborate and conspicuous ritual behaviors that are usually irrational and bizarre is a similarly intense and extraordinary experience. Such are compulsions. The sustained experience of obsessions and/or compulsions comprises the psychopathology of DSM-III-defined obsessive compulsive disorder, variously referred to as obsessional neurosis, compulsion neurosis, and obsessional disorder.

The classification of obsessive compulsive disorder as an anxiety disorder derives from the psychoanalytic concept of the disorder as a particular form of psychoneurosis; that is, a set of symptoms unconsciously intended to defend a person against the experience of anxiety. This formulation has carried conviction for two reasons. First, the experience of obsessive thoughts and the effort to resist compulsive acts are generally associated with subjective anxiety. Second, obsessive and compulsive symptoms appear to provide convincing evidence of unconscious and taboo mental activity erupting into consciousness despite the efforts of mental defense mechanisms.

Obsessive compulsive disorder has been considered to be conceptually and empirically related to the affective disorders (Coryell, 1981b; Gittleson, 1966; Goodwin & Guze, 1984; Lewis, 1936; Nemiah, 1984; Videbech, 1975), to schizophrenia (Blacker, 1966; Hare, Price & Slater, 1972; Lewis, 1936; Lo, 1967), to organic brain disease (Behar, et al., 1984; Lewis, 1936; McKeon, Roa & Mann, 1984) and, more intuitively, to phobic and other anxiety disorders (Goodwin & Guze, 1984; Insel, 1984; Kringlen, 1965; Nemiah, 1984). Cummings and Frankel (1985) and Green and Pitman

(1986) have reviewed impressive evidence for a relationship between obsessive compulsive disorder and Tourette's disorder. This stereotyped movement disorder was described by the French physician Gilles de la Tourette in 1885. It begins in childhood with involuntary facial movements or tics, and progresses to include vocal grunts, shouts, and sudden, jerky body movements. It is generally of lifelong duration, is more common in boys than girls, and can be helped by medication (Barabas, 1988).

Jenike (1986) has emphasized the blurred boundary between obsessive compulsive disorder and certain obsessional and delusional hypochondriacal disorders. Hypochondriasis is defined by DSM-III as follows: "The essential feature is . . . an unrealistic interpretation of physical signs or sensations as abnormal, leading to preoccupation with the fear or belief of having a serious disease. A thorough physical evaluation does not support the diagnosis of any physical disorder that can account for the physical signs or sensations or for the individual's unrealistic interpretation of them, although a coexisting physical disorder may be present" (American Psychiatric Association, 1980, p. 249).

The pathophysiologic vulnerability underlying obsessive compulsive disorder may share elements of both the anxiety and affective disorders (Insel et al., 1982; Zahn, Insel, & Murphy, 1984).

Obsessive compulsive disorder has been traditionally regarded as rare, chronic, disabling, and resistant to treatment. This perspective is supported by 50 years of published clinical research reports (Goodwin, Guze, & Robins, 1969; Lewis, 1936, 1957; Nemiah, 1984; Salzman & Thaler, 1981; Templer, 1972). As Nemiah pointed out, "It is one of the ironies of clinical psychiatry that, although the obsessive compulsive disorder illuminates the psychoanalytic concept of psychodynamic conflict perhaps better than any other psychoneurosis, its symptoms generally remain impervious to psychoanalytic treatment" (Nemiah, 1984. p. 9). However, encouraging studies of the use of behavioral (Baer & Minichiello, 1986; Foa & Steketee, 1984; Foa, Steketee, & Ozarow, 1985) and pharmacologic (Ananth, 1985; Insel & Mueller, 1984; Jenike, 1986) treatment approaches to obsessive compulsive disorder have recently appeared.

DIAGNOSIS

The *Diagnostic and Statistical Manual of Mental Disorders, Third Edition* (DSM-III) defines obsessions as "recurrent, persistent ideas, thoughts, images, or impulses that are ego-dystonic, that is, they are not experienced as voluntarily produced, but rather as thoughts that invade consciousness and are experienced as senseless or repugnant. Attempts are made to ignore or suppress them. Compulsions are repetitive and seemingly purposeful behaviors that are performed according to certain rules or in a stereotyped fashion. The behavior is not an end in itself, but is designed to produce or to prevent some future event or situation. However, the activity is not connected in a realistic way with what it is designed to produce or prevent, or may be clearly excessive" (American Psychiatric Association, 1980, p. 234).

The DSM-III criteria for the diagnosis of obsessive compulsive disorder specify that either obsessions or compulsions be present, that they "are a significant source of stress to the individual or interfere with social or role functioning" and that they are "not due to any other mental disorder, such as Tourette's Disorder, Schizophrenia, Major Depression or Organic Mental Disorder" (American Psychiatric Association, 1980, p. 235). Obsessions and compulsions that arise in association with Tourette's disorder, schizophrenia (see chapter 3), or major depressive disorder (see chapter 4) are considered by DSM-III not to be due to obsessive compulsive disorder. Obsessions or compulsions that precede the development of a major depression are considered to represent obsessive compulsive disorder and both diagnoses are made.

Obsessive compulsive disorder does not include all forms of compulsive behavior. Compulsive eating, drinking, gambling, and sexuality are not included, but are rather assigned other diagnoses by DSM-III. An important criterion for their exclusion is that they are (generally) inherently pleasurable behaviors, while the compulsive behavior included in obsessive compulsive disorder is not rewarding in and of itself, but is carried out to prevent some form of imagined disaster or to neutralize worry about realistic or potential difficulties—such as financial or health worries. They are also distinguished from true obsessions, which are experienced as irrational and alien. As is the case with the diagnosis of phobia, the diagnosis of obsessive compulsive disorder requires only one symptom: a single obsession or compulsion is sufficient.

DSM-III also includes compulsive personality disorder, a diagnosis given to individuals afflicted with a stiff, cold personality and perfectionist attention to detail and formality, but who do not suffer from true obsessions or compulsions. There seems little danger that the diagnostic criteria for obsessive compulsive disorder would be confused with those for compulsive personality disorder.

The 1987 revision of DSM-III (DSM-III-R) more carefully and fully defines and demarcates requisite symptoms from symptoms not part of the disorder. Thus, specific examples of obsessions, such as repeated blasphemous throughts by a religious person or thoughts of killing a loved child by a parent, are given. The criterion that "the person recognizes that the obsessions are the product of his or her own mind, not imposed from without (as in thought insertion)" (American Psychiatric Association, 1987, p. 247) has been added to more clearly demarcate obsessions from schizophrenic symptoms. It is likely that the greater clarity and specification of symptoms in DSM-III-R will reduce the number of "borderline" cases in future epidemiologic studies employing the revised criteria and will produce a slight lowering of prevalence rates from those reported here, which are based on the less clearly defined DSM-III criteria.

MEASUREMENT OF OBSESSIVE COMPULSIVE DISORDER BY THE DIAGNOSTIC INTERVIEW SCHEDULE

The DIS contains two basic questions about obsessions and three concerning compulsions. The first question asks if the respondent has had any unpleasant, persistent thought, such as " . . . that you might harm or kill someone you love." If the respondent says no, a second question gives two other examples of obsessions—that one's hands are dirty despite repeated washings, and that absent relatives may have been killed or injured. For an obsessive thought to be counted as due to obsessive compulsive disorder, it must have persisted for at least three weeks and to have continued despite the person's repeated efforts to get rid of it. The age of onset and recency of any obsession is also determined. If the first question about obsessions is answered affirmatively, the second question about obsessions is not asked.

The initial question about compulsions inquires whether the respondent has had " . . . to do something over and over again" despite resisting the behavior and considering it irrational. Repeatedly checking locked doors or gas jets or washing hands are offered as examples. A negative answer leads to a second question about having to carry out actions—such as getting dressed—in a particular order, and of having to repeat the entire sequence if the order is interrupted. A third question concerning compulsive counting (despite resistance) is asked of all respondents. In addition, the recency and age of onset of all reported compulsions are ascertained.

For every symptom of the disorder reported as positive, the respondent is asked if it was severe enough to report to a physician or other professional, caused the person to take medication two or more times, or significantly interfered with the respondent's life activities. Only if one of these severity criteria is met is the symptom counted as being due to obsessive compulsive disorder. Also, to be counted as due to the disorder, a symptom must not have resulted from medical illness or injury, or the use of alcohol, drugs, or medication.

Although DSM-III contains rules by which the presence of one disorder hierarchically excludes the presence of another disorder when there are symptoms of both, the prevalence rates reported here, except as indicated, are for diagnoses made without exclusions. The diagnoses that hierarchically "exclude" obsessive compulsive disorder (Tourette's disorder, schizo-phrenia, major depressive episode, organic mental disorder) have been already discussed. Tourette's disorder is not investigated in the ECA study. The ECA estimate of organic mental disorder does not permit dating the onset of any impairment detected (see chapter 12), thus precluding evaluation of the sequence of its co-occurrence with obsessive compulsive disorder.

PREVALENCE

Reliable epidemiologic data concerning obsessive compulsive disorder in commuity populations has been totally lacking—a situation reflected by the DSM-III comment of "no information" regarding its prevalence.

Surveys have given estimated prevalence rates of obsessive compulsive disorder ranging from 0.9% to 4% in psychiatric patient populations (Coryell, 1981; Kringlen, 1965; Lo, 1967; Rasmussen & Tsuang, 1984, 1986). The estimated prevalence of the disorder in the general population is often quoted in English-language reviews as being 0.05% (Nemiah, 1985). This figure represents an extrapolation from prevalence studies among patient populations. The extrapolation from patient populations is questionable because symptoms of obsessive compulsive disorder may often only mildly impair daily functioning and not compel the sufferer to seek treatment. It is perhaps for this reason that the five-site ECA lifetime prevalence for obsessive compulsive disorder of 2.6% is so much greater than anticipated from prior clinical studies.

Studies of patients with obsessive compulsive disorder find that the majority experience both obsessions and compulsions (Jenike, Baer, & Minichiello, 1986; Rasmussen & Tsuang, 1984, 1986). Our findings in the community contrast sharply with this pattern. Among the household respondents with a lifetime history of obsessive compulsive disorder (N = 462), 55% had experienced obsessions, 53% reported compulsions, and only 9% reported both. However, a higher proportion of institutional respondents (22%) who had the disorder (N = 109) at some time during their lifetime reported experiencing both obsessions and compulsions. Thus, it is probable that those who report both classes of symptoms may have a more severe and disturbing form of the disorder.

The apparent independence of the two kinds of symptoms suggested the possibility that they might represent two distinct disorders, each with its own risk factors and associated features. To examine this possibility we carried out separate analyses of the demographic characteristics and risk factors for obsessions and compulsions. However we found no significant differences between the two groups. We also found no differences in use of health or mental health services associated with symptom type.

ONSET AND DURATION

Clinical studies find that patients with obsessive compulsive disorder are typically young, and that they report having had the disorder for many years (Kringlen, 1965; Pollit, 1957; Rasmussen & Tsuang, 1984, 1986). These findings suggest that it is a disorder with an early age of onset and prolonged duration.

The ECA data confirm these clinical findings (Figure 9–1). The first symptoms of obsessive compulsive disorder are most likely to appear in childhood (20%) or adolescence (29%). Just under two-thirds (64%) of those with obsessive compulsive disorder report onset before 25, and almost three-fourths (74%) develop the disorder before the age of 30. However, one in twelve of those afflicted report an onset after age 50.

Among persons who have had obsessive compulsive disorder at some time in their life, but not in the prior year, the mean reported duration of the disorder is 7.2 years. One out of five (20%) of those who have had the disorder sometime in their life report a duration of more than ten years. Thirty percent have had the disorder for a brief period of less than one year (Figure 9–2).

The disorder has a relatively low remission rate (Table 9–1). Not only have more than two-thirds of those who have ever in their lives met DSM-III criteria for obsessive compulsive disorder reported having the disorder within the past year, about half of those ever positive have suffered from it in the past 30 days. Thus obsessive compulsive disorder tends toward

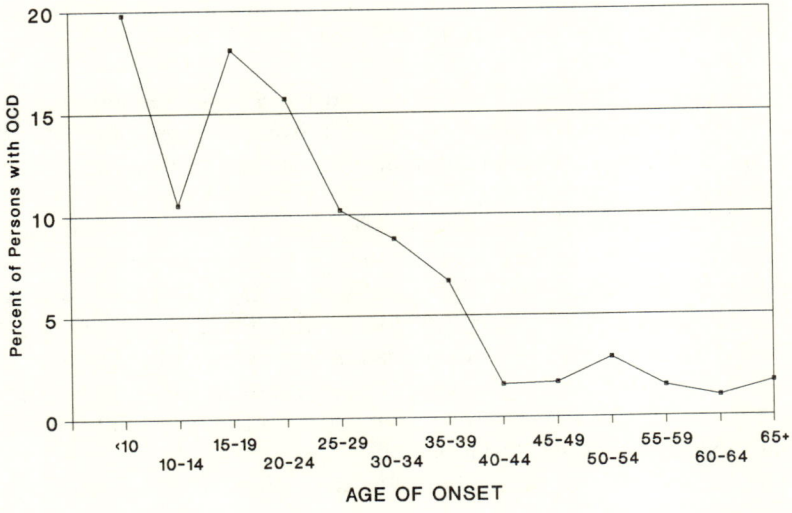

Figure 9–1 Age of Onset of Obsessive Compulsive Disorder (OCD)

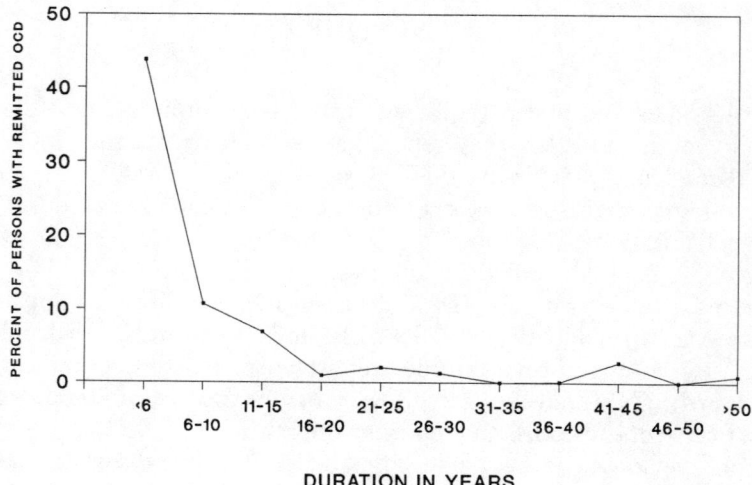

Figure 9–2 Duration of Obsessive Compulsive Disorder (OCD) Among Persons with Remitted OCD

chronicity. The apparently higher remission rate among Hispanic respondents is not statistically significant.

CORRELATES
OF OBSESSIVE COMPULSIVE DISORDER

GENDER, AGE, AND ETHNICITY

Rasmussen and Tsuang (1984, 1986) reported a slight female preponderance (53%) among 1,630 patients compiled from their own and later studies, and Black reported a similar female preponderance in a summary of 11 studies (1974).

The ECA data (Table 9–1) also indicate a greater prevalence of obsessive compulsive disorder among women than men (as is clearly the case for the anxiety disorders in general). Other analyses of these data show that when marital status, employment status, job status, ethnicity and age are controlled, there is no remaining difference in prevalence rates for men compared to women (Karno et al., 1988). The relationship between gender and obsessive compulsive disorder appears to be complexly related to these other social and economic factors of life.

The highest lifetime rates, about 4%, are reported by women under 45 who are of white/other ethnic origin (Table 9–2). The lowest lifetime rates are reported by Hispanic males over 45. Among Hispanic males only one of

Table 9-1 Obsessive Compulsive Disorder Prevalence by Gender and Ethnicity

| | Prevalence in Percent (SE) | | | |
	One-Month	One-Year	Lifetime	Remission[a]
Total	1.33 (0.12)	1.65 (0.13)	2.56 (0.16)	36
Ethnicity:				
White/other	1.36 (0.12)	1.70 (0.15)	2.63 (0.18)	35
Black	1.41 (0.38)	1.63 (0.41)	2.31 (0.48)	29
Hispanic	0.77 (0.39)	0.98 (0.44)	1.82 (0.59)	46
Men:	1.13 (1.60)	1.42 (0.18)	2.03 (0.21)	30
White/other	1.12 (0.17)	1.43 (0.19)	2.03 (0.23)	30
Black	1.16 (0.51)	1.36 (0.55)	1.99 (0.67)	32
Hispanic	0.74 (0.54)	1.02 (0.64)	1.81 (0.85)	44
Women:	1.52 (0.18)	1.86 (0.19)	3.04 (0.25)	39
White/other	1.57 (0.20)	1.94 (0.22)	3.19 (0.28)	31
Black	1.62 (0.55)	1.85 (0.59)	2.59 (0.69)	29
Hispanic	0.81 (0.56)	0.94 (0.06)	1.83 (0.83)	49

[a]Lifetime minus one-year divided by lifetime prevalence: , (Lt − 1 Yr)/Lt.

138 aged 45–64 and none of the 60 over age 65 reports lifetime obsessive compulsive disorder. The small subsample sizes vitiate statistical significance in this finding. For the total male and female samples, lifetime prevalence is highest in the 30–44 age cohort, slightly lower in the 18–29 cohort, and significantly lower among those within the 65 and over age group. One-year prevalence shows a similar age pattern.

It is possible that older respondents tend to forget or minimize symptoms of obsessive compulsive disorder, particularly when they have occurred many years earlier. It is also possible that the disorder has been truly less prevalent within that generation of respondents. Our own purely intuitive belief is that the former explanation is more likely correct.

EDUCATION

The clinical literature has reported that high levels of educational attainment characterize patients afflicted with obsessive compulsive disorder (Goodwin & Guze, 1984; Rasmussen and Tsuang, 1984). This finding is not borne out by ECA community data.

Figure 9–3 demonstrates a saw-tooth relationship between the lifetime prevalence of obsessive compulsive disorder and educational attainment. Obsessive compulsive disorder is more common among those who have not

Table 9–2 Obsessive Compulsive Disorder Prevalence by Gender, Age, and Ethnicity in Percent (SE)

	Men			Women			Total		
	One-Year	Lifetime	Remission	One-Year	Lifetime	Remission	One-Year	Lifetime	Remission
Age:									
18–29	1.84 (0.35)	2.35 (0.40)	20	2.63 (0.42)	3.50 (0.48)	22	2.23 (0.27)	2.92 (0.31)	21
30–44	1.89 (0.39)	2.80 (0.47)	29	2.23 (0.41)	3.79 (0.53)	34	2.06 (0.28)	3.31 (0.36)	32
45–64	0.76 (0.25)	1.33 (0.33)	38	1.24 (0.30)	2.91 (0.46)	54	1.01 (0.20)	2.16 (0.29)	49
65+	0.75 (0.36)	1.05 (0.43)	26	0.93 (0.34)	1.24 (0.39)	20	0.85 (0.25)	1.16 (0.29)	22
Total	1.42 (0.18)	2.03 (0.21)	27	1.86 (0.19)	3.04 (0.25)	34	1.65 (0.13)	2.56 (0.16)	31
White/ Other:									
18–29	1.68 (0.38)	2.18 (0.43)	21	2.90 (0.50)	3.90 (0.57)	23	2.29 (0.31)	3.03 (0.36)	22
30–44	2.21 (0.46)	3.08 (0.55)	26	2.32 (0.47)	4.00 (0.61)	35	2.26 (0.33)	3.55 (0.41)	31
45–64	0.71 (0.26)	1.34 (0.35)	42	1.27 (0.33)	3.02 (0.51)	55	1.00 (0.21)	2.22 (0.31)	51
65+	0.76 (0.39)	0.98 (0.44)	19	0.92 (0.36)	1.15 (0.40)	19	0.85 (0.26)	1.08 (0.30)	19
Total	1.43 (0.19)	2.03 (0.23)	27	1.94 (0.22)	3.19 (0.28)	35	1.69 (0.15)	2.63 (0.18)	32
Black:									
18–29	2.27 (1.16)	2.89 (1.31)	22	2.13 (1.07)	2.64 (1.18)	15	2.20 (0.79)	2.76 (0.88)	18
30–44	0.41 (0.57)	1.12 (0.94)	54	1.86 (1.11)	2.71 (1.34)	32	1.19 (0.66)	1.98 (0.84)	36
45–64	1.22 (1.08)	1.46 (1.18)	8	1.64 (1.12)	2.83 (1.45)	29	1.45 (0.78)	2.22 (0.96)	22
65+	0.99 (1.50)	2.31 (2.27)	56	1.42 (1.47)	1.66 (1.59)	14	1.25 (1.07)	1.92 (1.32)	29
Total	1.36 (0.55)	1.99 (0.67)	28	1.85 (0.59)	2.59 (0.69)	22	1.63 (0.41)	2.31 (0.48)	25
Hispanic:									
18–29	2.18 (1.41)	2.71 (1.57)	20	0.69 (0.83)	1.06 (1.03)	35	1.46 (0.84)	1.92 (0.95)	23
30–44	0.19 (0.52)	2.14 (1.70)	88	2.16 (1.63)	3.14 (1.95)	31	1.23 (0.89)	2.66 (1.30)	49
45–64	0.07 (0.38)	0.07 (0.38)	0	0.00 (—)	1.52 (1.63)	100	0.04 (0.18)	0.82 (0.86)	96
65+	0.00 (—)	0.00 (—)	N/A	0.00 (—)	1.36 (2.45)	100	0.00 (0.44)	0.81 (1.46)	100
Total	1.02 (0.64)	1.81 (0.85)	39	0.94 (0.60)	1.83 (0.83)	49	0.98 (0.44)	1.82 (0.59)	44

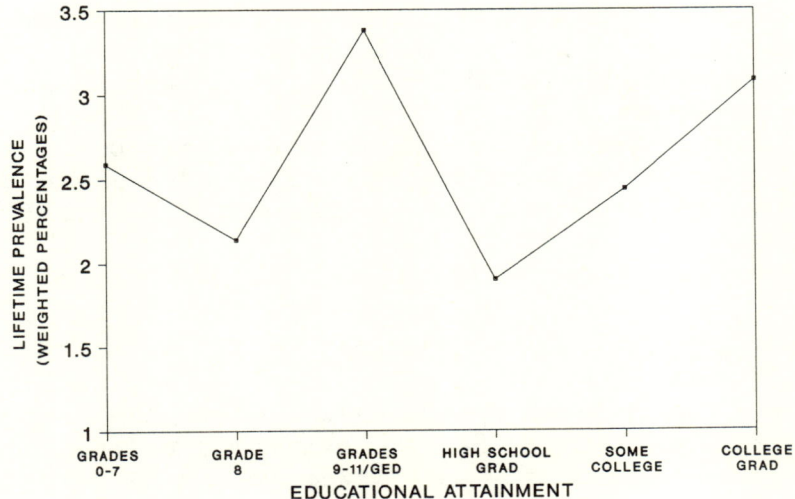

Figure 9–3 Lifetime Prevalence of Obsessive Compulsive Disorder (OCD) by Education

completed a given level of schooling than those who have. For example, lifetime prevalence is 3.4% among those with some high school, but only 1.9% among those who graduated. The exception is college graduates, whose lifetime prevalence (3.1%) is higher than that of respondents who attended college but did not graduate (2.4%).

MARITAL STATUS, MARITAL HISTORY, AND HOUSEHOLD SIZE

As summarized by Rasmussen and Tsuang (1984), prior clinical reports indicated that persons afflicted with obsessive compulsive disorder were particularly subject to marital maladjustment. This was generally considered to be a consequence of the rigid personality patterns thought to characterize those prone to the disorder.

The ECA data do not support this clinical finding. There is no statistically significant association of marital status with one-year prevalence of obsessive compulsive disorder. However, divorced and separated persons have the highest rates (2.5%), with the married and widowed (1.5% each) lowest and the never married intermediate (1.7%).

Black respondents show a different pattern, with maximum rates in the widowed group (2.7%), lowest rates among the married (1.1%), and intermediate rates among the separated/divorced (1.7%) and never married (2.0%). When age is controlled, these high rates for widowed respondents are apparent in individuals 45 to 64 years old, with maximum rates for those 65 and older appearing in the widowed group. Among 30- to 44-year-olds there is little variability in rates of obsessive compulsive disorder as a function of marital status.

The one-year prevalence of obsessive compulsive disorder for those in stable marriages (1.2%) is nonsignificantly lower than for those divorced or separated once (2.2%) or more than once (2.7%) or who have cohabited without marrying (2.1%).

Household size is unrelated to obsessive compulsive disorder.

EMPLOYMENT STATUS AND INCOME

Current unemployment is not related to obsessive compulsive disorder, and among those employed, we found no association with level of income. Nor did we find a consistent relationship between type of occupation or job status and obsessive compulsive disorder, when controlling for age, gender, and ethnicity. Nonetheless, the underemployed, defined as those who were unemployed at least six months out of the prior five years, reported a higher one-year prevalence of obsessive compulsive disorder than others (3.5% versus 1.2%), a statistically significant finding. The generally early onset and relatively long duration of the disorder argue for the likelihood that symptoms of the illness tend to meaningfully impair occupational capacity.

WELFARE STATUS AND INSTITUTIONAL RESIDENCE

The ECA study evaluated two indicators of distressed life circumstances in relation to obsessive compulsive disorder. In the case of welfare status, welfare recipients were more than twice as likely as nonwelfare recipients to report having the disorder during the prior year (3.3% versus 1.5%), a statistically significant finding.

Institutional residents had rates three times as high as household residents (4.9% versus 1.6%), although the relatively small number of institutional residents prevents this finding from being statistically significant. Figure 9-4 reveals the dramatically higher prevalence rates of obsessive compulsive disorder in psychiatric hospitals compared to household settings and a substantially elevated rate in those incarcerated; however, again because of the relatively small number of respondents in prison or inpatient psychiatric hospitals, these differences are not statistically significant.

SITE

No geographic variations in the prevalence of obsessive compulsive disorder have been suggested in the clinical literature. However, two sites,

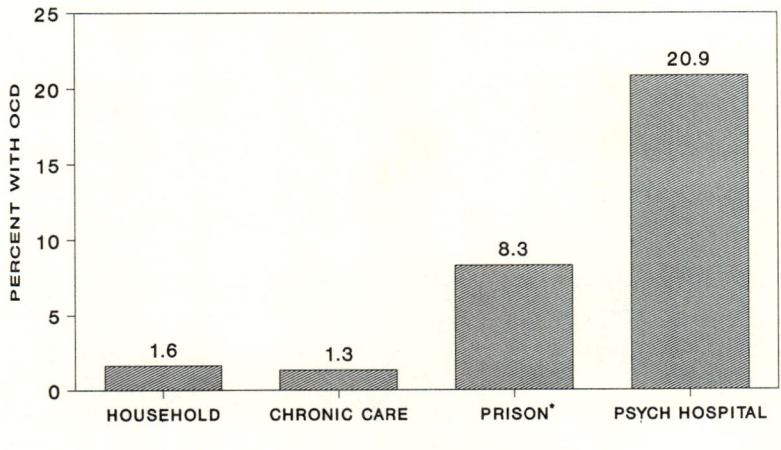

Figure 9–4 Prevalence of Obsessive Compulsive Disorder (OCD) in the Last Year, in Each Type of Residence

Baltimore and Durham, show relatively high rates compared to St. Louis and Los Angeles (Table 9–3). New Haven falls about in the middle. Other than the lower prevalence among Hispanic respondents affecting the Los Angeles rates, the reasons for these site differences are unknown. They are, however, similar to findings for phobia (see chapter 7), indicating that these two sites have increased rates of other anxiety disorders as well.

The remission rate for Los Angeles ranges from 2.5 to almost 3 times greater than that for Baltimore, St. Louis, and Durham. These significant

Table 9–3 Obsessive Compulsive Disorder: Site Differences in Prevalence (Weighted to Local Populations), in Percent (SE)

	One-Month	One-Year	Lifetime	Remission
New Haven	1.20 (0.21)	1.64 (0.24)	2.54 (0.30)	35
Baltimore	1.66 (0.26)	2.17 (0.29)	2.89 (0.33)	25
St. Louis	1.14 (0.26)	1.39 (0.29)	1.94 (0.34)	28
Durham	2.10 (0.30)	2.34 (0.32)	3.29 (0.37)	29
Los Angeles	0.74 (0.17)	0.79 (0.18)	2.14 (0.29)	63

differences reflect in part the ethnic (46% Hispanic) composition of the Los Angeles sample, but also reflect other and unknown site influences.

There is no difference in the prevalence rate for obsessive compulsive disorder among the total sample population resident in rural settings compared to those in urban settings.

USE OF HEALTH AND MENTAL HEALTH SERVICES

Active (one-year) obsessive compulsive disorder is significantly more prevalent among those who visited any health care or psychiatric setting in the past six months than among those who have not made such a visit (Figure 9-5).

A similar pattern is observed among those who have been hospitalized in either a medical or psychiatric hospital within the past year. The dramatically high rate of the disorder among those recently in psychiatric hospitals (Figure 9-5) suggests either that the disorder is often disabling, or that it is associated with other disabling mental disorders (see below).

Household residents with active obsessive compulsive disorder have more often sought care from a mental health specialist in the past six months than have those with phobic disorders (17.8% versus 6.8%) and they have equally as often sought mental health care from a general medical provider (10.9% versus 9.2%). In contrast, they have received less mental health care than those with active panic disorder, 26.4% of whom saw a

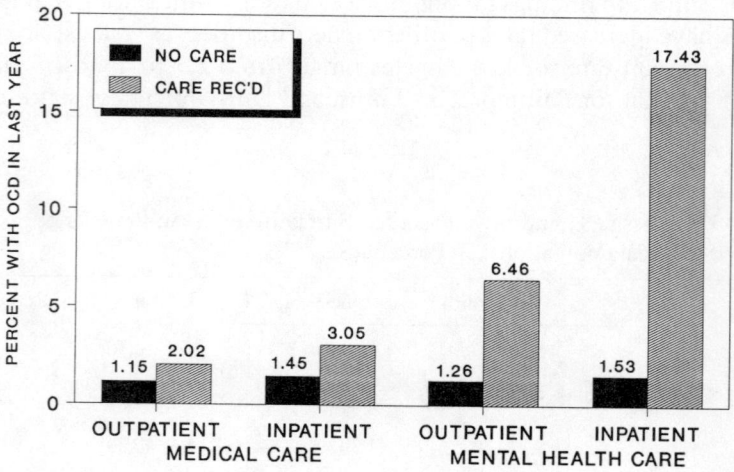

*In the past 6 months for outpatient care
and the past year for inpatient care

Figure 9-5 Prevalence of Obsessive Compulsive Disorder (OCD) Among Persons Receiving Medical and Mental Health Care*

mental health specialist and 19.3% of whom saw a general medical provider for mental health reasons.

Thus, obsessive compulsive disorder lies in the midrange among the anxiety disorders in regard to how frequently its sufferers seek professional care. However, because we do not know the specific symptoms or reasons that caused ECA respondents to seek professional care, we cannot conclude that symptoms of obsessive compulsive disorder rather than nonspecific symptoms of distress or symptoms of another mental disorder led to their utilization of health care resources.

COMORBIDITY

Because of clinical observations that obsessive compulsive disorder is commonly associated with other mental disorders (Rasmussen & Tsuang, 1984, 1986), we expected to find considerable comorbidity for our affected sample. And, indeed, three out of four persons with the disorder had at least one additional disorder.

Because obsessive compulsive disorder is considered secondary to other disorders in DSM-III, we were interested in whether it did in fact usually begin in the context of another disorder (Table 9–4).

In cases of obsessive compulsive disorder occurring along with depression or alcohol dependence, obsessive compulsive disorder was about equally likely to begin before as at the same time or after the other disorder. The exclusion rule of DSM-III states that in cases of obsessive compulsive disorder beginning before depression, both diagnoses should be made, whereas persons with major depression who subsequently develop obses-

Table 9–4 Comorbidity of Obsessive Compulsive Disorder (OCD) with Other Disorders: Order of Occurrence

Other Disorders	OCD Positives (Out of 468) with Each Other Disorder		Percent With OCD Occurring First in Respondents with Both Diagnoses
	N	%	
Major depressive episode	113	31.7	56.9
Panic disorder	57	13.8	40.1
Phobia	224	46.5	24.7
Schizophrenia	56	12.2	39.8
Alcohol abuse or dependence	114	24.1	52.7
Drug abuse or dependence	76	17.6	62.4

sions and/or compulsions are to be diagnosed as suffering from major depressive illness only. Both diagnoses are always to be given when the comorbid condition is an alcohol disorder.

The presumption of a close relationship between obsessive compulsive disorder and schizophrenia has largely derived from the superficial similarity of the obsessional symptoms of the former and the experience of "alien" thoughts that often characterizes the latter. The victims of schizophrenia generally disown their alien and bizarre thoughts, which are regarded as inserted or transmitted into their minds from another source or person, whereas persons suffering from obsessions recognize the obsessional thought as their own, even if irrational and unwanted. This symptom similarity and others—for example, victims of schizophrenia may carry out ritualized behavior superficially similar to compulsions—have for many decades caused speculation as to some inherent relationship between the two disorders. We found that 12% of the obsessive compulsives meet criteria for schizophrenia, about 12 times the rate in the population as a whole. But it was not clear which was the dominant diagnosis: in 60% of cases of schizophrenia comorbid with obsessive compulsive disorder, schizophrenia was the prior-occurring disorder; in the remainder, the obsessive compulsive disorder began equally early or earlier. Because DSM-III omits any mention of sequence criteria or a time limit on the excluding diagnosis of schizophrenia with regard to obsessive compulsive disorder, even those ECA respondents who experienced obsessions or compulsions before the reported onset of their schizophrenic symptoms would be diagnosed solely as schizophrenic if DSM-III exclusion criteria were strictly observed.

When panic disorder was present along with obsessive–compulsive disorder, the pattern was similar to schizophrenia: in 60% of cases with both disorders the obsessive compulsive disorder was clearly preceded by panic attacks. Phobia, the disorder that most frequently co-occurs with obsessive compulsive disorder, was also the disorder most likely to precede it: it did so 75% of the time.

Finally, drug abuse/dependency was the disorder that most often began *after* obsessive compulsive disorder in comorbid cases. This supports the hypothesis that this disorder, in instances of comorbidity, may be brought about by efforts to self-medicate and anesthetize the often very distressing symptoms of obsessions and compulsions.

CONCLUSION

The ECA study has provided the first epidemiologic evidence concerning the prevalence of obsessive compulsive disorder among the general population. The most important finding is that the lifetime prevalence of this disorder, as measured by the Diagnostic Interview Schedule (DIS), is about 50 times that estimated from earlier studies carried out among samples of psychiatric patients. Indeed, the ECA data indicate that obsessive compulsive disorder is a relatively common disorder, having afflicted about 1 in 40 persons.

It is quite possible that a substantial portion of the obsessive compulsive disorder reported by ECA respondents does not produce very significant suffering or impairment, despite the minimal severity criteria required. This may be the case, in large part, for the 30% of those with the disorder who have had it for less than a year.

Obsessive compulsive disorder tends to begin early in life (about half the cases began before age 20), and when it terminates, it typically has endured almost seven years. It is most common among women 18–44 who are of white/other ethnic origin and rarest among Hispanic males over 45. It is clearly more prevalent among the underemployed than the fully employed, the separated or divorced than the married, those on welfare than those self-supporting, those who reside in institutional settings rather than private households, and those who seek treatment for mental health problems than those who do not.

When comorbid with schizophrenia, it usually appears second. When comorbid with drug abuse, it usually precedes it, suggesting that self-medication of symptoms may be common among those who suffer from obsessive compulsive disorder.

In light of both its high prevalence and its positive association with indicators of distressed life circumstances (welfare status, underemployment, disrupted marital status) and health and mental health care utilization, obsessive compulsive disorder is of major public mental health importance. Public awareness of the high prevalence of obsessive compulsive disorder may encourage those who suffer from it to overcome feared social stigmatization and make public their wishes and needs for professional evaluation and specialized care.

10 Somatization Disorder

MARVIN SWARTZ / RICHARD LANDERMAN /
LINDA K. GEORGE / DAN G. BLAZER /
JAVIER ESCOBAR

THE DIAGNOSIS OF SOMATIZATION DISORDER

Somatization disorder is the presentation of multiple physical complaints in multiple organ systems for which no organic cause can be found (American Psychiatric Association, 1980). The disorder, originally termed hysteria, has its historical roots in antiquity (Goodwin & Guze, 1979), dating back at least to the time of Hippocrates. The Egyptians and Greeks believed that many unusual and unexplained symptoms in women were attributable to the displacement of the uterus and that cure might be effected by return of the uterus to its correct position. By the Middle Ages and thereafter, similar unexplained polysymptomatic presentations were attributed to supernatural or evil influences such as witches or demons. Hysteria referred to both multiple unexplained symptoms and/or single pseudoneurological symptoms such as "hysterical" paralysis. The pseudoneurological symptoms were of considerable interest to Charcot and Freud in the late 1800s (Goodwin & Guze, 1984) and have since been termed conversion symptoms. The polysymptomatic syndrome, usually including a sample of unexplained neurological symptoms, was first clearly delineated by Briquet in 1899 (Goodwin & Guze, 1979) and subsequently refined by Cohen, Purtell, and Robins and their collaborators in the early 1950s (Cohen et al., 1953; Purtell, Robins, & Cohen, 1951; Robins, Purtell, & Cohen, 1952).

The DSM-III (1980) diagnostic category of somatization disorder derives from this work by Cohen, Purtell, and Robins and from work by Perley and Guze (1962) at the Washington University School of Medicine, who eventually named it Briquet's syndrome (Goodwin & Guze, 1979). The interest of these investigators was to define a number of relatively distinct psychiatric disorders with characteristic phenomenologies or symptomatic presentations, natural histories, prognoses, treatment responses, and family histo-

220

ries. Somatization disorder, as defined by DSM-III (American Psychiatric Association, 1980), is a prototype of this diagnostic approach and is a direct descendant of the earlier concept of the disorder, which has been refined by the Washington University group over the past three decades.

The essential feature of somatization disorder is the presentation of recurrent and multiple somatic (physical) complaints of several years' duration for which medical attention has been sought but which do not derive from a specific physical disorder. By definition, somatization disorder begins before age 30 and has a chronic but fluctuating course (American Psychiatric Association, 1980). In past studies of hysteria or Briquet's syndrome, excellent diagnostic stability (Perley & Guze, 1962), a high degree of reliability (Spitzer et al., 1978), and good validity (Guze & Perley, 1963) have been obtained.

Despite the low prevalence of the disorder, the high propensity of individuals with somatization to seek medical care has led to the recognition of a consistent clinical picture. The disorder is found almost exclusively among women and is more common among those women who are less educated. According to DSM-III criteria, women must have 14 out of 37 somatization symptoms to obtain the diagnosis; the corresponding symptom threshold for men is 12 of the 33 symptoms that pertain to males as well as females (Table 10–1). DSM-III-R has fixed the diagnostic threshold at 13 symptoms for both sexes while maintaining the previous symptom list (American Psychiatric Association, 1987).

Individuals with somatization disorder typically use health services frequently and in large volume and also tend to have multiple hospitalizations and surgeries. Among women, menstrual symptoms and sexual indifference are prototypic symptoms. These symptoms are so common that Goodwin and Guze (1979) suggest caution in making the diagnosis of somatization disorder if menstrual and sexual histories are normal. Marital discord, separation, and divorce are also common in somatization disorder (Guze & Perley, 1963).

Individuals with somatization disorder often report psychological or affective symptoms as well as somatic complaints. According to DSM-III, anxiety and depressed mood are extremely common, and many seek health care because of depressive symptoms, including suicide threats and attempts. Antisocial behavior, occupational difficulties, and interpersonal problems are common, and hallucinations (particularly of hearing one's name called) are often reported. Drug and alcohol abuse are commonly associated difficulties (American Psychiatric Association, 1980).

There is no evidence of excessive mortality among persons with somatization disorder when compared with the normal population (Coryell, 1981a), nor on the other hand, of improvement or remission over time. Although somatizing patients seek much medical care, many never see a psychiatrist. Thus it is difficult to estimate their number based on the

Table 10–1 How the DIS Covers DSM-III Criteria for Somatization Disorder

DSM-III Criteria	DIS Questions
A. A history of physical symptoms of several years' duration, beginning before the age of 30.	I'm going to mention the problems you have told me about. . . . What's the earliest age you first had one of these problems?
B. Complaints of at least 14 symptoms for women and 12 symptoms for men from the 37 symptoms below:	Have you ever had a lot of trouble with:
1. Abdominal pain	Abdominal or belly pain (not counting times when you are menstruating)?
2. Pain in back	Back pain?
3. Pain in joints	Pain in joints?
4. Pain in extremities	Pain in your arms or legs other than in the joints?
5. Chest pain	Chest pain?
6. Painful menstruation	Excessively painful menstrual periods?
7. Pain on urination	Pain when you urinate (pass your water)?
8. Pain in genital area (other than during intercourse)	Burning pain in your mouth or around your private parts?
9. Other pain (not including headaches)	Pain anywhere else?
10. Vomiting spells (other than during pregnancy)	Vomiting (when you are not pregnant)?
11. Severe vomiting throughout pregnancy or causing hospitalization during pregnancy	Vomiting all through pregnancy or hospitalized for vomiting during pregnancy?
12. Nausea	Nausea—feeling sick to your stomach but not actually vomiting?
13. Diarrhea	Loose bowels or diarrhea?
14. Bloating (gassy)	Excessive gas or bloating of your stomach or abdomen?
15. Intolerance of (e.g., made sick by) a variety of foods	Foods that you couldn't eat because they made you ill?
16. Trouble walking	Walking?

Table 10-1 continues

Table 10–1 continued

DSM-III Criteria	DIS Questions
	Have you ever been:
17. Urinary retention or difficulty urinating	Completely unable to urinate for 24 hours or longer (other than after childbirth of surgery)?
18. Blindness	Blind in one or both eyes, where you couldn't see anything at all for a few seconds or more?
19. Deafness	Deaf, where you've completely lost your hearing for a period of time?
20. Paralysis	Paralyzed—that is, completely unable to move a part of your body for at least a few minutes?
21. Palpitations	Bothered by palpitations, that is, your heart beating so hard that you could feel it pounding in your chest?
22. Dizziness	Bothered by dizziness?
23. Muscle weakness	Bothered by periods of muscle weakness—when you could not lift or move things you could normally lift or move?
24. Difficulty swallowing	Bothered by a feeling that there was a lump in your throat?
25. Belief that he or she has been sickly for a good part of life	Sickly for a majority of your life?
26. Loss of consciousness or fainting	Unconscious for any (other) reason?

Table 10-1 continues

Table 10–1 continued

DSM-III Criteria	DIS Questions
	Have you ever had:
26. (continued)	Fainting or falling-out spells where you felt weak or dizzy and then passed out?
27. Seizures or convulsions	Seizures or convulsions of any kind since you were 12 where you were unconscious but your body jerked?
28. Memory loss	Amnesia—that is, a period of several hours or days where you couldn't remember anything afterwards about what happened during that time?
29. Double vision	Problems that seem strange, like double vision or unusual spells?
30. Excessive menstrual bleeding	Excessive bleeding with your menstrual periods?
	Has there ever been:
31. Loss of voice	A time when you lost your voice for 30 minutes or more, and couldn't speak above a whisper?
32. Lack of pleasure during intercourse	A period of several months in your life when having sex was not pleasurable for you (even when it wasn't painful)?
33. Blurred vision	Has your vision ever become blurred for some period, when it wasn't just due to needing glasses or changing glasses?
34. Menstrual irregularity	Other than your first year of menstruation, have your menstrual periods ever been irregular?
35. Sexual indifference	Has your sex life been important to you or could you have gotten along as well without it?
36. Pain during intercourse	Have sexual relations even been physically painful for you?
37. Shortness of breath	Have you ever gotten short of breath when you had not been exerting yourself?

population of psychiatric patients. The study of these cases in community populations is therefore particularly important.

The ECA program estimated the prevalence of somatization disorder both in its present diagnostic categorization in DSM-III as well as in its previous categorizations—hysteria and Briquet's disorder. The prevalence of somatization disorder (SD) ranged from less than 0.05% to 0.38% across ECA sites (Karno et al., 1987, Myers et al., 1984, Swartz et al., 1986a). The highest prevalence of somatization disorder was at the Durham site. Sociodemographic and symptomatic features of Durham community respondents diagnosed with somatization disorder strongly resembled the features described in clinical populations (Swartz et al., 1986a). They tended to be female, unmarried, and nonwhite. They mostly lived in rural areas and were less educated than average. Also associated with the diagnosis were reports of poor physical health, nervousness, depression, and some psychotic and suicidal symptoms, as well as drug abuse problems and sexual difficulties.

Because past studies have differed in their diagnostic criteria, it has been unclear how similar cases identified by different diagnostic systems would be. In a previous publication from the ECA study, patients positive according to three diagnostic systems—Feighner et al. (1972), RDC (Spitzer et al., 1978), and DSM-III—were compared (Swartz et al., 1987). Among four ECA sites, 100 respondents with somatization disorder according to at least one of the three definitions were identified and the concordance of the three diagnoses examined. Briquet's disorder (the RDC term) identified the largest number of respondents, and hysteria (the Feighner term) identified the fewest. Despite different numbers identified, each system chose respondents with similar sociodemographic and associated features. It appeared that differences between systems were chiefly in severity thresholds for the disorder.

An alternate way of examining community data on somatizing respondents is to suspend judgment about the criteria for "caseness." Such an approach allows us to examine the "natural" categorization of somatizing syndromes that emerge from symptom reports. Using this approach we can determine if a syndrome or symptom profile resembling somatization disorder "naturally" emerges from symptom reports. We ask whether symptoms reported cluster in a manner comparable to the presumed clinical syndrome of somatization disorder. In a study of Durham respondents, the natural clustering of somatic symptoms was examined and a symptom profile strongly resembling DSM-III somatization disorder emerged (Swartz et al., 1986b).

Somatization disorder somewhat resembles hypochondriasis, which is an exaggerated attention to physical problems or the belief that normal physical signs or sensations are abnormal (Kenyon, 1964; Pilowsky, 1970). In exploring whether this diagnosis could be made with the ECA data, Escobar and co-workers (1987a) examined the distribution and predictive validity of somatic symptom counts below the threshold of somatization disorder. An abridged construct was conceived more or less serendipitously in a clinical study; a criterion score of 4 or more of the DIS symptoms serving somatization disorder was used to identify male somatizing respondents and a score of 6 was used for females (Escobar et al., 1987a, 1987b). This construct may be akin to such concepts as somatization "trait," hypochondriasis/somatization syndrome, or "below threshold" somatization disorder. In the present chapter this criterion score will be referred to as "somatization syndrome."

Previous studies in Los Angeles and Puerto Rico (Escobar et al., 1989) revealed a prevalence of somatization syndrome that was 30 to 150 times greater than the prevalence of somatization disorder. Thus, while somatization disorder is rare, its symptoms are not. Sixty to 80% of the normal population will experience at least one symptom in a given week (Kellner, 1975, 1985).

This higher prevalence allowed comparison of somatizing patterns across ethnic and age groups, a comparison not possible using full DSM-III criteria because of somatization disorder's rarity. The syndrome was found to be associated with the sociodemographic factors of low socioeconomic status, female gender, older age, and a Hispanic ethnic background, as in previous studies (Barsky & Klerman, 1983; Lin, Carter, & Kleinman, 1985).

The syndrome is also associated with high use of medical services and high indices of disability. A substantial portion (20–84%) of patients presenting to physicians are felt to have somatic complaints for which no organic cause can be found (Kellner, 1965, 1985; Kessel, 1960; Mayou, 1976, 1978). Somatizing patients have been estimated to account for up to 50% of ambulatory health costs in the U.S. (Barsky & Klerman, 1983; Kellner, 1985).

The concept of somatization syndrome will be further explored in this chapter. Where numbers of cases allow, prevalence and correlates of somatization disorder, somatization syndrome, and mean somatic symptom counts will be compared.

PREVALENCE OF SOMATIZATION DISORDER AND SOMATIZATION SYNDROME

SOMATIZATION DISORDER

Prevalence in the ECA study is determined by the proportion of individuals reporting enough symptoms of somatization disorder on the Diagnostic

Interview Schedule (DIS) to meet the DSM-III requirements for the diagnosis. To meet criteria, individuals must have had at least one symptom of the disorder prior to the age of 30 and, over their lifetimes, must have accumulated 12 of 33 symptoms if they are men and 14 of 37 symptoms if they are women. The symptoms need not overlap in time. Given that full criteria have been met, the recency of the diagnosis is determined by the last appearance of at least one of these symptoms.

The DIS is designed to accept as symptoms of somatization disorder, only symptoms that are severe and not explained by physical illness or by drug and/or alcohol abuse. This unique characteristic of the DIS—that it attempts to distinguish whether symptoms are totally or partially psychogenic in origin—means that symptoms accepted are more specific to somatization disorder than are symptoms counted in previous community surveys. Nonetheless, a community survey, lacking a clinical examination and access to medical records, cannot definitively assess whether or not somatic symptoms have a physical basis.

At the Durham site, the initial decision on whether a positively reported symptom was exclusively due to a physical disorder and/or drugs (including alcohol) was based on the standard probe structure of the DIS. However, if the lay interviewer had doubts about the origin of a symptom, a brief summary of the response was reviewed by a physician, who made the final determination of whether a symptom ought to be counted toward the diagnosis of somatization disorder. This additional medical editing, which did not occur at other sites, made it more likely that symptoms considered by the respondent to be medically explained would be scored as possibly psychogenic in Durham. This difference in method may have contributed to higher rates of somatization disorder in Durham.

The lifetime prevalence of somatization disorder in the total ECA sample is only 0.13% (Table 10-2a). The disorder is significantly more common among blacks (0.45%) than others, and among women (0.23%) than men (0.02%). Black women, because of the independent contributions of race and sex, demonstrate especially high rates (0.78%). Among males, the disorder is uncommon in all ethnic groups. Somatization disorder is clearly a predominantly female disorder, with a female to male ratio of over 10:1, but it is also a black disorder, with a black to nonblack ratio of over 4:1. However, it is rare even in black women compared with other disorders investigated.

Somatization disorder is a chronic disorder; remission is uncommon. Of the total group with a lifetime diagnosis (Table 10-2a), over 90% report symptoms within the past year, rendering a remission rate of less than 8%. This confirms the clinical observation (Guze & Perley, 1963) that the disorder usually takes a chronic, albeit fluctuating course. The proportion active in the last year and in the last month are identical. Due to this identity, one-month recencies will not be further discussed.

Table 10–2a Prevalence of Somatization Disorder by Race and Sex,[a] in Percent (SE)

	One-Month		One-Year		Lifetime	
Total	0.12	(0.04)	0.12	(0.04)	0.13	(0.04)
Non-black	0.08	(0.03)	0.09	(0.03)	0.10	(0.03)
Black	0.43	(0.21)	0.43	(0.21)	0.45	(0.22)
Male	0.02	(0.02)	0.02	(0.02)	0.02	(0.02)
Non-black	0.02	(0.02)	0.02	(0.02)	0.02	(0.02)
Black	0.06	(0.12)	0.06	(0.12)	0.07	(0.12)
Female	0.21	(0.07)	0.21	(0.07)	0.23	(0.07)
Non-black	0.15	(0.06)	0.15	(0.06)	0.17	(0.06)
Black	0.74	(0.37)	0.74	(0.37)	0.78	(0.38)

[a]Race and sex both have significant effects, ($p < .05$) on all measures of prevalence.

SOMATIZATION SYNDROME

Approximately 11.6% of the population meet criteria for lifetime somatization syndrome (defined as four or more symptoms among men and six or more symptoms among women) (Table 10–2b). This prevalence is roughly 100 times greater than somatization disorder's. When active somatization syndrome is defined in parallel fashion to somatization disorder—one symptom present among respondents who ever met criteria—the prevalence in the last year is 11.5%. Less than 9% of individuals with lifetime somatization syndrome have been in total remission for the last year—rendering a picture of chronicity very similar to that of somatization disorder.

As was true for somatization disorder, sex and race are significantly associated with somatization syndrome. Among blacks, the prevalence of lifetime somatization syndrome is almost a third higher (15%) than among other groups (Table 10–2b). Rates for females are moderately higher. Sex and race are similarly related to the active (one-year) syndrome.

Of particular interest clinically are people who have the somatization syndrome cross-sectionally, that is, people who have had at least four (for men) or six (for women) different symptoms within the last year. The one-year cross-sectional prevalence is roughly 4%. This group presents the prototypical picture of concurrent symptoms in multiple body systems unexplained by physical illness. We should expect impairment to be particularly common in such persons. In this chapter those identified as having an active somatization syndrome will be those meeting a cross-sectional diagnosis. Because two sites did not determine the recency of individual

Table 10-2b Prevalence of Somatization Syndrome and Somatic Symptom Count by Race and Sex[a]

	One-Year[b]					Lifetime[c]				
		Syndrome		Symptom Count			Syndrome		Symptom Count	
Group	N	%	(SE)	Mean	(SE)	N	%	(SE)	Mean	(SE)
Total	11,006	3.98	(0.26)	0.93	(0.02)	14,237	11.62	(0.40)	2.02	(0.03)
Non-black	8,048	3.63	(0.27)	0.90	(0.02)	10,004	11.21	(0.42)	1.99	(0.03)
Black	2,958	6.98	(1.05)	1.21	(0.09)	4,193	15.09	(1.40)	2.29	(0.12)
Male	4,746	3.83	(0.37)	0.60	(0.03)	6,106	8.68	(0.51)	1.21	(0.03)
Non-black	3,575	3.36	(0.37)	0.58	(0.03)	4,472	8.31	(0.53)	1.18	(0.04)
Black	1,171	8.05	(1.67)	0.83	(0.11)	1,634	12.00	(1.88)	1.42	(0.13)
Female	6,260	4.12	(0.37)	1.24	(0.04)	8,131	14.30	(0.61)	2.76	(0.05)
Non-black	4,473	3.88	(0.38)	1.20	(0.04)	5,572	13.89	(0.64)	2.73	(0.05)
Black	1,787	6.08	(1.34)	1.52	(0.13)	2,559	17.66	(2.01)	3.01	(0.18)

[a]Sex and race both have significant effects ($p < .05$) on lifetime somatization syndrome and one-year and lifetime symptom counts; race, but not sex, also has a significant effect on one-year somatization syndrome.

[b]Based on data from three sites (New Haven and St. Louis excluded), weighted to national demographic distributions.

[c]Based on data from four sites (New Haven excluded), weighted to national demographic distributions.

229

symptoms, these results will be based on the other three sites, weighted to represent the nation.

Female sex is associated with most measures of somatization syndrome, although the association is less dramatic than in the case of somatization disorder. Because of this weaker association with gender, females do not have more of *all* measures of somatization syndrome (for example, active somatization syndrome in Table 10–2b), but the trend in subsequent analyses consistently demonstrates an elevation of somatization syndrome in females.

Sex and race also have significant effects on mean somatic symptom counts (Table 10–2b). Data for these analyses were available from four ECA sites. The average number of somatic symptoms ever experienced was 2.02, with an average of .93 experienced in the last year. The average ever experienced is significantly higher among blacks than nonblacks (2.29 versus 1.99), but the effect of sex is more dramatic, with women reporting an average of 2.76 symptoms versus 1.21 symptoms for men. It must be recalled that four more somatic symptoms are available for females (three menstrual symptoms plus vomiting during pregnancy) than for men, so that symptom counts for women would be expected to be somewhat higher. However, the ratio of female to male symptoms is over 2:1, while the ratio of available symptoms is only 1.1:1, showing that sex differences in somatic symptom counts cannot be "explained away" by uniquely female somatic symptoms. In a multivariate study in Durham that deleted uniquely female somatic symptoms (Swartz et al., 1989), the effect of female sex remained significant even when sociodemographic controls such as residence and education were introduced. The elevation in somatic symptoms was particularly marked among urban females. Thus, by all measures, somatization appears to be a more common expression of psychic distress among females than males.

Up to this point we have divided race into blacks and nonblacks, with Hispanics, whites, Asians, and American Indians included in the non-black group. Overall, the lifetime rate for Hispanics is very close to the rate for the remainder of the nonblack group, 0.08% versus 0.10% (Table 10A–1 in this chapter's Appendix). Hispanic rates for lifetime somatization syndrome and mean lifetime somatic symptom counts are also very similar to counts for other nonblacks (Table 10A–2). Because overall rates for Hispanics are not different from those of non-Hispanic whites, they will be grouped with other nonblacks in subsequent analyses.

AGE OF ONSET

Among individuals with the disorder, the age of onset of somatization disorder is determined by the age at which the first somatic symptom was reported.

By definition, somatization disorder must have an onset prior to the age of 30, but most somatization disorder respondents report a much earlier onset. Forty percent of individuals with somatization disorder report onset of the disorder at age 10 or earlier. A surprising 55% of individuals report an onset at age 15 or less. Thus, somatization among individuals with somatization disorder is an early development, underscoring the embeddedness of the disorder in the individual's character. Somatization disorder begins early, is chronic and unremitting, and appears to be a deeply ingrained adaptation to life.

REGIONAL VARIATIONS

Lifetime rates of somatization disorder are approximately four times higher in Durham than in the other sites (Table 10–3a). The rates for men are fairly constant across sites other than Durham, where the rate for men is 0.13%. The cross-site prevalence for women are more variable across sites. The Los Angeles rate is remarkably low (0.05%). Rates for women are 0.16% in Baltimore, 0.28% at St. Louis, and 0.29% at New Haven. Once

Table 10–3a Prevalence of Somatization Disorders by Sex and Site[a]
(Weighted to Local Population)

Site	N	One-Year		Lifetime	
		%	(SE)	%	(SE)
New Haven	5,106	0.13	(0.07)	0.16	(0.08)
Male	2,175	0.01	(0.03)	0.01	(0.03)
Female	2,931	0.23	(0.12)	0.29	(0.14)
Baltimore	3,584	0.09	(0.06)	0.09	(0.06)
Male	1,444	0.00	(0.01)	0.00	(0.01)
Female	2,140	0.16	(0.11)	0.16	(0.11)
St. Louis	3,228	0.15	(0.09)	0.15	(0.10)
Male	1,360	0.01	(0.04)	0.02	(0.05)
Female	1,868	0.28	(0.18)	0.28	(0.18)
Durham	4,141	0.42	(0.13)	0.44	(0.14)
Male	1,702	0.13	(0.11)	0.13	(0.11)
Female	2,439	0.66	(0.23)	0.71	(0.24)
Los Angeles	3,508	0.03	(0.03)	0.03	(0.03)
Male	1,717	0.00	(—)	0.00	(—)
Female	1,791	0.05	(0.05)	0.05	(0.06)

[a]Site has a significant effect, ($p < .05$) on prevalence independent of the significant effect of sex.

again the rate in Durham is highest, 0.71%, a rate approximately two and one-half times the average across sites.

Cross-site differences in somatization syndrome and mean somatic symptom count follow the trends established for somatization disorder. The syndrome rate is highest in Durham (20.1%) and lowest in Los Angeles (9.3%) (Table 10–3b). Lifetime rates at other sites vary between 9.3% and 10.4%, with rates for men between 5.8% and 7.8% and for women between 11.7% and 12.7%. Mean lifetime symptom counts also follow this trend with mean symptom counts ranging from 1.7% to 2.0% at sites other than Durham and 2.8% in Durham. In each site women generally reported twice as many symptoms as men.

ARE REGIONAL DIFFERENCES REAL?

The higher rates of somatization disorder, syndrome, and mean symptom count in Durham than in other sites could reflect the confounding effect of differences in demographic composition across sites. Because significant relationships with somatization are found for race and sex, and as we shall see later for low educational level (Table 10–8), regional differences might be a function of differences in the distribution of these characteristics across sites. From Tables 10–3a and 10–3b it can be seen that differences between sites are not attributable to differences in sex distributions because they persist when one controls for the effect of sex. We also found that significant differences between sites remain when controls are introduced for education and race. Site differences do decrease by 10% to 30% when these controls are introduced, but remain significant. Thus, the high rate in Durham cannot be "explained away" by its large black population or its population's relatively low educational level.

Recall that a special medical edit, whereby symptoms claimed to have been physically explained were sometimes reclassified as psychogenic, occurred only in Durham. This probably contributed to the higher prevalence of somatization disorder in Durham. However, when the editing procedure was uniformly "relaxed" in all sites by calling all medically attributed symptoms possibly psychogenic, the higher rate in Durham persisted and prevalence did not rise appreciably.

Not all possible controls have been introduced, and the differences between sites may still be explained by other unexamined sociodemographic characteristics. However, none of the demographic factors that significantly affected somatization rates in this study can fully account for elevated rates in Durham. Thus somatization, whether represented in mean somatic symptom counts, somatization syndrome, or somatization disorder, appears to be a distinctive idiom of distress in Durham as compared to other sites.

Table 10–3b Prevalence of Somatization Syndrome and Somatic Symptom Count by Sex and Site[a] (Weighted to Local Population)

| | One-Year | | | | | Lifetime | | | | |
| | | Syndrome | | Symptom Count | | | Syndrome | | Symptom Count | |
Group	N	%	(SE)	Mean	(SE)	N	%	(SE)	Mean	(SE)
Baltimore	3,587	3.84	(0.38)	0.88	(0.03)	3,587	9.48	(0.58)	1.68	(0.05)
Male	1,445	3.42	(0.54)	0.56	(0.04)	1,445	6.82	(0.74)	1.00	(0.05)
Female	2,142	4.19	(0.54)	1.15	(0.05)	2,142	11.69	(0.86)	2.25	(0.08)
St. Louis	—	—	—	—	—	3,231	10.41	(0.74)	1.97	(0.06)
Male	—	—	—	—	—	1,360	7.79	(0.95)	1.15	(0.06)
Female	—	—	—	—	—	1,871	12.71	(1.11)	2.70	(0.10)
Durham	4,146	7.25	(0.54)	1.35	(0.05)	4,146	20.06	(0.83)	2.84	(0.07)
Male	1,703	8.35	(0.85)	0.95	(0.06)	1,703	16.25	(1.13)	1.79	(0.08)
Female	2,443	6.32	(0.69)	1.68	(0.07)	2,443	23.28	(1.19)	3.73	(0.10)
Los Angeles	3,511	2.40	(0.31)	0.72	(0.03)	3,511	9.32	(0.58)	1.78	(0.05)
Male	1,719	1.47	(0.35)	0.39	(0.03)	1,719	5.80	(0.67)	0.99	(0.04)
Female	1,792	3.27	(0.50)	1.02	(0.05)	1,792	12.63	(0.93)	2.53	(0.08)

[a]Site has a significant effect ($p < .05$) on syndrome and symptom count independent of the significant effect of sex.

233

Durham also differed from other sites in having higher rates of phobias, schizophrenia, obsessive-compulsive disorder, and cognitive impairment (Burnam et al., 1987a) and unusually low rates of antisocial personality disorder, drug abuse/dependence, and alcohol abuse/dependence. Thus, the most striking regional differences in rates of disorder are in the anxiety/somatiform spectrum, disorders that have in common the expression of psychic distress in the form of visceral or somatic symptomatology as opposed to the direct expression of affect in acting-out disorders (substance abuse and antisocial personality disorder) or intellectual expression of cognitive-existential distress (depression, dysthymia, etc.).

A high rate of somatization has also been found in a study using the DIS in Puerto Rico (Canino et al., 1987). The overall rate of somatization disorder in Puerto Rico is 0.7%, even higher than the 0.44% in Durham. Somatization syndrome is also elevated in Puerto Rico (Escobar et al., 1989). Although the disorder and the syndrome are predominantly female in Durham and at other ECA sites, rates for males and females are equal in Puerto Rico. These results underscore unique subcultural and cultural aspects of somatization.

RURAL PLACE OF RESIDENCE

In Durham, the only site with a substantial rural population, comparing urban with rural areas showed a nonsignificant trend toward a higher level of somatization disorder in rural areas (Table 10–4a). This slight increase in rural areas is equally evident for men and women.

Table 10–4a Prevalence of Somatization Disorder by Sex and Urban/Rural Residence[a] (Durham Site Data, Weighted to Local Population)

Group	Sample Size	Prevalence in Percent (SE)	
		One-Year	Lifetime
Total	3,835	0.39 (0.13)	0.41 (0.13)
Urban	1,889	0.28 (0.15)	0.28 (0.15)
Rural	1,946	0.52 (0.23)	0.58 (0.24)
Male	1,508	0.11 (0.10)	0.11 (0.10)
Urban	783	0.08 (0.11)	0.08 (0.11)
Rural	725	0.15 (0.19)	0.15 (0.19)
Female	2,327	0.62 (0.22)	0.66 (0.23)
Urban	1,106	0.46 (0.26)	0.46 (0.26)
Rural	1,221	0.81 (0.38)	0.90 (0.40)

[a]No significant urban/rural effect.

Table 10–4b Prevalence of Somatization Syndrome and Somatic Symptom Count by Sex and Urban/Rural Residence[a] (Durham Site Data, Weighted to Local Population)

Group	One-Year				Lifetime			
	Syndrome		Symptom Count		Syndrome		Symptom Count	
	%	(SE)	Mean	(SE)	%	(SE)	Mean	(SE)
Total	7.12	(0.54)	1.34	(0.04)	19.89	(0.83)	2.82	(0.07)
Urban	6.89	(0.71)	1.38	(0.06)	21.85	(1.15)	2.94	(0.09)
Rural	7.41	(0.83)	1.27	(0.07)	17.38	(1.20)	2.67	(0.11)
Male	8.21	(0.85)	0.93	(0.06)	16.03	(1.13)	1.77	(0.08)
Urban	7.16	(1.05)	0.89	(0.07)	16.81	(1.52)	1.75	(0.10)
Rural	9.66	(1.41)	0.99	(0.09)	14.95	(1.70)	1.80	(0.13)
Female	6.20	(0.68)	1.67	(0.07)	23.15	(1.20)	3.71	(0.10)
Urban	6.65	(0.95)	1.82	(0.09)	26.35	(1.69)	4.00	(0.14)
Rural	5.66	(0.97)	1.49	(0.10)	19.27	(1.66)	3.36	(0.16)

[a]Sex and residence have a significant interactive effect ($p < .05$) on one-year and lifetime symptom count. Residence has a significant effect (independent of sex) ($p < .05$) on lifetime syndrome.

Curiously, in light of this nonsignificant trend for somatization disorder, urban dwellers have a significantly higher level of lifetime somatization syndrome than do rural residents (Table 10–4b). The effect of residence on the syndrome appears to be stronger among women than men. Mean lifetime symptom counts are also higher in urban areas, but a significant interaction of sex and residence exists whereby men are slightly more symptomatic in rural areas and women more symptomatic in urban areas.

These findings do not suggest a strong association between somatization disorder and place of residence. However, milder indices such as somatization syndrome and somatic symptom counts *are* associated with urban residence.

AGE

Most clinicians expect somatization to be more common among older respondents. However, age does not have a significant effect on the prevalence of somatization disorder when those younger than 45 are compared with those 45 and older (Table 10–5a). Age also had little impact on somatization syndrome or symptom count, whether lifetime or active (one-year) (Table 10–5b).

MARITAL STATUS

Because marital status can change, the association between current marital status and active (one-year) somatization is investigated. Widowed individuals have the highest rates of somatization disorder (0.40% for both sexes), followed by the divorced and separated (0.24%) (Table 10–6a). This result approaches significance among females.

Divorced, separated, and widowed individuals demonstrate significantly elevated rates of current somatization syndrome and mean symptom counts (Table 10–6b). Among females, the most elevated rates are found among the divorced and separated, followed by the widowed and married. Among males, rates are equally elevated for the widowed and the divorced or separated. For both sexes, those never married have the lowest rates, and loss of a spouse appears to be associated with somatization.

EDUCATION

Significantly higher lifetime and one-year rates of somatization disorder are found among those who did not graduate from high school. The less educated predominate in a ratio of 4:1. This effect is evident for both sexes, but

Table 10–5a Prevalence of Somatization Disorder by Age
for Sex and Race Groups[a]

Group	Prevalence in Percent (SE)			
	One-Year		Lifetime	
Total:	0.12	(0.04)	0.13	(0.04)
Age less than 45	0.11	(0.05)	0.13	(0.05)
45 or older	0.14	(0.06)	0.14	(0.06)
Non-black	0.09	(0.03)	0.10	(0.03)
Age less than 45	0.07	(0.04)	0.09	(0.04)
45 or older	0.10	(0.05)	0.10	(0.05)
Black	0.43	(0.21)	0.45	(0.22)
Age less than 45	0.41	(0.26)	0.42	(0.26)
45 or older	0.46	(0.36)	0.52	(0.39)
Male:	0.02	(0.02)	0.02	(0.02)
Age less than 45	0.02	(0.03)	0.02	(0.03)
45 or older	0.03	(0.04)	0.03	(0.04)
Non-black	0.02	(0.02)	0.02	(0.02)
Age less than 45	0.02	(0.03)	0.02	(0.03)
45 or older	0.02	(0.03)	0.02	(0.03)
Black	0.06	(0.12)	0.07	(0.12)
Age less than 45	0.00	(0.02)	0.01	(0.06)
45 or older	0.18	(0.34)	0.18	(0.34)
Female:	0.21	(0.07)	0.23	(0.07)
Age less than 45	0.20	(0.09)	0.24	(0.09)
45 or older	0.22	(0.10)	0.23	(0.10)
Non-black	0.15	(0.06)	0.17	(0.06)
Age less than 45	0.12	(0.07)	0.16	(0.08)
45 or older	0.18	(0.10)	0.18	(0.10)
Black	0.74	(0.37)	0.78	(0.38)
Age less than 45	0.78	(0.48)	0.78	(0.48)
45 or older	0.68	(0.59)	0.77	(0.63)

[a]No significant age effect.

is more prominent among women where rates of the disorder are higher
(Table 10–7a). Thus, in addition to the significant effects of sex and race,
low education is an independent predictor of the diagnosis. Similarly,
somatization syndrome is significantly more prevalent among the less educated, particularly the less educated women (Table 10–7b). Mean somatic
symptom counts are also significantly higher among less educated respondents.

SOMATIZATION DISORDER
AND OTHER PSYCHIATRIC DISORDERS

In the ECA, having one diagnosis substantially increases the likelihood of
meeting criteria for another disorder (Boyd et al., 1984). Somatization disor-

Table 10–5b Prevalence of Somatization Syndrome and Somatic Symptom Count by Age for Sex and Race Groups[a]

Group	One-Year[b] Syndrome %	(SE)	One-Year Symptom Count Mean	(SE)	Lifetime[c] Syndrome %	(SE)	Lifetime Symptom Count Mean	(SE)
Total:	3.98	(0.26)	0.93	(0.02)	11.62	(0.40)	2.02	(0.03)
Age less than 45	3.85	(0.34)	0.94	(0.03)	11.74	(0.53)	2.00	(0.04)
45 or older	4.17	(0.41)	0.93	(0.04)	11.46	(0.62)	2.04	(0.05)
Non-black	3.63	(0.27)	0.90	(0.02)	11.21	(0.42)	1.99	(0.03)
Age less than 45	3.50	(0.35)	0.90	(0.03)	11.48	(0.56)	1.98	(0.05)
45 or older	3.80	(0.41)	0.90	(0.04)	10.86	(0.63)	2.00	(0.05)
Black	6.98	(1.05)	1.21	(0.09)	15.09	(1.40)	2.29	(0.12)
Age less than 45	6.44	(1.26)	1.19	(0.11)	13.69	(1.67)	2.16	(0.14)
45 or older	7.96	(1.89)	1.24	(0.16)	17.62	(2.49)	2.51	(0.22)
Male:	3.83	(0.37)	0.60	(0.03)	8.68	(0.51)	1.21	(0.03)
Age less than 45	3.31	(0.45)	0.53	(0.03)	8.80	(6.67)	1.19	(0.04)
45 or older	4.63	(0.65)	0.71	(0.05)	8.49	(0.81)	1.23	(0.06)
Non-black	3.36	(0.37)	0.58	(0.03)	8.31	(0.53)	1.18	(0.04)
Age less than 45	2.93	(0.45)	0.51	(0.03)	8.71	(0.71)	1.18	(0.04)
45 or older	3.99	(0.63)	0.68	(0.05)	7.71	(0.81)	1.18	(0.06)
Black	8.05	(1.67)	0.83	(0.11)	12.00	(1.88)	1.42	(0.13)
Age less than 45	6.33	(1.84)	0.70	(0.11)	9.49	(2.09)	1.21	(0.12)
45 or older	11.48	(3.40)	1.08	(0.24)	16.95	(3.76)	1.82	(0.29)
Female:	4.12	(0.37)	1.24	(0.04)	14.30	(0.61)	2.76	(0.05)
Age less than 45	4.38	(0.51)	1.34	(0.05)	14.62	(0.83)	2.80	(0.07)
45 or older	3.79	(0.53)	1.11	(0.05)	13.91	(0.91)	2.71	(0.08)
Non-black	3.88	(0.38)	1.20	(0.04)	13.89	(0.64)	2.73	(0.05)
Age less than 45	4.07	(0.53)	1.30	(0.05)	14.23	(0.87)	2.77	(0.07)
45 or older	3.64	(0.55)	1.08	(0.05)	13.48	(0.94)	2.68	(0.08)
Black	6.08	(1.34)	1.52	(0.13)	17.66	(2.01)	3.01	(0.18)
Age less than 45	6.54	(1.75)	1.61	(0.17)	17.38	(2.53)	2.99	(0.23)
45 or older	5.31	(2.07)	1.37	(0.21)	18.12	(3.34)	3.04	(0.30)

[a] No significant effect of age.
[b] Based on data from three sites (New Haven and St. Louis excluded).
[c] Based on data from four sites (New Haven excluded).

Table 10–6a Prevalence of Somatization Disorder by Sex and Marital Status[a]

Group	One-Year Prevalence	
	%	(SE)
Total:	0.12	(0.04)
Married	0.06	(0.03)
Widowed	0.40	(0.23)
Divorced/Separated	0.24	(0.16)
Never married	0.12	(0.07)
Male:	0.02	(0.02)
Married	0.01	(0.02)
Widowed	0.08	(0.25)
Divorced/Separated	0.04	(0.10)
Never married	0.05	(0.06)
Female:	0.21	(0.07)
Married	0.11	(0.06)
Widowed	0.47	(0.27)
Divorced/Separated	0.37	(0.25)
Never married	0.22	(0.15)

[a]Marital status has no significant effect.

der fits this observation (Table 10–8a). Somatization syndrome, and perhaps somatization disorder as well, is often conceptualized as a secondary feature of another psychiatric disorder such as depression or anxiety. In fact, clinicians may often neglect to diagnose somatization disorder because they consider the co-occurring diagnosis to be more "treatable" than somatization disorder or because the co-occurring diagnosis represents a change in state against a persisting background of somatic complaints. Thus, the data available in the ECA sample are useful in examining the co-occurrence of other psychiatric disorders with somatization disorder free of clinical or sampling bias.

All diagnoses covered are more prevalent among somatization disorder respondents than in the general population. In fact, every respondent with somatization disorder met criteria for at least one other lifetime diagnosis. Their prevalence ratio for some co-occurring core diagnosis is 2.9 (prevalence of another diagnosis among somatization disorder respondents divided by the prevalence of a disorder among those without somatization disorder). The most common and significantly associated disorders among somatization disorder respondents are phobic disorders (69%, prevalence ratio 5.5), major depression (55%, prevalence ratio 10.7), panic disorder (38%, prevalence ratio 24.8), alcohol abuse (23%, prevalence ratio 1.7), schizophrenia (21%, prevalence ratio 21.9), and dysthymia (19, prevalence ratio 5.7). The relationship with drug abuse/dependence (14%, prevalence

Table 10-6b Prevalence of Somatization Syndrome and Somatic Symptom Count by Sex and Marital Status[a]

	One-Year Prevalence			
	Syndrome[b]		Symptom Count[c]	
Group	%	(SE)	Mean	(SE)
Total	3.99	(0.26)	0.93	(0.02)
Married	3.68	(0.34)	0.88	(0.03)
Widowed	4.61	(0.96)	1.12	(0.09)
Divorced/Separated	6.81	(0.96)	1.27	(0.08)
Never married	3.09	(0.45)	0.81	(0.04)
Male	3.83	(0.37)	0.60	(0.03)
Married	3.43	(0.47)	0.58	(0.03)
Widowed	6.25	(2.63)	0.83	(0.15)
Divorced/Separated	6.98	(1.51)	0.80	(0.10)
Never married	3.21	(0.61)	0.56	(0.04)
Female	4.14	(0.37)	1.23	(0.04)
Married	3.92	(0.50)	1.18	(0.05)
Widowed	4.25	(1.02)	1.18	(0.10)
Divorced/Separated	6.69	(1.24)	1.61	(0.11)
Never married	2.92	(0.67)	1.14	(0.07)

[a]Current marital status has a significant effect ($p < .05$) on one-year syndrome and symptom count, independent of sex.
[b]Based on data from three sites (New Haven and St. Louis excluded), weighted to national distributions.
[c]Based on data from four sites (New Haven excluded), weighted to national distributions.

Table 10-7a Prevalence of Somatization Disorder by Sex and Education[a]

	One-Year		Lifetime	
Group	%	(SE)	%	(SE)
Total	0.12	(0.04)	0.13	(0.04)
Non-high school graduate	0.24	(0.09)	0.25	(0.09)
High school graduate	0.06	(0.03)	0.08	(0.04)
Male	0.20	(0.02)	0.02	(0.02)
Non-high school graduate	0.07	(0.07)	0.08	(0.07)
High school graduate	0.00	(—)	0.00	(—)
Female	0.21	(0.07)	0.23	(0.07)
Non-high school graduate	0.38	(0.15)	0.40	(0.15)
High school graduate	0.12	(0.06)	0.15	(0.07)

[a]Education has a significant effect ($p < .05$) on one-year and lifetime disorder independent of the significant effect of sex.

Table 10-7b Prevalence of Somatization Syndrome and Somatic Symptom Count by Sex and Education[a]

| | One-Year[b] | | | | Lifetime[c] | | | |
| | Syndrome | | Symptom Count | | Syndrome | | Symptom Count | |
Group	%	(SE)	Mean	(SE)	%	(SE)	Mean	(SE)
Total								
Non-high school graduate	3.99	(0.26)	0.93	(0.02)	11.61	(0.40)	2.02	(0.03)
High school graduate	5.82	(0.53)	1.15	(0.04)	14.56	(0.75)	2.30	(0.06)
	3.01	(0.28)	0.82	(0.03)	9.98	(0.47)	1.86	(0.04)
Male								
Non-high school graduate	3.82	(0.37)	0.60	(0.03)	8.66	(0.51)	1.21	(0.03)
High school graduate	5.63	(0.75)	0.78	(0.05)	11.29	(0.98)	1.41	(0.07)
	2.84	(0.40)	0.51	(0.03)	7.26	(0.59)	1.10	(0.04)
Female								
Non-high school graduate	4.14	(0.37)	1.23	(0.04)	14.28	(0.61)	2.75	(0.05)
High school graduate	5.99	(0.74)	1.49	(0.07)	17.42	(1.10)	3.08	(0.10)
	3.15	(0.40)	1.10	(0.04)	12.51	(0.72)	2.57	(0.06)

[a]Education has a significant effect ($p < .05$) on one-year and lifetime syndrome and symptom count independent of the significant effect of sex.
[b]Based on data from three sites (New Haven and St. Louis excluded), weighted to national distributions.
[c]Based on data from four sites (New Haven excluded), weighted to national distributions.

Table 10–8a Prevalence of Other Psychiatric Disorders Among Respondents with Somatization Disorder

Other Psychiatric Disorders	Percent with Other Disorders		Prevalence Ratio[a]
	Somatization Disorder	No Somatization Disorder	
Antisocial personality	5.44	2.50	2.18
Manic episode	5.35	0.30	17.83
Drug abuse/dependence	14.20	2.79	5.08
Alcohol abuse/dependence	22.61	13.51	1.67
Schizophrenia	21.45*	0.98	21.89
Panic disorder	37.77*	1.52	24.84
Obsessive/compulsive disorder	29.95*	2.52	11.88
Dysthymia	18.69*	3.25	5.75
Major depressive episode	55.10*	5.12	10.76
Phobic disorder	68.90*	12.49	5.52
Cognitive impairment	3.86	0.65	5.94
Any diagnosis	100.00*	33.97	2.94

*Significant at $p < .05$.

[a]Prevalence ratio is the prevalence among respondents with somatization disorder divided by the prevalence among respondents without somatization disorder.

ratio 5.1) and mania (5.3%, prevalence ratio 17.8) are not significant. These data suggest that somatization disorder is never uncomplicated but intersects with schizophrenia, anxiety, affective, and alcohol abuse disorders.

The specific comorbidities may differ by sex simply because certain diagnoses are more common among members of one sex than the other. However, in the case of somatization disorder, so few cases are found among males that comorbidity for somatization disorder respondents largely reflects comorbidity among females. Among females, results are the same as results for the total sample.

Comorbidity is best examined by looking at prevalence ratios, because they control for the fact that diagnoses vary in prevalence. Prevalence ratios show that the diagnoses most strongly associated with somatization disorder are panic, schizophrenia, mania, obsessive compulsive disorder, and major depression. The association with panic and major depression makes intuitive sense. Many symptoms of panic, depression, and somatization overlap, and indeed the Feighner diagnostic criteria for the disorder included anxiety and depressive symptoms as criterion symptoms. The association with schizophrenia is unclear. Perhaps schizophrenics do have multiple (and perhaps bizarre) somatic preoccupations. Alternatively, perhaps respondents with somatization disorder, who by definition endorse a plethora of somatic complaints, will also endorse other symptoms at a high rate. Whether approximately 21% of somatization disorder respondents are truly schizophrenic must be resolved by more in-depth clinical evaluation. The association of somatization disorder with mania and obsessive compulsive disorder is similarly difficult to explain.

Like somatization disorder, somatization syndrome is associated with a high rate of various psychiatric disorders. The disorders most often associated with somatization syndrome are the same ones most often associated with the disorder. Results for the two sexes are similar (Table 10-8b). In both sexes, all diagnoses except cognitive impairment in females are significantly associated with somatization syndrome. Some other diagnosis is found in 65% of women with somatization syndrome (prevalence ratio 2.4). The most commonly associated diagnoses are phobias (38%, prevalence ratio 2.7), major depression (25%, prevalence ratio 6.7), dysthymia (16%, prevalence ratio 6.3), alcohol abuse/dependence (9.6%, prevalence ratio 2.6), and obsessive compulsive disorder (9.3%, prevalence ratio 4.6). Among men, some other diagnosis is found in 70% (prevalence ratio 2.1). The most common lifetime diagnoses are alcohol abuse/dependence (41%, prevalence ratio 1.8), phobias (33%, prevalence ratio 4.1), major depression (15%, prevalence ratio 8.4), dysthymia (11%, prevalence ratio 8.2), and antisocial personality disorder (10%, prevalence ratio 2.5).

Ordering the association of lifetime diagnoses and somatization syndrome by the size of their prevalence ratios provides a different picture. The three diagnoses most strongly associated with somatization syndrome for both men and women are mania, schizophrenia, and panic disorder, as they were for somatization disorder.

Major depression, dysthymia, and obsessive-compulsive disorder consistently form the second group of associated diagnoses for both. The large number of disorders found to overlap with the somatization syndrome suggests that somatization may be an associated feature of any severe psychopathology.

While a relationship was found between somatization syndrome and antisocial personality disorder, that association was no more striking than relationships of somatization syndrome with other disorders. This is surprising, since Robins and co-workers (1952) found that among a group of men with "hysteria," approximately 14% had psychopathic personalities, while no controls demonstrated psychopathy. Guze (1964) and his coworkers (Guze, Woodruff, & Clayton, 1971a, 1971b) found an association between antisocial personality disorder and conversion or somatic symptoms and found an elevated rate of childhood delinquency among adult women with hysteria. Among a group of female felons with psychopathy, Cloninger and Guze (1970) found that 40% met criteria for hysteria. Other work by Spalt (1980) and Guze, Goodwin, and Crane (1969) has supported the relationship between antisocial personality disorder and hysteria among women but not men. These earlier studies were looking at correlates of hysteria and Briquet's syndrome. Perhaps the differences in their symptom patterns

Table 10–8b Prevalence of Other Psychiatric Disorders Among Respondents with Somatization Syndrome, by Sex[a]

| | Percent with Other Disorders | | | | | |
| | Females with: | | | Males with: | | |
Other Psychiatric Disorders	Somatization Syndrome[b]	No Somatization Syndrome	Prevalence Ratio[c]	Somatization Syndrome[b]	No Somatization Syndrome	Prevalence Ratio[c]
Antisocial personality	2.50	0.66	3.79	10.47	4.15	2.52
Manic episode	2.31	0.15	15.40	2.50	0.18	13.89
Drug abuse/dependence	5.35	1.60	3.34	8.14	2.85	2.86
Alcohol abuse/dependence	9.57	3.65	2.62	41.07	23.22	1.77
Schizophrenia	3.92	0.30	13.07	6.03	0.33	18.27
Panic disorder	8.91	0.95	9.79	8.28	0.43	19.26
Obsessive/compulsive disorder	9.35	2.04	4.58	9.52	1.39	6.85
Dysthymia	15.88	2.51	6.33	10.78	1.31	8.23
Major depressive episode	25.48	3.78	6.74	15.33	1.83	8.38
Phobic disorder	38.47	14.32	2.69	33.05	8.26	4.06
Cognitive impairment	0.85	0.52	1.63	1.73	0.54	3.20
Any diagnosis	64.84	26.66	2.43	69.61	33.93	2.05

[a]All other disorders significantly more common in those with somatization syndrome ($p < .05$) except cognitive impairment in females.
[b]Based on data from four sites (New Haven excluded) weighted to national distributions.
[c]Prevalence ratio is the prevalence among respondents with somatization syndrome divided by the prevalence among respondents without somatization disorder.

from the DSM-III definition of somatization explains the different results. In addition, unbiased community samples in the ECA study may account for differences when compared to the selected samples used in earlier studies.

WHICH COMES FIRST?

Having noted that all respondents with a lifetime diagnosis of somatization disorder had other lifetime disorders, we may question whether somatization disorder is a risk factor for other diagnoses or vice versa.

Among respondents with a lifetime history of both somatization disorder and phobia, the somatization began first in 54% and in approximately 42% phobia began first (Table 10–9). The order of onset is not known in approximately 4%. Among those with major depression, somatization began first in approximately 89% whereas major depression began first in approximately 2.5%. The order of onset is unknown in approximately 9%. Among those with somatization and obsessive compulsive disorder, somatization began first in approximately 61% while obsessive compulsive disorder began first in 35%, with an unknown order of onset in approximately 4%. In somatization and panic disorder, somatization began first in approximately 35% while panic began first in approximately 41% with an unknown order of onset in approximately 24%.

Clinicians have often noted that depressed persons complain of somatic symptoms, and have considered these symptoms to be somatic expressions of their depressions. However, these results suggest that in the minority of depressed persons who meet criteria for somatization disorder, the depression rarely precedes the first symptom of the somatization disorder. Thus, it is unlikely that the somatic symptoms are a consequence of the major depression. More likely, individuals with somatization disorder develop secondary major depressions in the course of their illnesses.

Other co-occurring diagnoses demonstrate similar patterns in their relationships to somatization disorder. Interestingly, when panic and somatization disorder co-occur, approximately one-quarter of respondents experience the onset of both disorders within the same year. This suggests a close relationship between the two disorders and/or an overlap in symptom profiles. In fact, both syndromes have in common unexplained somatic symptoms and may not be nosologically distinct syndromes.

Considering the group of co-occurring diagnoses together, roughly half of respondents have an onset of somatic symptomatology first, while the remainder have the onset of another disorder first, or the order is unknown. Thus somatization disorder can neither be viewed as a complication of other psychiatric disorders nor can other disorders typically be seen as complications of somatization disorder.

Table 10–9 Order of Onset Between Somatization and Four Other Disorders When Both Occurred

Somatization and Other Disorders	Somatization Symptom Occurred First (%)	Symptom of Other Disorder Occurred First (%)	Order of Onset Known (%)	Total (%)
Somatization with phobia (N=41)	54.01	42.2	3.8	100.0
Somatization with obsessive compulsive disorder (N=21)	61.3	35.0	3.7	100.0
Somatization with depression (N=29)	88.9	2.4	8.7	100.0
Somatization with panic (N=21)	34.9	40.9	24.2	100.0

In sum, the data on comorbidity and age of onset refute the notion that somatization disorder is a "secondary" disorder attendant on the development of a "primary" disorder such as major depression. Although "masked" depression, in which somatic symptoms obscure the mood changes, may be common, the severe somatization disorder diagnosis appears to have a complicated longitudinal course of its own.

SOMATIZATION DISORDER
AND INDICATORS OF IMPAIRMENT

In a cross-sectional study such as the ECA survey, we can examine the relationship between the disorder and various sociodemographic and other social concomitants. Whether these social cocomitants are risk factors for or consequences of the disorder is difficult to determine without longitudinal data. Because somatization disorder is a chronic condition with an early onset, many indicators of functioning are probably a result of the disorder. In any case, whether causes or effects, social concomitants are useful measures of associated functional impairment.

Because somatization disorder is a more severe disorder than somatization syndrome, we expect more severe impairment to be present among somatization disorder respondents. However, given the rarity of the disorder, its indicators of impairment are difficult to study. In the next two sections, indicators of impairment are more fruitfully examined among respondents with active somatization syndrome and compared in relation to trends among respondents with somatization disorder.

Employment. Most individuals with active somatization syndrome are able to work, but they do demonstrate significant vocational impairment. Approximately 39% were not employed full-time at the time of interview, and a third had been unemployed at least six months in the past five years. Comparable figures for those without the syndrome were 27% currently unemployed and 15% unemployed six months or more. Trends for individuals with somatization *disorder* also indicate marked employment difficulties (Table 10–10). About half of them had been unemployed at least six months in the past five years. Information about current unemployment was unstable because of the small number with somatization disorder, but rates of unemployment were extremely high—75%.

Income. Data on income are available only for respondents working full-time. Roughly two-thirds of working individuals with current somatization syndrome report incomes below $15,000, compared to about 50% of other respondents. Low earnings are also found among working respondents with somatization disorder.

Welfare. Approximately 20% of respondents with current somatization

Table 10–10 Unemployment and Underemployment Among Respondents with Somatization Disorder and Somatization Syndrome[a]

Group	Not Employed Full-Time[c]			Unemployed at Least Six Months in Past Five Years		
	N	%	(SE)	N	%	(SE)
Active (One-Year) Somatization Disorder						
No	14,319	37.05	(0.54)	11,654	13.49	(0.51)
Yes	21	[75.15]	(19.76)	46	49.59	(21.67)
Active (One-Year) Syndrome[b]						
No	6,942	26.76	(0.70)	7,153	14.91	(0.52)
Yes	285	39.33	(4.22)	465	33.03	(3.09)

[a] All results are significant at $p < .05$ level (except where cell size is below 25, as shown by [ ]).
[b] Based on data from three sites (New Haven and St. Louis excluded) weighted to national distributions.
[c] Baltimore site only includes part-time workers as employed.

248

syndrome are currently receiving welfare assistance, a significantly high rate. An even higher rate, 50%, is found for those with current somatization disorder, a result which is highly statistically significant. About 10% of respondents with neither syndrome nor disorder receive some form of welfare assistance. Thus, while about twice as many respondents with somatization syndrome received state assistance, about five times as many respondents with somatization disorder require assistance when compared to those with neither syndrome nor disorder.

Institutionalization. Significantly high rates of institutionalization are found among respondents with somatization disorder (Table 10-11). Of those with a current diagnosis of somatization disorder, approximately 9% were found in institutions, including psychiatric hospitals, nursing homes, and prisons, compared with only 0.5% of those without somatization disorder. Among institutionalized persons with current somatization disorder, about two-thirds (6.6%) are in chronic care facilities (nursing homes or boarding care homes). The remaining third are divided between jails or residential treatment centers for drugs and alcohol addiction (1.2%) and psychiatric hospitals (1.4%). Thus the preponderance of those institutionalized are in chronic care settings, indicating considerable levels of disability, but rates are elevated in residents of all types of institutions.

Approximately 2% of those with current somatization syndrome are found in institutions. Institutionalized persons with current somatization syndrome are distributed like those with somatization disorder—approximately two-thirds (1.2%) in chronic care facilities and the remainder divided between jail or residential substance abuse treatment centers (0.4%) and inpatient psychiatric settings (0.3%). Compared to those free of somatization syndrome, respondents with somatization disorder were approximately 18 times as likely to be institutionalized and respondents with the syndrome were approximately four times as likely to be institutionalized.

TREATMENT

In view of the fact that "doctor shopping" is one of the hallmarks of somatization disorder, it was expected that a high proportion of respondents with current somatization disorder would report use of outpatient general health services for physical conditions. In fact, approximately 95% have visited a health care provider in the last six months (Table 10-12) and nearly 45% have been hospitalized in the past year. Among those with current somatization syndrome, use of outpatient general health services is also quite high. Approximately three-quarters of respondents with somatization syndrome report use of services in the past six months and some-

Table 10–11 Somatization Disorder and Somatization Syndrome: Institutionalization[a]

Group	N	Chronic Care Facility[b]		Jail or Residential Treatment[c]		Inpatient Psychiatric Facility[d]	
		%	(SE)	%	(SE)	%	(SE)
Active (One-Year) Somatization Disorder							
No	19,503	0.33	(0.06)	0.16	(0.04)	0.04	(0.02)
Yes	64	6.60	(7.75)	1.23	(3.44)	1.40	(3.67)
Active (One-Year) Somatization Syndrome[e]							
No	10,607	0.31	(0.08)	0.12	(0.05)	0.03	(0.02)
Yes	637	1.23	(0.73)	0.40	(0.42)	0.34	(0.39)

[a] All differences statistically significant at $p < .01$.
[b] Include nursing homes, chronic hospitals, and boarding care homes.
[c] Include prison, jail, and residential substance-abuse treatment centers.
[d] Include psychiatric hospitals and mental retardation facilities.
[e] Based on data from three sites (New Haven and St. Louis excluded) weighted to national distributions.

Table 10–12 Somatization Disorder and Somatization Syndrome: Utilization of General Health Services[a]

Group	Used Outpatient Services Past Six Months			Used Inpatient Services Past Twelve Months		
	N	%	(SE)	N	%	(SE)
Active (One-Year) Somatization Disorder						
No	19,496	57.34	(0.51)	19,435	12.56	(0.34)
Yes	64	95.25	(6.54)	64	44.87	(15.52)
Active (One-Year) Somatization Syndrome[b]						
No	10,605	55.64	(0.67)	10,543	11.54	(0.43)
Yes	636	77.05	(2.81)	634	26.98	(2.96)

[a]All differences statistically significant at $p < .01$.
[b]Based on data from three sites (New Haven and St. Louis excluded), weighted to national distributions.

251

what more than a quarter report hospitalization in a general medical ward. In contrast, among those who did not meet criteria for somatization syndrome, 57% report use of outpatient health services in the past six months and 13% were hospitalized within the past year. These differences are statistically significant.

Individuals with somatization disorder do not use general health services as a substitute for mental health services; rather they use both in great abundance. Of those with the current diagnosis, 56% were seen in an outpatient mental health setting in the last six months, in comparison with 7.6% of those without the disorder (Table 10–13). Of those with a current somatization syndrome, 34% were seen in outpatient mental health services. Those with current somatization disorder also had a high rate of inpatient psychiatric hospitalization; 16.5% were hospitalized for psychiatric reasons in the past year. Of those with current somatization syndrome, 2% were hospitalized for psychiatric reasons. Both groups differ from those without a somatization syndrome, whose rate of hospitalization was less than 0.5%. Thus, respondents with somatization disorder are nearly eight times as likely to use outpatient mental health services and thirty times as likely to use inpatient psychiatric services as is the general population, and those with somatization syndrome are nearly five times as likely to seek outpatient and four times as likely to receive inpatient care as the general population.

Given the comorbidity associated with somatization disorder and syndrome, health service use is not necessarily for somatization symptoms but may be for symptoms of the co-occurring disorder. With the present data, it is impossible to identify which disorders were addressed in treatment beyond a rough distinction between general medical and mental health visits.

CONCLUSION

Somatization disorder is an uncommon psychiatric disorder. Only 0.13% of individuals have met DSM-III criteria for the disorder over their lifetimes. Those affected are unlikely to remit; almost all still had at least one symptom of the disorder present in the past year. Since it also begins young (usually before age 15), it is a disorder of unusually long duration. Perhaps this is why the impairment is so severe.

Although the disorder is uncommon, its prevalence is strongly associated with certain sociodemographic characteristics. Women are about ten times as likely as men to meet criteria for the diagnosis. Blacks are about four times as likely as whites or Hispanics to meet criteria. Those with less than a high school education are twice as likely to have the diagnosis of somatization disorder, an effect that is constant across the sexes. A threefold in-

Table 10-13 Somatization Disorder and Somatization Syndrome: Utilization of Mental Health Services[a]

Group	Used Outpatient Services in Past Six Months		Used Inpatient Services in Past Twelve Months	
	%	(SE)	%	(SE)
Active (One-Year) Somatization Disorder				
No	7.55	(0.27)	0.78	(0.09)
Yes	56.42	(15.47)	16.52	(11.59)
Active (One-Year) Syndrome[b]				
No	7.59	(0.36)	0.30	(0.07)
Yes	34.00	(3.16)	2.19	(0.98)

[a] All differences statistically significant at $p < .01$.
[b] Based on data from three sites (New Haven and St. Louis excluded) weighted to national distributions.

253

crease is found among the widowed and a twofold increase among the divorced and separated. Individuals in the Durham area demonstrate rates four times higher than in other regions surveyed. In part, this reflects higher rates in the rural counties surrounding Durham, where the disorder increases twofold. Among these high risk groups, for example, rural black females, the disorder rises to 1.5%, a rate close to their overall rates for disorders such as major depression (Blazer et al., 1985). Given the serious impairment associated with somatization disorder, it becomes an important source of morbidity in these demographic groups.

Sociodemographic correlates of somatization disorder may be viewed as putative risk factors for the disorder. Thus sex, race, place of birth, or rearing are possible risk factors. Given the early onset of somatization disorder, low educational level, which may be a risk factor for disorders with later onset, might as often be a consequence as a risk factor for somatization disorder, as is marital disruption.

Three-quarters of somatization disorder respondents do not work full-time; many are underemployed as well. When they do work, they occupy low status occupations and earn relatively little. Their poor work success probably explains the high proportion receiving welfare.

One out of ten somatization disorder respondents were in an institution at the time of the interview, one out of six had been in a psychiatric hospital during the past year, and nearly half had been hospitalized in a general hospital during the past year. Almost every somatization disorder respondent had a recent general medical visit, and over half had used specialty mental health services in the past six months, indicating very high utilization of general medical and psychiatric services. Although somatization disorder may be uncommon, treatment episodes for the disorder are not. Given the likely chronicity, comorbidity, and associated functional impairment that accompany the disorder, it represents a relatively severe and persistent disorder.

Comorbidity and functional impairment are substantial. All respondents with lifetime somatization disorder have another lifetime psychiatric disorder, a threefold increase in the risk of comorbidity compared to those without somatization disorder. The most common co-occurring diagnoses are phobic disorder, major depression, panic disorder, obsessive-compulsive disorder, alcohol abuse/dependence, and schizophrenia. Risk ratios are highest for panic disorder, schizophrenia, mania, obsessive-compulsive disorder, and major depression, indicating their more specific association with somatization disorder.

In contrast to somatization disorder, somatization syndrome is a common condition of milder severity. On the whole, this lower level of somatization is associated with sociodemographic characteristics, impairment, elevated treatment seeking, and comorbidity similar to those for somatization disorder, but associations are weaker.

Some level of somatic symptomatology unexplained by identifiable physical illness is found throughout the population. The similar correlates for somatic symptoms, somatization syndrome, and somatization disorder might indicate that disorder and syndrome are merely separated by quantitative differences in symptom levels and levels of impairment. Nonetheless, certain features suggest that somatization disorder and below-threshold somatization are qualitatively different. First, below-threshold somatization is higher among urban residents while somatization disorder shows a trend toward higher rates in rural settings. Second, below-threshold somatization is highest among the separated and divorced, whereas the widowed had highest rates of somatization disorder. The association of the syndrome with urban residence and marital discord suggests that it may be a stress-related phenomenon with a somatic presentation. Somatization disorder appears to be relatively unrelated to indices of recent stress and instead shows a severe lifelong pattern of impairment.

The broader phenomena of somatization, mean somatic symptom counts and somatization syndrome, appear to be related to aspects of culture not reducible to simple sociodemographic characteristics (Kirmayer, 1984; Kleinman, 1982). Previous studies of cultures in which psychic distress is expressed somatically have been hampered by the lack of comparable methodology. However, it does appear that somatization decreases with increasing western/industrial acculturation. As new cross-cultural studies using the DIS are completed in the near future, more rigorous comparisons of somatization and culture will be possible.

Table 10–A1 Prevalence of Somatization Disorder by Race

Group	One-Month %	(SE)	One-Year %	(SE)	Lifetime %	(SE)
Total	0.12	(0.04)	0.12	(0.04)	0.13	(0.04)
White/Other	0.09	(0.03)	0.09	(0.03)	0.10	(0.04)
Black	0.43	(0.21)	0.43	(0.21)	0.45	(0.22)
Hispanic	0.08	(0.13)	0.08	(0.13)	0.08	(0.13)

Table 10–A2 Prevalence of Somatization Syndrome and Number of Somatic Symptoms by Race

| | One-year[a] | | | | Lifetime[b] | | | |
| | Syndrome | | Symptom Count | | Syndrome | | Symptom Count | |
Group	%	(SE)	Mean	(SE)	%	(SE)	Mean	(SE)
Total	3.98	(0.26)	0.93	(0.02)	11.62	(0.40)	2.02	(0.03)
White/Other	3.67	(0.28)	0.91	(0.02)	11.24	(0.43)	2.00	(0.24)
Black	6.98	(1.05)	1.21	(0.09)	15.09	(1.40)	2.29	(0.12)
Hispanic	3.07	(0.99)	0.81	(0.09)	10.75	(1.67)	1.85	(0.14)

[a]Based on data from three sites (New Haven and St. Louis excluded), weighted to national distributions.
[b]Based on data from four sites (New Haven excluded), weighted to national distributions.

11 Antisocial Personality

LEE N. ROBINS / JAYSON TIPP / THOMAS PRZYBECK

THE DIAGNOSIS

Antisocial personality is a disorder that begins in childhood with a variety of behavior problems at home and in school and continues into adult life with failure to conform to social norms in many areas including work, family, and other interpersonal relationships. Persons with the disorder tend to be aggressive and impulsive and are thought to lack normal capacities for love, guilt, and cooperation with authority figures. Many of them come into conflict with the legal system.

Antisocial personality is the only diagnosis from Axis II of the *Diagnostic and Statistical Manual* (American Psychiatric Association, 1980) investigated in the ECA study. Axis II contains the personality disorders and the specific developmental disorders of childhood. By design, no childhood disorders were included in the ECA study. Antisocial personality was the only personality disorder included, because it alone had both clearly defined criteria and a substantial body of previous work with which ECA results could be compared. Axis II categories have been separated onto a separate axis to "ensure that consideration is given to the possible presence of disorders that are frequently overlooked when attention is directed to the usually more florid Axis I disorders." This statement from the Manual (p. 23) suggests that the personality disorders will frequently (but not always) have one or more diagnoses from Axis I associated with them. We shall see whether that is the case for antisocial personality.

Personality disorders, unlike Axis I disorders, are assumed to begin in childhood, and presumed to continue into adult life and persist for a long time. The Manual introduces the personality disorders by saying, "The manifestations of Personality Disorders are generally recognizable by adolescence or earlier and continue throughout most of adult life, though they often become less obvious in middle or old age. . . . The diagnosis of a Personality Disorder should be made only when the characteristic features

258

are typical of the individual's long-term functioning and are not limited to discrete episodes of illness" (p. 305). Although this is a statement about personality disorders in general, antisocial personality is the only one for which either onset in childhood (3 symptoms before age 15) or continuity of symptoms over time is specifically required. Written with the clinician facing a new patient in mind, the rules for diagnosing antisocial personality require that there never have been as many as 5 consecutive years without symptoms between age 15 and the "present." This criterion had to be modified in the ECA project to make it appropriate to an epidemiological study that surveys persons who have recovered from past disorders as well as the currently symptomatic. We required instead that there have been some symptoms in the age period 18 to 25, to insure that there has been no long hiatus between the symptoms required before age 15 and those present in adult life.

Antisocial personality is characterized by the violation of the rights of others and a general lack of conformity to social norms. It has been a troubling diagnosis to the psychiatric community and its critics. Some have argued that it is an attempt to "medicalize" bad behavior; others that it focuses on the wrong patient, that is, that these behaviors express the alienation of the disadvantaged and are symptoms of a sick society rather than a sick patient. We have argued previously (Robins, 1978) that antisocial personality meets three important criteria for a psychiatric disorder: (1) its symptoms are highly intercorrelated, making it a coherent syndrome, not just an assemblage of various types of deviance; (2) it has been shown to have a genetic component (Schulsinger, 1972); and (3) it occurs in and is recognized by every society, no matter what its economic system, and in all eras, showing that it is not purely an indication of a modern "sick" society. Although its prevalence varies with time and place, the same can be said of almost every psychiatric and nonpsychiatric disorder.

The revision of criteria for the diagnosis of antisocial personality in DSM-III-R (American Psychiatric Association, 1987) as compared with DSM-III has been substantial for childhood symptoms, and very modest for adult symptoms. In both versions, the diagnosis requires 3 childhood problems out of a possible 12 before age 15 and 4 adult problems out of a possible 9 (in DSM-III) or 10 (in DSM-III-R). Both require continuity of symptoms and occurrence other than in the context of mania and schizophrenia and mental retardation.

While the *number* of childhood symptoms remains the same, the specific childhood symptoms have been revised. The role of childhood aggression has been expanded so that instead of accounting for only one of the 12 possible symptoms (the DSM-III symptom was fighting) there are now 5 additional symptoms related to aggressiveness, including weapon use, cruelty to animals, cruelty to people, forcing sex on others, and stealing with confrontation. Fire-setting has been separated from other forms of vandalism. Conduct problems dropped to allow this expansion of forms of aggression and vandalism include early substance use, casual sex, breaking rules at home and school, school expulsion, official delinquency, and academic underachievement. These changes in the child variables are likely to increase the excess of male over female rates of antisocial personality, because they expand the role of violence and diminish the role of school problems, drug use, and early sexual activity, areas in which girls' rates more nearly approximate boys'.

The number of adult symptoms has increased by one in DSM-III-R with the addition of "lack of remorse." This addition was a response to criticisms that the DSM-III criteria failed to describe the underlying psychological deficits that were the essence of the disorder, concentrating instead exclusively on their observable behavioral expression. It was felt that inability to experience empathy and guilt or to profit from experience were essential to the diagnosis and that basing the diagnosis purely on observable behaviors gave too large a role to criminality (Frances, 1979; Millon, 1981). Other adult topics remain the same: work problems, marital problems, child neglect, violence, transiency, illegal behaviors, sexual behavior, and lying, although the content of three of these topics has been slightly altered. In addition, these behaviors are now counted as adult behaviors if they occur after age 15; in DSM-III, they counted only if they occurred after 18.

THE COMMON ADULT SYMPTOMS
OF ANTISOCIAL PERSONALITY

If the criticism were warranted that the diagnosis of antisocial personality according to DSM-III criteria was simply a medicalizing of criminality, we would expect to find that most persons with that diagnosis had a criminal history, and that most persons with a criminal history earned that diagnosis. This turned out not to be the case (Table 11–1). In fact, less than half (47%) of those positive for the DSM-III diagnosis have a significant record of arrest (defined as two or more arrests other than for a moving traffic violation or any felony conviction). Rather than criminality, the adult symptoms that typify the antisocial personality are job troubles (found in 94%), violence (found in 85%), multiple moving traffic offenses (found in 72%), and severe marital difficulties (desertion, multiple separations or divorces, multiple infidelities, found in 67%).

Not only are most antisocial persons noncriminal, only a minority (37%) of those arrested met criteria for antisocial personality. Thus, criminality was neither necessary nor sufficient for the diagnosis.

Nor was any other adult symptom pathognomonic. Only about one-quarter of those who admitted child neglect, vagrancy, or lying a great deal

Table 11-1 Adult Symptoms of Antisocial Personality

	Percent of Those with Antisocial Personality Who Have the Symptom			Percent of Those with the Symptom Who Meet Diagnostic Criteria for Antisocial Personality			
Adult Symptoms	Total (N=628) %	Male (N=517) %	Female (N=111) %	N %	Total %	Male %	Female %
Job troubles	94	94	95	3,706	7	11	3
Violence	85	85	83	1,984	13	18	6
4+ traffic offenses	72	79	44	1,858	11	11	6
Severe marital problems	67	60	97	2,349	11	19	5
Vagrancy	51	49	57	754	23	28	14
Multiple non-traffic arrests	47	55	17	841	37	40	18
Persistent lying	44	44	45	820	23	32	11
Child neglect	12	12	12	184	29	42	13

met the criteria (Table 11-1), and even fewer qualified among those who reported fighting, traffic offenses, marital problems, or a poor work history. Clearly no adult behavior problems occur solely in persons meeting criteria for antisocial personality. What is distinctive about persons with the disorder is the broad spread of their behavior problems in both childhood and adult life.

Symptom patterns were similar for men and women meeting diagnostic criteria for antisocial personality, although men exceeded women in both traffic and nontraffic arrests, as they do in the population at large, while antisocial women exceeded antisocial men in marital difficulties.

SYMPTOM COVERAGE
AND PREVALENCE ESTIMATES

Assessing the presence of antisocial personality requires asking about illegal behaviors and behaviors that could be considered embarrassingly personal. Probably for this reason, no previous surveys provide estimates of its prevalence in the general population, although there have been estimates made in many special populations expected to have rates higher than the general population's, including prisoners (Guze et al., 1969; Hare, 1983), psychiatric clinic patients, and psychiatric emergency room attenders (Robins et al., 1977), patients of substance abuse treatment centers (Hesselbrock et al., 1985; Lewis et al., 1983a), former child guidance clinic patients (Robins, 1966), adoptees (Crowe, 1974), the recently divorced (Briscoe et al., 1973) and relatives of criminals (Cloninger & Guze, 1973).

The interview used in the ECA study had to be approved by the federal government's Office of Management and Budget (OMB), as required for all surveys carried out under a government contract or as a cooperative agreement. That office refused approval of questions about illegal occupations, such as fencing stolen goods, pimping, prostitution, and selling drugs, about infidelity and promiscuity, about financial irresponsibility, and about age at first sexual intercourse. The questions they disapproved were omitted by most sites but included at St. Louis by adding them into the 30-minute discretionary section not sponsored by the government and available to each site. In two sites an additional question was omitted because it concerned child beating, and the investigators thought interviewers would be obliged to turn names of those who responded positively over to the state agency on child abuse, violating the promised confidentiality.

The absence of the disapproved questions means that the prevalences for antisocial personality reported here will be underestimates. We can judge how much undercounting was caused by the excluded questions by comparing St. Louis prevalence estimates with and without the banned questions. Based only on the approved questions, St. Louis had a somewhat higher rate of lifetime disorder, 3.4%, than other sites. When the banned questions were added, the St. Louis rate rose to 5.1%, an increase of 53%. When all five sites were combined and weighted to represent the country as a whole, the overall lifetime rate was 2.6% Applying the 53% increase found in St. Louis to this figure gives an estimate for the country of 4.0% of the population having ever warranted a diagnosis of antisocial personality (Table 11–2).

Because the degree of undercounting varied by ethnic, age, and sex group in St. Louis, we also estimated its effects on national estimates separately for these demographic subpopulations. However, because St. Louis did not have many Hispanics, we could not estimate how great the loss was for them.

Correcting for the missing questions increased the already striking associations of antisocial personality with sex and age. The male:female ratio rose from 5.6 to 7.3, and the age 18–29:44–64 ratio rose from 2.7 to 4.3, the age 30–44:44–64 ratio rose from 2.5 to 3.1. The similarity in rates for blacks and whites remained after correction for the omitted questions.

In the remainder of this chapter, we use only the questions that were approved by OMB and consequently asked in all sites. As we have shown,

Table 11-2 Effect of Excluded Adult Questions on Estimates of Lifetime Prevalence of Antisocial Personality

	(A) Lifetime Prevalence (%) in St. Louis Based on Questions Asked in All Sites	(B) Lifetime Prevalence (%) in St. Louis Based on Questions Asked in All Sites Plus Excluded Questions	(C) Proportional Increase (B/A) in Estimate Explained by Added Questions	(D) Lifetime Prevalence (%) in U.S. Based on Questions Asked in All Sites (5-site Data)	(E) Estimated U.S. Lifetime Prevalence (D × C) if Excluded Questions Had Been Asked in All Sites
Total	3.4	5.1	1.53	2.6	4.0
Male	5.8	9.4	1.62	4.5	7.3
Female	1.2	1.5	1.25	0.8	1.0
White	3.2	4.8	1.50	2.6	3.9
Black	4.3	7.0	1.63	2.3	3.7
18–29	5.2	9.3	1.79	3.8	6.8
30–44	5.0	6.6	1.32	3.7	4.9
45–64	1.4	1.6	1.14	1.4	1.6
65+	0.2	0.6	3.00	0.3	0.9

263

the rates produced will be underestimates, but there will be little distortion of the relationships between antisocial personality and its correlates.

COURSE

AGE OF ONSET OF CHILDHOOD SYMPTOMS

By definition, antisocial personality must begin before age 15. However, the age of onset is typically much earlier than that. The average age, defined as the age of the first childhood symptom, falls between the 8th and 9th birthdays for both men and women and for all age groups with sufficient numbers to provide stable estimates. (We do not have enough cases in men over 65 or women over 45 for accurate estimation.) Rarely do persons with antisocial personality report onsets before age 5, and by age 11, 80% of all future cases have had a first symptom.

REMISSION AND DURATION

Antisocial personality is placed on Axis II because it is supposed to be a chronic disorder, more or less lifelong. However, about half of those who ever qualified for the disorder have had none of its symptoms in the last year (active cases occur in 1.2% of the population, while 2.6% have qualified in their lifetime, (Table 11–3). This finding of about half having recovered applies to all three ethnic groups and both sexes. Remission probabilities increase with age. While less than 40% of those affected and under age 30 have been symptom-free for a year, almost all of those over 45 have been. These results confirm the findings of an early follow-up of child-guidance patients, who were in their early forties at follow-up (Robins, 1966). That study noted that this supposedly "interminable" disorder often remitted in the fourth decade of life. The ECA study now extends that finding into later age ranges, and shows that as persons with antisocial personality age, more and more of them go into remission. These results help to explain why crime is a "young man's game," with most offenders disappearing from arrest records by their midthirties. It is not just that criminals become cleverer about hiding their misdemeanors as they age. Rather, aging is accompanied by a decrease in the spectrum of antisocial behaviors, including crime.

   The fact that antisocial personality remits with age does not mean that it should not be considered a chronic disorder. Among those with no symptoms in the past year, the average duration from first to last symptom was 19 years. Thus, although not typically lifelong, it is a disorder with a protracted duration.

Table 11–3 Prevalence of Antisocial Personality

	Prevalence in Percent (SE)			Remission[a]
	Lifetime	One-Year	One-Month	
Total	2.6 (0.16)	1.2 (0.11)	0.5 (0.07)	54
Males	4.5 (0.31)	2.1 (0.22)	0.9 (0.14)	53
Females	0.8 (0.13)***	0.4 (0.09)***	0.2 (0.06)***	50
Whites	2.6 (0.18)	1.2 (0.12)	0.5 (0.08)	54
Blacks	2.3 (0.48)	1.1 (0.33)	0.4 (0.21)	52
Hispanics	3.4 (0.80)	1.6 (0.56)	0.7 (0.38)	53
<30	3.8 (0.36)	2.3 (0.28)	0.9 (0.17)	39
30–44	3.7 (0.38)	1.5 (0.25)*	0.8 (0.17)	59
45–64	1.4 (0.23)***	0.2 (0.09)***	0.1 (0.07)***	86
65 + years	0.3 (0.15)***	0.0 (0.5)*	0.0 (0.05)	100

*p < .05; ***p < .001.
[a]Remission = Lifetime prevalence minus one-year prevalence divided by lifetime prevalence: (Lt − 1 Yr)/Lt.

PROGRESSION FROM CHILD TO ADULT SYMPTOMS

Overall, only 26% of children who have met the childhood criteria for antisocial personality have also met the adult criteria (Table 11–4). (St. Louis results show that a higher rate of those meeting childhood criteria would meet adult criteria if all the adult items had been covered. We estimate the correct figure to be 31%, still less than one-third.) This relatively low rate of persistence of antisocial behavior into adult life is consistent with results of an earlier study, which showed that among children with three or more antisocial symptoms, only 27% met criteria for antisocial personality as adults (Robins, 1966). Most antisocial children recover without developing the diagnosis of antisocial personality.

Number Versus Type of Childhood Problem. The likelihood of meeting adult diagnostic criteria increases as the number of childhood conduct problems increases, from 18% with the minimum three conduct problems to 46% when there were at least six conduct problems. This gradual increase suggests that conduct problems can function as a dimensional variable. Indeed, there is no sharp break in their relation to adult antisocial symptoms at the minimum of three required symptoms (Figure 11–1). The number of childhood symptoms was found to account for 30% of the variance in whether the diagnosis will be positive.

Table 11–4 Levels of Childhood Antisocial Symptoms and Risk of Meeting Criteria for Antisocial Personality

	Percent with Antisocial Personality When Level of Childhood Symptoms:			
	3	4 or 5	6+	Total 3+
Total sample	18	26	46	26
Sex:				
Male	19	27	49	27
Female	17	21	33	21
Ethnic group:				
White	19	25	46	26
Black	15	25	46	19
Hispanic	22	30	46	29
Age group:				
18–29	14	21	43	22
30–44	24	37	51	34
45–64	22	26	[49][a]	27
65+	15	3	—[b]	12

[a]Brackets indicate a cell size of 25–29.
[b]Dash indicates a cell size below 25.

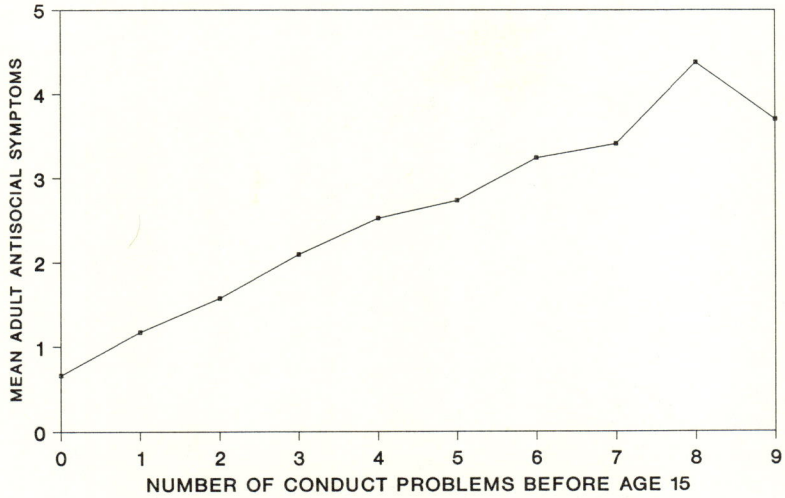

Figure 11-1 Child and Adult Antisocial Symptoms
Data from 3 ECA Sites—St. Louis, Durham, Los Angeles

No individual childhood behavior problem is a particularly good predictor of antisocial personality. Indeed, none added as much as 1% to the explained variance once the number of problems was taken into account. The best single childhood predictor was running away (Table 11-5, col. 1). Twenty-nine percent of all runaways before age 15 met criteria for the disorder. Next best predictors were delinquency (25%) and vandalism (21%). But the importance of these symptoms resides mainly in their being indicators that a child is likely to have at least three childhood behavior problems.

Progression from Child to Adult Problems by Age, Sex, and Ethnicity. More men than women met the childhood criteria for antisocial personality, and younger cohorts of both men and women more often met these criteria than their elders (Figure 11-2). Indeed as many women under 30 met criteria as did men 45–64.

Although the two sexes remain far apart, there is some evidence that women are beginning to catch up with men in meeting these childhood criteria. In the youngest group they are closer than they would have been had the youngest group followed the trajectory of change found in older groups (Figure 11-3). In Figure 11-3, the trajectory established by the 45–64 year olds compared to the 65 + group is shown by the dashed line; the trajectory established by the 30–44 year olds compared to the 45–64 year olds is shown by the dotted line. The youngest women's level of conduct problems lies above either trajectory, while the youngest men show approximately the same increase as did the previous cohort. Despite

Table 11–5 Prevalence of Antisocial Personality in Persons with Specific Childhood Symptoms, by Sex, Age, Ethnic Group

Behavior Problems before 15	All Ages		Under Age 45	Men under 45				Women under 45			
	N	%	%	All %	White %	Black %	Hispanic %	All %	White %	Black %	Hispanic %
Runaway	628	29	31	41	42	36	40	15	14	15	—[a]
Delinquent	682	25	26	29	31	19	29	13	13	19	—[a]
Vandalism	713	21	23	24	24	21	33	13	15	[3][b]	—[a]
Early substance use	628	18	18	23	22	19	24	8	8	11	—[a]
Fighting	1,324	17	20	23	23	25	22	10	12	6	11
Expelled/Suspended	1,527	16	16	19	21	6	23	8	8	8	9
Truant	1,669	16	17	22	22	18	22	9	9	12	9
Discipline problem	1,558	16	17	20	20	18	25	11	11	7	14
Lying	2,147	13	15	20	22	13	15	8	9	6	5
Stealing	2,830	11	13	15	15	12	20	7	7	12	6
Underachievement	1,460	10	12	16	16	14	31	5	5	7	7

[a]N = < 25.
[b]N = 25–29.

268

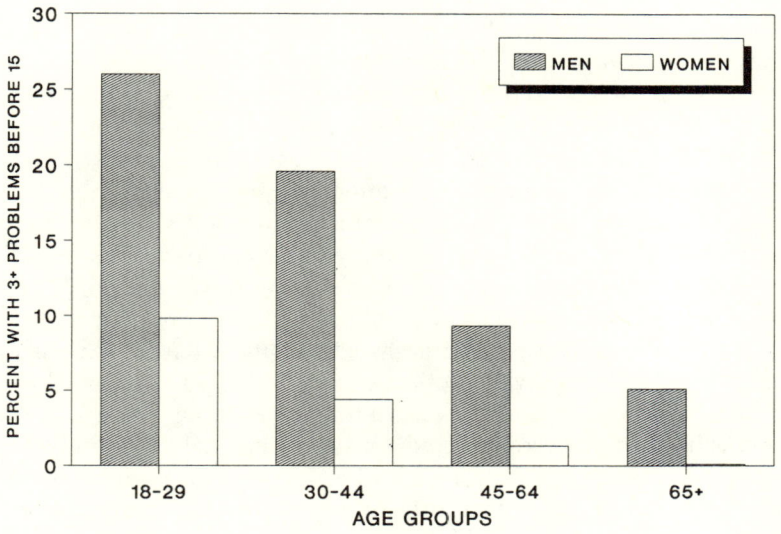

Figure 11-2 Cohort Differences in Conduct Problems

this trend toward convergence of female toward male rates, the remaining substantial difference in rates means that parity is unlikely to occur in the near future.

Given the increase in the frequency of conduct problems among the young, and particularly among young women, one might expect their conduct problems to have become less prognostic of adult symptoms. If "every-

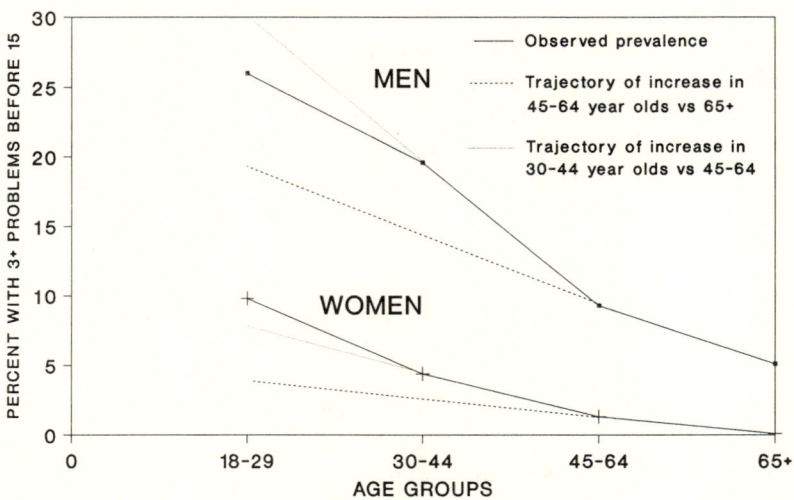

Figure 11-3 Convergence of Sexes in Having Three or More Conduct Problems

one is doing" a disapproved behavior, that behavior might be expected to be less an indicator of an underlying tendency toward deviance. But the evidence says otherwise. Each behavior problem was at least as prognostic of meeting full diagnostic criteria in persons under 45 as in the total population (Table 11-5, col. 2 versus col. 1).

Every conduct problem was more common in men than women. One might expect that the same problem occurring in a girl would be more ominous than in a boy, just because it is more unusual. To see whether this was so, we looked at the outcome of problems by sex (Table 11-5). We considered only persons under 45 years of age because conduct problems were so rare in older persons, particularly older women. Rather than being more ominous in girls, behavior problems predicted future antisocial personality better in boys. For example, running away from home was the childhood behavior that best predicted antisocial personality for both men and women below age 45. However, 41% of males who had been childhood runaways later met criteria for antisocial personality, compared to only 15% of females. When males and females shared any particular symptom, the males were two or three times more likely than the females to develop antisocial personality. Because the number of child and adult symptoms is so much higher in males than females, the presence of any conduct problem is a much better indicator in males than females that there will be at least the two other childhood problems plus the four adult symptoms needed to qualify for antisocial personality.

Childhood behavior problems were about equally prognostic for blacks and whites, although each symptom except fighting was slightly more prognostic of antisocial personality for white than black males. The only significant difference was found for expulsion or suspension from school, a childhood experience with little prognostic significance for black males. For black females, however, it was as prognostic as for whites. Since black men reported more school suspensions than did whites or Hispanics, but no more conduct problems overall, it is possible that black boys were suspended with little provocation, making their suspensions a poor indicator of their predisposition to antisocial behavior.

RISK FACTORS

CURRENT AND FUTURE COHORT DIFFERENCES

Antisocial personality, like several other disorders in this volume, appears to have been on the increase in recent cohorts, since young people had higher rates than their elders even though the older groups have had more years in which to carry out the behaviors that warrant the diagnosis (Table 11-3).

The eventual excess of antisocial personality in the youngest cohort is underestimated in a cross-sectional study like the ECA because the largest number of new cases can be expected to appear in this group. There are two reasons: first, symptoms of antisocial personality rarely appear for the first time after young adulthood and, therefore, new ones can be expected only in the two younger groups; and second, the youngest cohort contains a larger proportion of persons at risk of developing the disorder than the second youngest. That is, more of the youngest cohort have met childhood criteria than any other age group (Figure 11–2), and of those meeting childhood criteria, more of the youngest than those 30 to 44 are still at risk of developing the adult criteria (78% compared to 66%, Table 11–4). We can estimate their likely short-term future prevalence by extrapolating from the second youngest group's rate of meeting adult criteria once they meet childhood criteria. By the time the youngest cohort reaches 30 to 44 years of age, if the same proportion of those with three or more childhood symptoms meets adult criteria as among the current 30–44 year olds, their lifetime prevalence rate will be 6.4%, compared with the rate of 3.7% in the cohort now 30–44 years old.

MALE AND FEMALE DIFFERENCES
BY ETHNIC GROUP AND AGE

We noted above that male rates of antisocial personality greatly exceed female rates. This was the case for every age and ethnic group (Table 11–6). However, the sex ratio is lower among the young than among the elderly, suggesting that there may be convergence over time, and is lower among blacks than whites. The sex ratio of lifetime rates is especially low for the youngest blacks (1.9). (There are equally low sex ratios in older Hispanics because Hispanic men share the pattern of highest rates in youngest cohorts with other ethnic groups, but there is no marked variation by age for Hispanic women. But overall rates of antisocial personality are so low in older Hispanics that their low sex ratio may not be meaningful.)

IS ETHNIC EQUALITY AN ARTIFACT?

No significant differences in rates of antisocial personality were found among the three ethnic groups. Yet minority groups are overrepresented in arrested and incarcerated populations. Since many inmates of penitentiaries warrant a diagnosis of antisocial personality (Guze et al., 1969; Hare, 1983), one might have expected minorities to have especially high rates of antisocial personality. Why did this not occur? We will seek explanations only for blacks, because the number of Hispanics is too small for intensive investigation.

Table 11–6 Prevalence of Antisocial Personality by Age, Sex, and Ethnicity in Percent (SE)

	Men			Women			Male to Female Ratio		
	One-Month	One-Year	Lifetime	One-Month	One-Year	Lifetime	One-Month	One-Year	Lifetime
Total	0.87 (0.14)	2.11 (0.22)	4.51 (0.31)	0.19 (0.06)	0.37 (0.09)	0.82 (0.13)	4.6	5.7	5.5
Age									
18–29	1.31 (0.30)	3.79 (0.50)	5.96 (0.62)	0.44 (0.17)	0.85 (0.24)	1.60 (0.33)	3.0	4.5	3.7
30–44	1.38 (0.34)	2.80 (0.48)	6.51 (0.71)	0.19 (0.12)	0.35 (0.17)	1.03 (0.28)	7.3	8.0	6.3
45–64	0.23 (0.14)	0.36 (0.17)	2.57 (0.45)	0.04 (0.06)	0.10 (0.09)	0.25 (0.13)	5.8	3.6	10.3
65+	0.08 (0.12)	0.08 (0.12)	0.69 (0.35)	0.00	0.00 a	0.04 (0.07)	b	b	17.3
Whites									
18–29	0.85 (0.15)	2.11 (0.24)	4.52 (0.34)	0.19 (0.07)	0.34 (0.09)	0.75 (0.14)	4.5	6.2	6.0
30–44	1.22 (0.32)	3.95 (0.57)	6.13 (0.71)	0.47 (0.21)	0.87 (0.28)	1.64 (0.38)	2.5	4.5	3.7
45–64	1.51 (0.39)	2.89 (0.53)	6.65 (0.79)	0.22 (0.10)	0.33 (0.18)	0.99 (0.31)	6.9	8.8	6.7
65+	0.17 (0.13)	0.32 (0.17)	2.57 (0.49)	0.00 a	0.04 (0.06)	0.13 (0.11)	b	8.0	19.8
	0.07 (0.12)	0.07 (0.12)	0.59 (0.35)	0.00 a	0.00 a	0.00 (0.03)	b	b	b
Blacks									
18–29	0.69 (0.40)	1.61 (0.60)	3.63 (0.90)	0.20 (0.19)	0.61 (0.34)	1.20 (0.48)	3.5	2.6	3.0
30–44	0.83 (0.71)	2.16 (1.14)	3.50 (1.44)	0.14 (0.27)	0.90 (0.70)	1.81 (0.98)	5.9	2.4	1.9
45–64	0.85 (0.82)	2.30 (1.35)	5.62 (2.06)	0.14 (0.30)	0.68 (0.68)	1.31 (0.94)	6.1	3.4	4.3
65+	0.45 (0.66)	0.49 (0.30)	2.25 (1.46)	0.44 (0.58)	0.44 (0.58)	0.82 (0.79)	1.0	1.1	2.7
	0.30 (0.82)	0.30 (0.82)	1.77 (1.99)	0.00 a	0.00 a	0.00 a	b	b	b
Hispanics									
18–29	1.26 (0.71)	2.81 (1.05)	5.64 (1.47)	0.19 (0.27)	0.40 (0.39)	1.20 (0.68)	6.6	7.0	4.7
30–44	2.50 (1.51)	4.61 (2.03)	7.05 (2.47)	0.49 (0.70)	0.64 (0.80)	1.07 (1.03)	5.1	7.2	6.6
45–64	0.60 (0.91)	2.78 (1.93)	6.75 (2.95)	0.01 (0.10)	0.02 (0.17)	1.25 (1.24)	60.0	139.0	5.4
65+	0.05 (0.30)	0.05 (0.30)	2.63 (2.20)	0.00 a	0.66 (1.08)	1.30 (1.51)	b	0.1	2.0
	0.00 a	0.00	0.98 (2.50)	0.00	0.00 a	1.36 (2.45)	c	c	0.7

aStandard error not calculated when percent = 0.00.
bNot computable because women's rate = 0.
cNo cases.

272

We noted previously that even if the excluded questions had been asked, there still would have been black–white equality (Table 11–2). Omitted questions, then, were not the explanation.

If the ECA had been a study restricted to household residents, the low rate for blacks might have been accounted for by many blacks with antisocial personality having been sent to prison, leaving the black community residents with low rates of antisocial personality. But the ECA sample includes prisoners, and our prisoner sample shows the expected high proportion of blacks. At interview, we found 1.8% of the black male sample below age 45 in prisons, jail, or in residential alcohol and drug treatment centers compared with .3% of white and hispanic men under 45 (Table 11–7). We report rates of incarceration only for men under 45 because few women are ever incarcerated, and prison populations contain very few older men. We include residential alcohol and drug treatment centers with jails and prisons because many of their clients are on probation or parole and are being offered treatment as an alternative to prison or jail.

There remains the possibility that blacks with antisocial personality are missed in our survey because they are neither in prison nor in households. The only part of the population not represented in the ECA sample is those with no fixed home address or living on military bases or overseas. The military are not likely to contain many persons qualifying for antisocial personality because serious criminal records are grounds for rejection and because discipline problems in service lead to discharge. But could the black cases of antisocial personality have been missed because they were

Table 11–7 Ethnicity and Current Incarceration, Controlling for Antisocial Personality and Number of Arrestable Behaviors[a]

	Percent of Those below Age 45 Incarcerated		
	White %	Black %	Hispanic %
Total	0.3	1.8	0.3
Antisocial personality			
Negative	0.2	1.1	0.2
Positive	2.7	14.6	1.8
Arrestable behaviors			
None	0.0	0.8	0.1
One	0.2	2.7	0.3
Two	1.1	5.2	2.1
Three	4.6	10.9	4.6

[a](1) Use of weapons, (2) spouse battering, (3) repeated use of heroin, cocaine, or amphetamines.

not attached to households? The U.S. Census reported that a serious un-dercounting of young black men had occurred in 1960, perhaps as great as 20%. The Census discovered the problem when they noticed that the number of black men in their thirties in 1970 was considerably larger than the number in their twenties in 1960. These should have been the same people, reduced in 1970 by those who died or emigrated between censuses. The larger number in 1970 had to mean that a substantial number of men in their twenties had been missed by census takers 10 years earlier. If men were missed when they had no fixed residence, but moved about among relatives and sexual partners, those missed should have had a high rate of antisocial personality, if for no other reason than the fact that transiency is one of the criterion symptoms for the diagnosis. If a large number of transient young black men were also missed in the ECA survey, their absence might account for the low rate of antisocial personality in black males. But we should have also found higher lifetime rates of antisocial personality in blacks than whites over 30, because the census found that blacks in that age group reappeared as household members. Table 11-6 shows this was not the case. The only age bracket in which black men exceed whites in rate of antisocial personality is the oldest (those over 65).

Another possible artifact could have been differential reporting, if blacks were less willing than whites to report antisocial behavior. However, more black than white men reported having been convicted of a felony (5.4% versus 2.1% of whites), confirming the well-known excess of convictions in blacks. No other question used to make the diagnosis of antisocial personal-ity appears more "sensitive," and so more likely to be denied.

It seems probable, then, that blacks truly do have more convictions than whites without a correspondingly higher rate of antisocial personality. We consider two possible explanations: (1) with or without qualifying for a diagnosis of antisocial personality, blacks more than others may commit acts likely to lead to arrest, and (2) blacks may be more liable to arrest and incarceration than whites with the same pattern of behaviors.

If the first hypothesis is correct, then antisocial symptoms experienced by blacks should differ from those experienced by whites in ways that could explain their being more often incarcerated. Among adult symptoms of antisocial personality other than arrests and felony conviction, blacks ex-ceeded whites in only two: prolonged unemployment and weapon use (Table 11-8). Both symptoms probably increased the risk of arrest, unem-ployment by creating the severe financial need that might prompt theft, and weapon use by increasing the likelihood of seriously injuring or killing others in the course of fighting. (It is not that more blacks fight; fighting as an adult is reported in about one-fifth of the men in each ethnic group.)

Blacks' higher rates of chronic unemployment and weapon use do not result in higher rates of antisocial personality overall because they are balanced by lower rates than whites' of other symptoms, in particular

Table 11–8 Ethnic Differences on Selected Adult Symptoms
of Antisocial Personality

Symptom	Males from Three Sites: St. Louis, Los Angeles Durham[b]			Prevalence Ratios[c] %	
	Whites %	Blacks %	Hispanics %	B:W	H:W
Legal					
4 or more moving traffic violations	27.5	26.3	18.2	1.0	0.7
2 or more non-traffic arrests	4.8	10.3	7.4	2.2	1.5
Felony conviction	2.1	5.4	2.2	2.6	1.0
Transiency					
1 month with no address	6.5	4.3	7.9	0.7	1.2
Travel about/no job[a]	5.8	4.3	13.9	0.7	2.4
Work					
Unemployed 6 or more months in 5 years	12.1	23.2	19.6	2.0	1.6
3 or more jobs in 5 years	28.3	20.6	22.9	0.7	0.8
Fired twice or more	6.2	6.4	6.1	1.0	1.0
Quit 3 or more times without job prospect	7.3	4.9	6.5	0.7	0.9
Absenteeism	8.0	10.9	6.4	1.4	0.8
Violence					
Fighting	17.8	20.3	17.4	1.1	1.0
Weapon use	4.9	10.7	3.9	2.2	0.8
Child abuse[a]	2.7	1.5	1.5	0.6	0.6
Spouse battering, if married	5.6	7.1	8.3	1.3	1.5

[a]Data not available for Durham.

[b]Baltimore and New Haven omitted because adult symptoms of antisocial personality were asked only of persons who had three or more childhood symptoms.

[c]Percentage with this symptom among blacks (B) or Hispanics (H) divided by the percentage with this symptom among whites (W).

repeatedly quitting jobs without another in prospect. The rarity with which blacks quit jobs impulsively makes sense in terms of the precariousness of black positions in the job market.

Our second hypothesis, that blacks may be arrested or convicted more readily than whites who commit the same acts, also may be correct. We looked at the arrest experience of men with and without the three behaviors that we thought would put them at greatest risk for arrest—weapon use, spouse battering, and use of amphetamines, heroin, or cocaine. Having none of these three behaviors, no whites but a small proportion of blacks (0.8%) were found in prison at the time of interview (Table 11–7). When all three behaviors were reported, whites were only half as likely to be found in prison as blacks (4.6% versus 10.9%). These results suggest discriminatory incarceration, although it is also possible that blacks had more frequent or more serious offenses than whites. We do not have the data necessary to control for the severity of the antisocial symptoms.

If our two hypotheses are correct—that blacks' particular pattern of problem behaviors makes them more likely to be imprisoned and that they also get imprisoned on less provocation than whites, we should expect to find that these particular problem behaviors are more common in blacks than whites who do *not* have antisocial personality diagnoses as well, and that a smaller proportion of black than white arrestees meet criteria for antisocial personality.

We did indeed find that fewer black than white weapon users qualified as antisocial personalities (21% versus 35% of whites). We also found that the use of weapons by blacks was less often preceded by the multiplicity of childhood behaviors that predict adult antisocial behavior. Only 38% of black weapon users met childhood criteria for conduct problems, compared with 55% of white weapon users. This suggests that there is a greater acceptance of weapon use in the black than in the white community, and that weapon use puts blacks without a serious predisposition to antisocial behavior at risk of imprisonment.

We also found, as expected, that black arrestees less often met criteria for antisocial personality than did white arrestees. Among blacks arrested twice or more, fewer than one-quarter met criteria for antisocial personality, while almost half of the whites and Hispanics with two or more arrests did so. Black arrestees' lower rates of antisocial behavior applied to both the childhood (37% versus 56% of whites) and the adult criteria (46% versus 60% of whites) of antisocial personality. Similarly, blacks with a felony conviction met all criteria for antisocial personality in only 35% of cases, while half of white felons did so (51%). Thus, arrested blacks, including those convicted of a felony, are more "normal" than whites with the same arrest history.

EDUCATION AND IQ

Most other disorders typically begin after education is complete, and educational level can therefore be interpreted as a risk factor. This is obviously not possible for antisocial personality, which usually begins at age eight or nine. Interpreting the relationship between educational level and antisocial personality is doubly difficult because underachievement, school discipline problems, truancy, and expulsion are childhood symptoms of the disorder, and all are associated with early school leaving.

As expected, then, lifetime rates of antisocial personality are lowest in college graduates (1.2%). However, there is no smooth association with amount of completed education. The highest rate occurs not among those with the least education (less than eight years, with a rate of 2.9%), but among those who entered high school but did not complete it (4.9%).

Men and women show similar associations between education and the diagnosis of antisocial personality (Figure 11–4), although women lack the elevation among those who did not finish 8th grade. Women who did not finish 8th grade have an even lower rate than do college graduates.

Because older people grew up at a time when it was commonplace to leave school as soon as one was old enough to work, early school leaving is less related to school problems for them than for younger people. A change in the organization of school levels has also occurred along with rising expectations about the number of school years that should be completed. American elementary schools used to end at 8th grade, high schools at 12th grade, and college at the 16th school year. Since the introduction of junior high schools and junior colleges, there are more graduation points at varying grade levels. This makes ambiguous for younger cohorts whether completion of a given year was at a graduation point.

For males over 45, highest rates of antisocial personality were found for persons who dropped out before completing 8th grade, that is, before graduating from elementary school; among those 30–44, highest rates were among those who finished eight years, but went no further. In their era of schooling, leaving at 8th grade is more likely to be a consequence of dropping out of junior high school than graduation from elementary school.

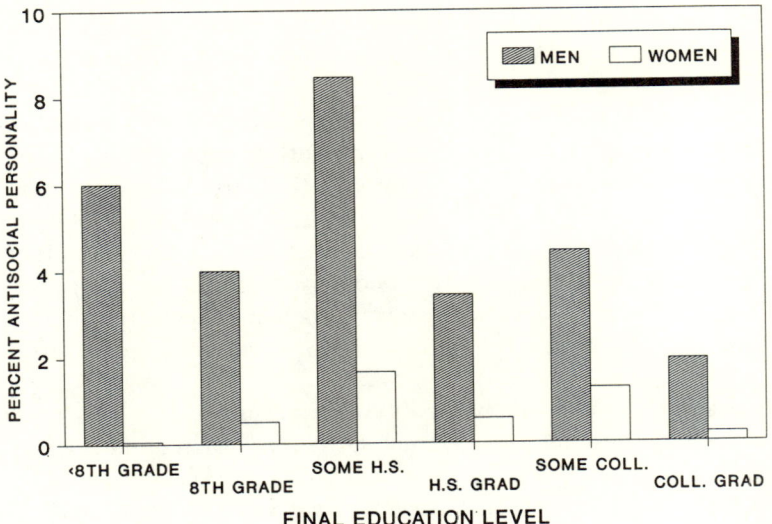

Figure 11-4 Education and Antisocial Personality

Among those under 30, highest rates occurred in those who left school after 9 to 11 years, presumably by dropping out of senior high school. It would appear that failing to complete the last unit of education entered is more strongly associated with antisocial personality than is the number of years completed.

Intelligence. A slightly lower than average IQ score has been repeatedly found to be associated with conduct problems in childhood and presumably, therefore, with later antisocial personality (Rutter & Madge, 1976). While the ECA project did not test IQ, the interview provides three clues to the intellectual capacity of the respondents. First, they are asked whether they had been held back more than one grade. Second, they are asked whether their school grades were poor, and if so whether the teacher thought they could have done much better. If they say the teacher thought they could have done much better, they are considered "underachievers." But if they had poor school success and were not underachievers, they presumably had a low IQ. Finally, respondents were given the Mini-Mental State Examination (MMSE), which was devised to detect dementia, but which has been shown to be correlated with educational level (Anthony et al., 1982). So far as we know, the question of whether that association is due to a lack of education or to low IQ, which prevents progress to the upper grades, has not been addressed. However, we found scores in the mildly or severely impaired range (seven or more errors) on the MMSE to be associated with both of our other presumed indicators of low IQ. Among those with scores in the impaired range, 11% had repeated grades and 9% reported poor grades but not "underachievement," compared with 4% and 1% respectively among those with greater success on the test. Because Alzheimer's disease is extremely rare before age 65, it is probable that most of the poor scores on the MMSE in younger people can be attributed to low IQ or lack of education.

Having one or more of these three possible indicators of retardation before age 45 was found to be associated with antisocial personality (Table 11–9). (We present results only for the young because the MMSE is a more appropriate measure of IQ for them, since they have almost no risk of being truly demented and they have had more educational opportunities than their elders.) More than 15% of young people with one or more of these three indicators of low IQ met diagnostic criteria for antisocial personality; in people with none of them, the rate was 3.3%, an almost fivefold difference.

The association of antisocial pesonality with presumed low IQ was far stronger for whites, both males and females, than for blacks and hispanics. This suggests either that antisocial personality is less related to low IQ in minorities or that these measures are much weaker indicators of IQ in minorities than in whites. We believe the latter alternative is the more probable.

Table 11-9 Possible Mental Retardation and Antisocial Personality in Persons Under 45 (New Haven Omitted)[a]

			Percent Diagnosed Antisocial Personality										
			White				Black				Hispanic			
	Total		Males		Females		Males		Females		Males		Females	
	N	%	N	%	N	%	N	%	N	%	N	%	N	%
Possible mental retardation[b]:														
No	6,667	3.3	1,774	5.4	1,959	1.4	838	4.0	1,323	1.6	474	6.1	392	1.0
Yes	737	15.6	161	28.2	83	6.2	140	9.7	108	2.7	89	15.0	71	3.1
Prevalence ratio[c]		4.7		5.3		4.4		2.4		1.7		2.5		3.1

[a] In New Haven, the question on repeating school grades was not asked.
[b] More than six errors in Mini-Mental State exam, held back two or more grades, or poor grades and teacher thought performed up to capacity.
[c] Prevalence of antisocial personality in those with possible mental retardation divided by prevalence of antisocial personality in those with no indicator of possible mental retardation.

279

RURAL–URBAN RESIDENCE

It is widely believed that increasing urbanization accounts in part for an increasing rate of antisocial behavior in the population. The explanations generally offered for this association are a combination of increased opportunities for theft, overcrowding that occasions irascibility and violence, and the breakdown of social controls with concomitant anonymity. Whether or not these explanations are correct, the ECA study does confirm the finding that urban areas have higher rates than rural areas in the two sites that have sufficient rural populations to examine, St. Louis and Durham. In St. Louis, we can compare rural and urban whites but not blacks, because there are few rural blacks in the Missouri ECA population. For white men, the lifetime rate of antisocial personality is 5.6% in urban St. Louis and 3.7% in the surrounding rural area; for white women, the respective figures are 1.2% and 0.5%. Among white men in Durham, the same pattern appears, with lifetime rates of 3.9% versus 2.3%. However, among white women living in Durham, the rates in both urban and rural areas are vanishingly small. Nor was an excess found for urban blacks.

SITE DIFFERENCES

Residents of St. Louis had higher lifetime rates of antisocial personality than did residents of Durham or New Haven (Table 11–10), while rates in Los Angeles and Baltimore fell between these.

We considered the possibility that these differences might be explained by demographic characteristics of the sites. For example, New Haven had the highest proportion of college graduates among the sites, and we have shown that higher education is associated with low rates of disorder.

To see whether these sites differences remained when we took demographic characteristics into account, we controlled on age and education (Table 11–11). We did not control on ethnicity because it had not been found significantly related to antisocial personality, or on sex, which although strongly related to diagnosis, does not vary geographically. Age and education remained important variables across sites, validating their choice as control variables. (The one exception was that education was unrelated to disorder in older persons in New Haven).

For older persons, there were no significant differences by site. However, site differences remained for the young. Among young people who did not graduate from high school, not only New Haven and Durham but also Los Angeles had a significantly lower rate than St. Louis. Among young people who completed high school, Durham's rate was lower than New Haven's, St. Louis's, and Los Angeles', and Baltimore's was lower than St. Louis's or Los Angeles'.

Table 11–10 Antisocial Personality: Site Differences (Weighted to Local Population Distribution)

	Prevalence in Percent (SE)			
	One-Month	One-Year	Lifetime	Remission
Durham	0.45 (0.14)	1.09 (0.22)	1.63 (0.26)	28 (7.62)
New Haven	0.32 (0.11)	0.75 (0.16)	2.00 (0.27)	62 (6.55)*
Baltimore	0.51 (0.14)	1.17 (0.22)	2.48 (0.31)	51 (6.50)*
Los Angeles	0.40 (0.13)	1.07 (0.21)	2.93 (0.34)	57 (6.33)*
St. Louis	0.80 (0.22)	1.71 (0.32)**	3.38 (0.44)***	45 (6.87)

*Significantly higher than Durham.
**Significantly higher than New Haven.
***Significantly higher than Durham and New Haven.

Table 11–11 Antisocial Personality by Site,[a] Controlling on Age and Education

Age: High School Graduate:	18–44						45 or Older					
	No			Yes			No			Yes		
	N	%	(SE)	N	%	(SE)	N	%	(SE)	N	%	(SE)
Durham	473	5.4	(1.23)	1,243	1.3	(0.35)	1,451	1.0	(0.44)	927	0.3	(0.24)
New Haven	368	4.9	(1.34)	1,388	2.6*	(0.45)	1,720	0.8	(0.39)	1,567	0.9	(0.33)
Baltimore	747	6.4	(1.06)	1,087	1.5	(0.42)	1,257	1.7	(0.45)	433	0.5	(0.41)
Los Angeles	778	6.0	(1.08)	1,514	3.0**	(0.53)	556	1.8	(0.65)	578	0.9	(0.42)
St. Louis	500	10.9***	(2.11)	1,304	3.2**	(0.64)	888	1.4	(0.61)	477	0.5	(0.40)

[a]Weighted to local population distributions
*Significantly higher than Durham.
**Significantly higher than Durham, Baltimore.
***Significantly higher than Durham, New Haven, and Los Angeles.

282

We are not certain why these regional differences were found for young people. St. Louis, with the highest rate, also had the lowest rate of non-response among the sites. Perhaps nonresponders are especially likely to have antisocial personalities, and their loss caused more underestimation outside of St. Louis. However, the lowest rate was in Durham and is likely to be related to its large rural population.

CURRENT LIFE-STYLES
ASSOCIATED WITH ANTISOCIAL PERSONALITY

In discussing risk factors for antisocial personality, we looked at their relation to lifetime prevalence because risk factors can have played a role in past as well as active cases. In examining the relation of antisocial personality to current life-styles, we will be looking at active cases, defined as having met criteria for the disorder plus having had at least one symptom in the year before interview. Overall, 1.2% of the sample could be called active cases, 2.1% of men and 0.4% of women.

Unlike other diagnoses, antisocial personality is diagnosed largely on the basis of what one might consider life-style. It is a disorder of persons with poor job performance, aggressive and illegal behaviors, and poor interpersonal relationships. Thus it is difficult to segregate the consequences of the disorder from its hallmarks.

MARITAL STATUS

Since a history of multiple divorces and separations is one of the criteria for antisocial personality, it is no surprise that the diagnosis is associated with marital status. Among men who are currently divorced or separated, 3.9% have active antisocial personality (that is, diagnosis ever positive and at least one symptom in the current year), and 9.1% have a past diagnosis. The corresponding figures for women are 0.9% and 2.3%. Lowest current rates of disorder are found for those currently married or widowed (1.6% for men and 0.3% for women), with single people falling between (2.8% for men, 0.5% for women).

A history of two or more divorces or separations if married or in a long-lasting cohabitation serves as a criterion symptom for antisocial personality. Because some of the currently married have had two or more divorces, and some of the currently divorced have had only one, marital *history* is more closely associated with antisocial personality than is current marital status. Among males with a history of two or more divorces, 6.1% have a diagnosis of active antisocial personality, as have 1.6% of multiply divorced women, and their lifetime diagnoses are respectively 15.4% and 3.0%.

A single divorce is not a criterion symptom for antisocial personality; yet those divorced only once have higher rates than those married but never divorced or single but never cohabiting. Highest rates of all are found in the never married who have cohabited; for males their rate of active disorder is 7.4% and for females 2.3%, even though cohabitation is not a criterion symptom.

Since open cohabitation has been common among blacks longer than among whites, its acceptability among them might be greater, making it a less striking correlate of antisocial personality for blacks. However, this was not the case for men (Figure 11–5). The rate of active antisocial personality in black men who have cohabited but never married is 7.8%, slightly higher than the rate for cohabiting white men (6.5%), and their lifetime rate is 13.5%, a slightly lower rate than for cohabiting white men (14.5%). On the other hand, multiple divorces and separations were more associated with antisocial personality among white and Hispanic than black men. For white men, the multiply divorced have rates of antisocial personality equal to or higher than the cohabitors (6.5% active and 17.1% lifetime), while for multiply divorced black men, the rate falls well below that for cohabitors (3.1% active and 6.6% lifetime). This suggests that among black men, even impermanent marriages are indicators of conformity, but this is not the case for ethnic groups who have more recently adopted cohabitation as an alternative to marriage.

While cohabitation is strongly associated with antisocial personality for men of all ethnic backgrounds, it is much less so for black than white women. Black women who have cohabited but not married have a lifetime rate of 3.3% versus 7.2% for whites, and an active rate of 1.4% versus 2.6% for whites. This suggests that factors other than the level of antisocial behavior, perhaps income, the antisocial history of their partner, and family traditions, determine the choice of cohabitation over marriage for more black than white women.

SOCIOECONOMIC STATUS

Because many women have not participated in the labor market continuously, many men under 30 have been in it only briefly, and many men over 65 may have left it through retirement, we will restrict the exploration of the relationship between antisocial personality and work history to men 30 through 64.

Chronic unemployment, that is, not working for six months or more in the last five years while not physically ill, is a symptom of antisocial personality, and therefore is inevitably higher in those with the diagnosis than in

MEN

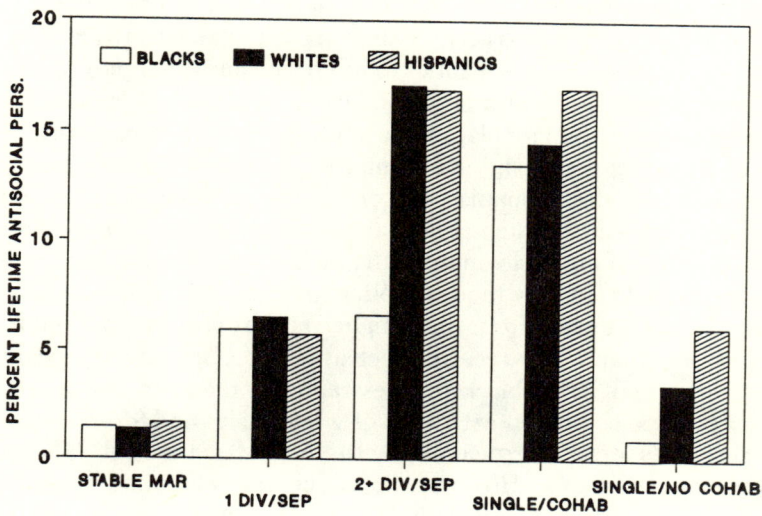

WOMEN

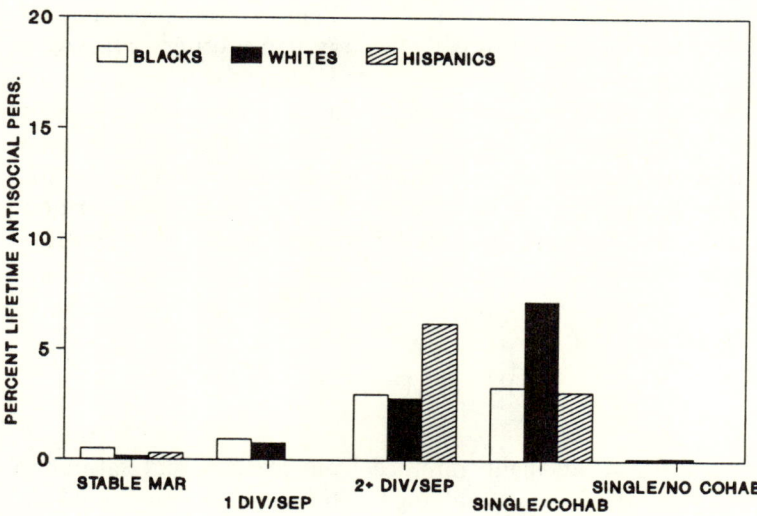

Figure 11-5 Marital History and Antisocial Personality

others. However, most persons with this history do not have the disorder. Of men 30–64 unemployed this much, 5.6% have active antisocial behavior, and 12.4% have met criteria at some time in their lives. Clearly, men do not have to have antisocial personalities to be chronically unemployed.

Underemployment serves as a better indicator of antisocial personality for white and Hispanic than for black men. The chances of having a current diagnosis of antisocial personality if chronically unemployed was 6.1% for white men and 6.8% for Hispanics, but only 2.9% for black men. Being black itself puts men at so much greater risk of long-term unemployment that the association of unemployment with antisocial personality is muted.

Those underemployed may require welfare assistance or disability payments. As we might expect from their higher rate of chronic unemployment, more blacks than whites received such assistance. Seventeen percent of black males and 30% of black females reported receiving welfare or disability payments, compared with 10% of white males and 9% of white females. Hispanics were intermediate, with 14% of males and 24% of females receiving assistance. However, no association was found between men's receiving disability or welfare payments and antisocial personality. This may reflect welfare policies that make it very difficult for an able-bodied man to qualify. For women, who can qualify through having dependent children, on the other hand, there was a striking relationship between welfare assistance and antisocial personality. Black women receiving payments had rates of antisocial personality twice as high as others, while white and Hispanic women receiving payments had rates four times as high as others. However, in all three ethnic groups, only 1% of women on welfare met criteria for current antisocial personality. Clearly welfare funds going to antisocial women form a tiny part of all welfare expenditures.

We explored relationships between antisocial personality and earnings, job level, and current unemployment for men 30 to 64. No significant relationships to antisocial personality were found.

TREATMENT

Persons with antisocial personality rarely seek medical care for treatment of its symptoms. Of all those ever qualifying for the diagnosis, only 14.5% had ever discussed any of its symptoms with a doctor. This failure to seek consultation for the symptoms of antisocial personality is confirmed by the finding that persons in whom antisocial personality was the only active diagnosis had an exceptionally low rate of mental health consultation for any reason; only 4% of them had had a visit related to mental health in the last six months, a rate no different from that of persons with no current diagnosis at all (Table 11–12). If they had a concurrent disorder, the treat-

Table 11–12 Recent Outpatient Mental Health Consultation by Persons with Antisocial Personality

	Percent with Mental Health Care in Last Six Months							
	Antisocial in Last Year				Not Antisocial in Last Year			
	No Other Active Disorder		Other Active Disorder		No Active Disorder		Active Disorder	
	N	%	N	%	N	%	N	%
Total	94	4	201	21	14,266	4	5,426	16
Ethnic group:								
White	42	3	104	20	9,992	5	3,182	17
Black	36	5	51	32	2,964	4	1,709	12
Hispanic	12	—a	40	14	1,117	3	441	10
Age:								
18–29	63	2	121	18	3,434	3	1,287	13
30–44	26	[7]b	64	23	3,398	6	1,211	23
Gender:								
Male	76	7	166	18	6,050	3	2,275	12
Female	18	—a	35	34	8,215	5	3,151	19

a$N < 25$.
b$N = 25$ to 29.

ment rate rose to 21%, a rate as high as that for persons with other psychiatric disorders but no antisocial personality, suggesting that it was the concurrent disorder rather than the antisocial personality that led to treatment. In all age, sex, and ethnic groups, antisocial personality alone did not add to the likelihood of receiving treatment.

Not surprisingly, given this low rate of outpatient mental health contact, persons with active antisocial personality did not differ from the general population in the likelihood of residing in mental hospitals, nursing homes, or chronic hospitals (0.3% did, as did 0.4% of the unaffected). The only forms of institutionalization elevated for persons with antisocial personality were imprisonment and residential treatment in alcohol and drug programs. But only a small proportion of persons with active antisocial personality were currently in these institutions (2.4% versus 0.1% of the unaffected sample.)

COMORBIDITY

Personality disorders were relegated to Axis II in DSM-III to encourage multiple diagnoses. In reporting on disorders which co-occur with antisocial personality, we look only at active cases and drop the exclusion rules in DSM-III, which state that "antisocial behavior is not due to either Severe Mental Retardation, Schizophrenia or Manic Episodes" (p. 321).

As suggested by the placement of antisocial personality on Axis II in DSM-III, it is rare for antisocial personality to be the only disorder present. Less than 10% of cases had no additional diagnoses. These results are similar to clinical samples, including patients in emergency rooms and outpatient clinics (Robins et al., 1977), where antisocial personality was the diagnosis least likely to occur in isolation; it did so in only 11% of the emergency room and 16% of the clinic samples.

It is well known that antisocial personality is associated with drug and alcohol abuse (Hesselbrock et al., 1985, Robins, 1977), and the current study confirms that fact. Men with active antisocial personality are three times as likely to abuse alcohol and five times as likely to abuse drugs as those without antisocial personality. These ratios are even higher for women: 13 times for alcohol and 12 times for drugs (Table 11–13).

Both of the diagnoses which serve as exclusion criteria for antisocial personality in DSM-III were also found to be strongly associated with it.

Table 11–13 Prevalence Ratios for Comorbidity Among Those with Active Antisocial Personality

Other Active Disorders	Prevalence Ratios[a]	
	Males	Females
Mania	10.3	20.9
Schizophrenia	6.9	11.8
Drug abuse	5.3	11.9
Obsessive compulsive	5.3	3.5
Alcohol	3.2	13.1
Depression	3.2	3.5
Dysthymia	2.8	3.2
Panic	2.2	4.5
Phobia	2.1	2.0

Note. Cognitive impairment is the only disorder without an elevated rate in persons with antisocial personality. Somatization disorder was too rare to investigate.

[a]Percent with this diagnosis in persons with antisocial personality divided by percent with this diagnosis in persons without antisocial personality.

With active antisocial personality, the risk for mania was 10 times the expected rate for men and 21 times for women; the risk for schizophrenia was 7 times the expected rate for men and 12 times for women. While we did not find previous reports of the co-occurrence of mania and schizophrenia with antisocial personality, the fact that they were specifically named as excluding diagnoses in DSM-III suggests that their co-occurrence must be a common clinical observation. Further, the strong association with schizophrenia is consistent with the evidence from previous studies that many schizophrenics had a premorbid history of conduct problems (Ricks & Berry, 1973; Robins, 1966). Although the prevalence ratios for these two disorders occurring along with antisocial personality are even higher than for drug abuse and alcoholism, the fact that mania and schizophrenia are both much rarer disorders that drug and alcohol abuse means that there are many more people in the population with both substance abuse and antisocial personality than with mania or schizophrenia and antisocial personality.

Persons with antisocial personality have elevated rates of all other diagnoses as well, except for cognitive impairment, which is virtually limited to the elderly. The traditional view of antisocial personalities (Cleckley, 1955) was that they lacked normal levels of fear and anxiety. However, later studies have found a broad assortment of nonantisocial symptoms accompanying antisocial personality (Robins, 1966; Robins et al., 1977), as does the present study, which finds that even the least associated disorder, phobia, occurs at twice the general population rate in persons with antisocial personality.

CONCLUSION

Antisocial personality typically begins about age eight with a variety of behavior problems at home and in school and is fully expressed by the late twenties or early thirties. Its most characteristic symptoms are job problems, marital difficulties, and violence. Only a minority have difficulties with the law, and only about half of all prison residents meet criteria for the disorder.

The disorder is predominantly male, but the male excess seems to have been reduced somewhat in recent years as rates for both sexes have increased, and women's increase has been somewhat greater. At least one reason for the increase may be the increasing urbanization of the population.

Although DSM-III places antisocial personality on Axis II, with the implication that it is a lifelong disorder, in fact the remission rate is high and goes up rapidly with age. Very few elderly persons have recent symptoms of the disorder.

Persons with the disorder have high rates of chronic unemployment, and women with the disorder have an increased risk of becoming financially dependent; however, they represent only a small proportion of women receiving welfare.

Blacks, whites, and Hispanics have similar rates of antisocial personality. Blacks and whites also share correlates and predictors of the disorder. However, the associations are generally weaker for blacks, because being black itself increases the risk of marital dissolution or failure to marry, unemployment, school dropout, arrest and incarceration, and dependency.

In concert with previous work, this study shows a strong association between antisocial personality and substance abuse. However, powerful associations with schizophrenia and mania were also found. Understanding whether these are truly concurrent disorders or only cases of schizophrenia and mania whose symptoms mimic antisocial personality, as the exclusion rules of DSM-III imply, requires more detailed study of their course than the current report can provide.

Antisocial personality is a serious and often incapacitating disorder that receives little treatment. However, current poor treatment success with this disorder argues against urging efforts at outreach. Nor are there demonstrated means at hand to prevent it. Yet, the high rate of spontaneous recovery from the conduct problems that are the childhood version of the disorder and its high rate of remission in the third and fourth decades of life suggests that it should be possible to discover how to promote earlier remission and in a larger proportion of those affected. Finding ways of treating or preventing antisocial personality is clearly of major concern because it has enormous costs to the family in terms of broken homes and nonsupport, to the state in terms of welfare and imprisonment, to the community in victims of crime and aggression, and to the affected person him or herself in terms of broken relationships, poverty, substance abuse, and other concurrent disorders.

12 Cognitive Impairment

LINDA K. GEORGE / RICHARD LANDERMAN /
DAN G. BLAZER / JAMES C. ANTHONY

ORGANIC MENTAL DISORDERS
AND COGNITIVE IMPAIRMENT

During the past decade, public awareness of and concern about the personal and social costs of dementing illnesses have increased dramatically. Alzheimer's disease, in particular, has been transformed from an unfamiliar syndrome to a major public health concern, as evidenced by increased research funding by government and strong advocacy programs in the private sector. Many dementing illnesses are most prevalent in later life. In light of the aging of the U.S. population, some observers worry about a virtual "epidemic" of dementing illnesses in the future (Kramer, 1980; Plum, 1979).

Dementing illnesses result from dysfunction of the brain. More generally, disorders resulting from aging of the brain, ingestion of substances that cause brain dysfunction, or brain dysfunction resulting from physical diseases are considered organic mental disorders (American Psychiatric Association, 1980). As such, they are a legitimate concern of psychiatric epidemiology and ECA investigators felt it important to consider organic mental disorders in their examination of psychiatric disorders in America. Assessment of organic mental disorders also is important because DSM-III attaches particular significance to them: the presence of organic mental disorder often precludes diagnoses of other psychiatric disorders (for example, schizophrenic and affective disorders) (American Psychiatric Association, 1980).

The topic of this chapter is cognitive impairment, which is the closest approximation to organic mental disorders that was possible in the ECA community and institutional surveys. Severe cognitive impairment is of major public health concern because a significant proportion of persons exhibiting severe cognitive impairment can be presumed to suffer from organic mental disorders (Folstein et al., 1985; Kay et al., 1985).

291

Using DSM-III, mental health professionals distinguish between *organic mental disorders* and *organic brain syndromes*. The latter refer to constellations of psychological and behavioral signs and symptoms observed without reference to their cause or the underlying disease. In contrast, organic mental disorders refer to specific syndromes for which etiology is known or can be reasonably presumed (American Psychiatric Association, 1980, p. 101). Thus, considerably more information is required for making diagnoses of organic mental disorders than for identifying organic brain syndromes. In DSM-III-R, the same logic is used but the term "organic brain syndromes" is replaced by "organic mental syndromes" (American Psychiatric Association, 1987).

DSM-III recognizes 10 organic brain syndromes and 47 organic mental disorders, with the latter classified into 13 categories (American Psychiatric Association, 1980). (See Table 12-1.) The specific DSM-III syndromes and disorders listed in Table 12-1 are not very important for purposes of this chapter; the table makes two relevant points, however. First, one can see that the organic mental disorders are, in fact, nearly identical to the organic brain syndromes, with the exception that cause or etiology of the syndrome is specified. Second, the table nicely documents the heterogeneity or variation among organic mental disorders.

Organic mental disorders share certain clinical features. At the most basic level, organic mental disorders involve impaired cognitive functioning. Common signs of impaired cognitive functioning are memory loss, disorientation to time and place, clouding of consciousness, impaired abstract thinking, and impaired judgment—although an individual with organic mental disorder may not exhibit all of these symptoms. Heterogeneity among and within organic mental disorders is generated by etiological factors which, in turn, affect associated features of the disorder (for example, mood disturbance, paranoid ideation, personality change, loss of impulse control), age at onset, permanence of the condition, and clinical course.

MEASURING COGNITIVE IMPAIRMENT

Although the *criteria* for differential diagnosis of organic mental disorders are reasonably well-specified, the *procedures* adequate for differential diagnosis are much less clear-cut. Precisely because of their cognitive dysfunction, persons suffering from organic mental disorders are poor sources of information about their symptoms and clinical histories. In addition, definitive clinical or laboratory tests do not exist for many of the organic mental disorders. Alzheimer's disease, for example, is a diagnosis of exclusion—that is, a diagnosis of Alzheimer's disease is made only after (1) clinical course has been observed over a substantial period of time, and (2) other,

Table 12-1 Organic Brain Syndromes and Organic Mental Disorders in DSM-III

Organic Brain Syndromes	*Organic Mental Disorders, continued*
Delirium	Opioid organic mental disorders (intoxication, withdrawal)
Dementia	Cocaine organic mental disorders (intoxication)
Amnestic syndrome	
Organic delusional syndrome	Amphetamine or similarly acting organic mental disorders (intoxication, withdrawal, delirium, delusional disorder)
Organic hallucinosis	
Organic affective syndrome	Phencyclidine (PCP) or similarly acting organic mental disorders (delirium, intoxication, mixed disorder)
Organic personality syndrome	
Intoxication	Hallucinogen organic mental disorders (hallucinosis, delusional disorder, affective disorder)
Withdrawal	
Atypical or mixed organic brain syndrome	Cannabis organic mental disorders (intoxication, delusional disorder)
	Tobacco organic mental disorder (withdrawal)
Organic Mental Disorders	Caffeine organic mental disorder (intoxication)
Dementias arising in the senium and presenium (primary degenerative dementia, multi-infarct dementia)	Other or unspecified substance-induced organic mental disorders (intoxication, delirium, hallucinosis, dementia, withdrawal, amnestic disorder, delusional disorder, affective disorder, personality disorder, atypical/mixed disorder)
Alcohol organic mental disorders (intoxication, withdrawal, withdrawal delirium, hallucinosis, amnestic disorder, associated dementia)	
Barbiturate or similarly acting sedative or hypnotic organic mental disorders (intoxication, withdrawal delirium, amnestic disorder)	Organic mental disorders due to physical diseases/conditions or in which the etiology is unknown (delirium, dementia, amnestic syndrome, organic delusional syndrome, organic hallucinosis, organic affective syndrome, organic personality syndrome, atypical or mixed organic brain syndrome)

more easily tested causal factors are ruled out (Henderson & Jorm, 1987; Rocca, Amaducci, & Schoenberg, 1986). Indeed, using presently available techniques the most definitive diagnosis of Alzheimer's disease can be made only at autopsy (Mortimer & Hutton, 1985; Rocca et al., 1986). Thus, it is not surprising that, even in carefully monitored clinic populations, autopsy results have confirmed only about 80% of the clinical diagnoses of Alzheimer's disease made prior to death (Henderson & Jorm, 1987).

Given the complexities involved in making diagnoses of organic mental disorders in clinical settings, identification of these disorders poses major challenges to epidemiologists conducting community studies. In most community studies, it is not feasible to observe clinical course over substantial periods of time and to administer the broad battery of clinical and laboratory tests that assist in differential diagnosis. Such was the case in the ECA program. ECA investigators thus found themselves unable to study specific organic mental disorders—or even specific organic brain syndromes—but nonetheless did not want to totally neglect organic brain dysfunction.

The approach taken in the ECA program—and in several other epidemiologic surveys (for example, Cornoni-Huntley et al., 1985; Kay et al., 1985)—was to include a measure of *current cognitive status*. More specifically, the Mini-Mental State Examination (MMSE) (Folstein et al., 1975) was included in the DIS (Robins et al., 1981b) and was administered to ECA participants.

The Mini-Mental State Examination (MMSE) was developed by Folstein and colleagues (1975) to serve as a short, easily scored test of cognitive status. Specifically, the MMSE measures orientation, memory, attention, ability to name, ability to follow verbal and written instructions, ability to write a sentence spontaneously, and ability to copy a figure. Folstein et al. purposely focused MMSE items on cognitive aspects of mental functioning; the instrument does not measure other abnormal mental experiences, such as forms of thinking, or mood. Moreover, the developers cautioned potential users that the MMSE is simply a measure of current cognitive status and not a diagnostic tool.

Available evidence suggests that the MMSE is psychometrically strong. Reliability data for the MMSE are especially strong. Test-retest reliability of the MMSE over intervals ranging from 24 hours to 28 days varies between .85 and .98 (Anthony et al., 1982; Folstein et al., 1975). Folstein et al. (1975) also report inter-rater reliability of .83.

Folstein et al. suggested that two kinds of data are particularly relevant to the validity of the MMSE as a measure of cognitive status. First, if the MMSE is valid, it should correlate strongly with other tests of mental functioning. Folstein et al. (1975) report that the MMSE correlates strongly with both the verbal and performance scores on the Wechsler Adult Intelligence Scale (WAIS) (correlations of .78 and .66, respectively). Given that the WAIS is a long and detailed test of mental functioning and the MMSE is a very short, 11-item index, the strength of these correlations is impressive evidence of the validity of the MMSE. Second, Folstein et al. (1975) suggested that MMSE scores should vary across groups of patients and nonpatients known to vary in cognitive status (note that this is different from claiming that the MMSE is a diagnostic tool). Strong evidence of such variability is provided by Folstein et al. (1975) for two samples.

The MMSE is one of several short instruments designed to measure cognitive status. Examples of other instruments used to measure cognitive status include the Mental Status Questionnaire (MSQ) (Kahn et al., 1960) and the Short Portable Mental Status Questionnaire (SPMSQ) (Pfeiffer,

1975). Use of the MMSE, rather than other available measures of cognitive status, has several advantages. First, the MMSE includes items that tap a broader range of cognitive abilities than other measures (that is, the MSQ and SPMSQ are restricted to measurement of memory and orientation). Second, the MMSE was developed and tested on age-heterogeneous samples whereas other instruments were designed to measure cognitive status in the elderly. Third, the psychometric properties of the MMSE are at least as good as—and probably somewhat better than—other measures.

Scoring of the MMSE takes place in two stages. First, each MMSE item is scored by the interviewer as correct or incorrect. The number of errors is summed, with a range of 0–30 points. Second, cut-points are used to classify scores into meaningful categories. Both of these scoring procedures are more complicated than they initially appear.

With regard to the scoring of items, the major issue of concern is how to handle nonresponse. Nonresponse refers to refusals to answer specific items on the MMSE ("I don't know" or "I can't" responses are scored as incorrect). The interviewer can never be sure whether respondents refuse to answer one or more items because they cannot answer them correctly or for other reasons. This is an important issue, however, because rates of cognitive impairment will vary, depending upon how nonresponse is scored.

Using data from the Durham ECA site, Fillenbaum et al. (1988a) divided a sample of 1,681 community residents age 60 and older into three groups, based on MMSE performance: (1) those with no or mild cognitive impairment, (2) those with severe cognitive impairment, and (3) those whose cognitive state was ambiguous because of nonresponse on one or more MMSE items. These three groups then were compared with regard to capacity to perform eight activities of daily living (for example, shopping, cleaning house). The results indicated that the group of respondents who were ambiguous with regard to cognitive status closely resembled the severely cognitively impaired with regard to self-care capacity. These authors thus recommend that nonresponse be scored as error.

In the analyses reported in this chapter, the effects of nonresponse were explored in some depth. As described below, we found that whether refusals were counted as errors or not substantially affected the prevalence of severe and mild cognitive impairment but did not alter the relationships between cognitive impairment and other characteristics. Consequently, basic prevalence data are reported using both methods of scoring MMSE items. In subsequent discussions of the correlates and consequences of cognitive status, however, results are based on the method of scoring the MMSE in which nonresponse is *not* counted as error. Though the analyses of Fillenbaum et al. are persuasive, we chose this scoring method because of its increased comparability with other research.

In their original description of the MMSE, Folstein et al. (1975) did not recommend cut-points for classifying categories of cognitive status. Two cut-points now are used with considerable consistency, however. Summing the number of errors, most investigators use the following cut-points: 13 or more errors = severe cognitive impairment; 7–12 errors = mild cognitive impairment; and 6 or fewer errors = no cognitive impairment. Validating the cut-points of the MMSE requires different data than are needed to validate the index as a measure of cognitive status. In the studies available to date, this issue has been examined by comparing MMSE categories to physician diagnosis. Kay et al. (1985) report that, combining mild and severe cognitive impairment, the sensitivity and specificity of the MMSE for dementia are 69% and 89%, respectively. For a combined category of delirium and dementia, Anthony et al. (1982) report that the MMSE has a sensitivity of 87% and a specificity of 82%. And, in a clinical followup of Baltimore ECA respondents, Folstein et al. (1985) report that 67% of the respondents with mild or severe cognitive impairment, as measured by these cut-points on the MMSE, had a diagnosable DSM-III organic mental disorder. Although the evidence concerning the utility of the cut-points for the MMSE is generally encouraging, several investigators question the distinction between mild and no cognitive impairment (Henderson & Jorm, 1987; Kay et al., 1985; Mortimer, Schuman, & French, 1981). In this chapter, three categories of cognitive status are examined, based on the cut-points described above: no impairment, mild impairment, and severe impairment.

One additional issue with regard to use of the MMSE merits brief note. Like all tests of mental, especially cognitive, functioning, it is important that the instrument used minimize cultural, socioeconomic, and educational bias. The degree to which the MMSE is biased has received limited attention in previous research. Available evidence suggests strong relationships between education and MMSE scores and modest relationships between race and MMSE scores (Weissman et al., 1985). In addition, Anthony et al. (1982) report that education and, to a lesser extent, age were significant predictors of "false positive" cognitive impairment scores on the MMSE (as compared to a physician's diagnosis of organic mental disorder). There is precedent for using education-specific and race-specific norms in scoring tests of cognitive status—such norms are used in scoring the SPMSQ, for example (Pfieffer, 1975). Anthony et al. (1982) suggest that such norms would not improve the performance of the MMSE, however.

The meaning of these findings is not clear-cut. Age, race, and education differences in MMSE scores do not necessarily indicate bias in the MMSE. Whether such differences represent measurement error or risk factors for cognitive impairment is a matter of interpretation. (For an excellent example of this debate, see Kittner et al., 1986, and related commentary by Berkman, 1986.) One could argue, for example, that failure in school (or failure to be schooled) is a risk factor for cognitive impairment in the modern U.S. Thus, using the MMSE as a measure of cognitive status, education-related errors need not represent bias. When the MMSE is used as an indicator of or screening tool for dementia, however, a somewhat different logic applies. In this context, education-related errors are problematic because they may be a source of false positives.

In this chapter, special attention is paid to the aassociations of age, race, and education with cognitive status, as measured by the MMSE. We will be particularly interested in the degree to which education accounts for age and race/ethnicity differences in MMSE performance.

Measuring cognitive impairment was as close as ECA investigators could come to estimating the prevalence of organic mental disorders and/or organic brain syndromes. Nonetheless, it should be noted that severe cognitive impairment can reflect a number of etiologies other than organic mental disorder. Consequently, the estimates of severe cognitive impairment reported in this chapter are higher than rates of specific organic mental disorders. It also should be recognized that the MMSE measures *current* cognitive status. Consequently, several distinctions usefully made in other chapters—including lifetime versus current disorder, age of onset, and rates of remission—cannot be examined in the context of cognitive impairment.

SAMPLING ISSUES

The fact that the ECA sample includes both community and institutional residents is particularly important for cognitive impairment. Although methods of measuring cognitive impairment vary widely across studies, previous research suggests that between 40% and 80% of all nursing home residents suffer from discernible cognitive impairment (for example, Butler and Lewis, 1977; Gottesman, 1977). Similarly, data from the National Nursing Home Survey suggest that at least half of all nursing home residents suffer from severe cognitive impairment (National Center for Health Statistics, 1979). Because the institutional population is so small in relation to the community population, the prevalences of most disorders examined in this volume are minimally affected by inclusion of the institutional sample. That is less true for cognitive impairment, however, because the proportion of institutional residents affected is so large.

It is important that the total burden of psychiatric disorder on the American population be examined. Given the high rates of cognitive impairment among institutionalized Americans, it is especially important that the ECA data include both institutional and community residents. It also should be noted, however, that this factor will make the findings in this chapter difficult to compare with results in previous studies because most previous studies are based only on community residents or only on institutional residents.

Previous research consistently documents that cognitive impairment, especially cognitive impairment so severe as to threaten personal independence, is concentrated among the very old (for example, Kay et al., 1985; Mortimer et al., 1981; Mortimer & Hutton, 1985; Weissman et al., 1985). This pattern also is characteristic of the ECA data. Consequently, most analyses reported in this chapter are restricted to ECA respondents age 55 and older. Because the prevalence of cognitive impairment is very low among persons younger than 55, it was not possible to generate stable estimates of prevalence and, especially, correlates of cognitive impairment for younger age groups.

It also is likely that severe cognitive impairment reflects very different etiologies for younger and older adults. More specifically, severe cognitive dysfunction is generally due to delirium, mental retardation, intoxication resulting from substance use, and head injury among young and middle-aged adults. Among older adults, the disease processes underlying the dementias are the primary causes of severe cognitive impairment and/or organic mental disorders. Because of age differences in etiology, demographic correlates and social consequences of cognitive impairment may vary by age—in which case, analyses based on the entire age range might blur or mask relationships of interest. In the interest of completeness, basic prevalence data are presented both for the entire ECA sample and for the subset of respondents aged 55 and older. More detailed analyses of the correlates and consequences of cognitive impairment, however, are restricted to the population aged 55 and older.

PREVALENCE AND DEMOGRAPHIC CORRELATES

In this section, major findings concerning the prevalence and demographic correlates of cognitive impairment are presented. Demographic factors examined include age, sex, race/ethnicity, education, geographic region, urban versus rural residence, and marital status. It is tempting to view these demographic factors as risk factors for cognitive impairment—that is, as factors implicated in the etiology of cognitive deficit. And, indeed, some demographic factors undoubtedly are etiologically relevant. For example, age is clearly a risk factor for dementia. Nonetheless, the ECA research design does not permit strong inferences about the etiological relevance of most demographic factors for cognitive impairment—primarily because information is unavailable about age of onset. Consequently, it is difficult to distinguish between risk factors for and consequences of cognitive impairment.

A conservative stance will be taken in this chapter; we will generally use the language of demographic correlates of cognitive impairment rather than that of demographic risk factors for cognitive impairment. To the extent possible, however, we will comment on the likelihood that the relationships examined are of potential etiologic significance. In addition, it should be noted that the relationships between demographic factors and cognitive impairment are important even in the absence of evidence of etiology. From a public health perspective, demographic correlates are important for identifying population subgroups at risk for cognitive impairment and for targeting services to those subgroups. (For a more detailed discussion of the distinction between etiologic and public health significance of disease correlates, see Kleinbaum et al., 1982.)

An initial concern is the prevalence of both mild and severe cognitive impairment in the United States. Table 12-2 provides total prevalence estimates for the U.S. adult population and for American adults aged 55 and older. Two features of the table merit brief comment. First, separate prevalences are presented for mild and severe cognitive impairment. Remember that these are current prevalences. Second, prevalence figures are presented for both scoring options of the MMSE (that is, counting only errors versus counting both errors and refusals as incorrect responses).

Depending on scoring method, the estimated prevalence of severe cognitive impairment for all American adults is .85% or 1.31%. Comparable figures for mild cognitive impairment are 4.16% and 5.74%. As expected, combining refusals with errors yields higher prevalences—54% higher for severe cognitive impairment and 38% higher for mild cognitive impairment. Obviously, choice of scoring method has important implications for conclusions about prevalence. Nonetheless, regardless of scoring method, severe cognitive impairment is relatively rare in the U.S. population, whereas mild cognitive impairment is relatively common.

For American adults aged 55 and over, the estimated prevalence of severe cognitive impairment is 2.26% or 3.30%, depending on the scoring

Table 12-2 Prevalence of Severe and Mild Cognitive Impairment in U.S. Adults Aged 18 or Older and 55 or Older

| Age Group | N | Severe Cognitive Impairment | | | | Mild Cognitive Impairment | | | |
| | | Errors Only | | Errors and Refusals | | Errors Only | | Errors and Refusals | |
		%	(SE)	%	(SE)	%	(SE)	%	(SE)
Total 18+	19,597	0.85	(0.09)	1.31	(0.12)	4.16	(0.21)	5.74	(0.24)
Total 55+	8,396	2.26	(0.25)	3.30	(0.29)	9.58	(0.49)	11.71	(0.53)

method used. Comparable figures for mild cognitive impairment are 9.58% and 11.71%. Again, the scoring method used has implications for prevalence estimates. Moreover, the prevalence of cognitive impairment is considerably higher among persons aged 55 and older than among all adults.

As noted earlier, cognitive impairment is expected to be considerably more prevalent among institutional residents than among adults dwelling in the community. As Table 12–3 indicates, this is indeed the case. (Note that this table is restricted to ECA respondents aged 55 and older.) Regardless of scoring method, severe cognitive impairment is much more prevalent among institutional residents (32.6% versus 2.3% and 43.1% versus 3.3%). The same pattern is found for mild cognitive impairment (28.3% versus 9.6% and 33.6% versus 11.7%). There also are substantial differences in its prevalence among types of institutions. No severe or mild cognitive impairment was found among prisoners, but the very small number of elderly prisoners makes this observation unstable. Both severe and mild cognitive impairment are most common among nursing home residents, where severe impairment affects one-third to almost one-half (depending on the scoring system) of those well enough to be tested. In addition, many of the persons not included in this report because they were

Table 12–3 Prevalence of Cognitive Impairment by Household and Institutional Residence, in Persons Age 55 or Older

| | Severe Cognitive Impairment | | | | Mild Cognitive Impairment | | | |
| | Errors Only | | Errors and Refusals | | Errors Only | | Errors and Refusals | |
Resident Status	%	(SE)	%	(SE)	%	(SE)	%	(SE)
Total population (100%)	2.3	(0.3)	3.3	(0.3)	9.6	(0.5)	11.7	(0.5)
Household population (98.4%)	1.9	(0.2)	2.8	(0.3)	9.2	(0.5)	11.4	(0.5)
Institutional population (1.6%)	32.6	(6.2)	43.1	(6.6)	28.3	(6.3)	33.6	(6.0)
Mental hospitals (0.02%)	13.0	a	25.3	a	26.9	a	38.1	a
Nursing homes (1.57%)	33.3	(6.4)	43.8	(6.7)	28.5	(6.4)	33.8	(6.1)
Prisons (0.01%)	b	a	b	a	b	a	b	a

aBecause of small cell size, standard error cannot be estimated.
bBecause of small cell size, prevalence cannot be reliably estimated.

not personally interviewable, not even to the extent of being able to respond to the MMSE, were found in nursing homes.

AGE, SEX, RACE/ETHNICITY, AND EDUCATION

Age, sex, race/ethnicity, and education are important indicators of social location—of one's place in American society. It is important to determine whether cognitive impairment is related to these basic demographic factors. Table 12-4 provides the estimated prevalence of severe and mild cognitive impairment by age, sex, race/ethnicity, and education for the U.S. adult population. Again, prevalence figures are presented for both scoring options of the MMSE. Another feature of this table also merits attention. Note that the total sample size always is smaller for mild than for severe cognitive impairment. This is because we examined cognitive impairment in a hierarchical fashion: comparing severe cognitive impairment to the combination of mild impairment plus no impairment, but comparing mild cognitive impairment only to no impairment. Thus, the denominators for all analyses of mild cognitive impairment exclude respondents with severe cognitive impairment. This approach is necessary for meaningful tests of statistical significance and is used in all subsequent tables.

Regardless of severity or scoring method, the prevalence of cognitive impairment is strongly related to age. Two age thresholds are associated with dramatic increases in prevalence: age 55 and age 75. Depending on the scoring method used, the prevalence of severe cognitive impairment is 1.4 to 2.5 times greater among persons aged 55–74 than among those 35–54. Severe cognitive impairment is even more common among persons aged 75 and older. Compared to persons aged 35–54, the prevalence of severe impairment is 9.5 to 16 times higher among those aged 75 and older, depending on the scoring method used. Mild cognitive impairment exhibits the same pattern. Age differences are very large and highly statistically significant.

There are no meaningful sex differences in the prevalence of mild or severe cognitive impairment. As expected on the basis of previous research, there are significant race/ethnicity differences in both severe and mild cognitive impairment. For severe impairment, regardless of the scoring method used, blacks have substantially higher prevalence than either Hispanics or whites. (The small group of persons who are neither white, black, nor Hispanic have been combined with whites. For reasons of convenience, this combined group will be referred to simply as white.) The pattern for mild cognitive impairment is different: regardless of scoring method, whites have much lower prevalence than either blacks or Hispanics, with the latter two groups exhibiting similar prevalences.

Education also is strongly related to cognitive impairment (Table 12-4).

Table 12–4 Prevalence of Cognitive Impairment by Age, Race/Ethnicity, and Education

		Severe Cognitive Impairment				Mild Cognitive Impairment in Those without Severe Impairment					
		Errors Only		Errors and Refusals			Errors Only			Errors and Refusals	
	N^a	%	(SE)	%	(SE)	N	%	(SE)	N	%	(SE)
Total	19,354	0.69	(0.09)	1.11	(0.11)	18,990	4.12	(0.21)	18,780	5.76	(0.24)
Age:											
18–34	6,863	0.24	(0.08)	0.32	(0.09)	6,842	1.13	(0.17)	6,828	2.31	(0.24)
35–54	4,283	0.29	(0.10)	0.69	(0.16)	4,249	3.12	(0.33)	4,217	4.80	(0.41)
55–74	5,911	1.01	(0.22)	1.63	(0.28)	5,783	7.54	(0.58)	5,711	9.72	(0.65)
75 and older	2,297	4.95	(0.96)	7.30	(1.15)	2,116	19.09	(1.79)	2,024	22.15	(1.91)
Sex:											
Male	8,258	0.68	(0.12)	1.09	(0.16)	8,104	3.90	(0.29)	8,015	5.56	(0.35)
Female	11,096	0.70	(0.12)	1.13	(0.15)	10,886	4.33	(0.29)	10,765	5.94	(0.34)
Race/Ethnicity:											
Black	4,682	2.04	(0.45)	2.99	(0.55)	4,530	9.62	(0.96)	4,443	12.32	(1.07)
Hispanic	1,598	0.60	(0.34)	1.31	(0.51)	1,582	7.94	(1.21)	1,565	14.43	(1.58)
White/Other	13,074	0.52	(0.08)	0.86	(0.10)	12,878	3.21	(0.20)	12,772	4.41	(0.23)
Education:											
< 9 years	4,692	3.57	(0.49)	5.09	(0.58)	4,400	19.24	(1.07)	4,268	24.12	(1.17)
9–11 years	4,171	0.58	(0.18)	1.02	(0.24)	4,125	3.87	(0.47)	4,088	5.52	(0.56)
12 years	4,627	0.07	(0.05)	0.25	(0.10)	4,613	1.62	(0.25)	4,586	2.69	(0.32)
> 12 + years	5,864	0.04	(0.04)	0.20	(0.08)	5,852	0.26	(0.09)	5,838	1.16	(0.18)

[a] Ns reflect some missing data for demographic variables.

For both mild and severe impairment and for both scoring methods, cognitive impairment is concentrated among persons with eight or fewer years of education. Indeed, depending on the scoring method used, severe cognitive impairment is approximately 5 times more common among persons with 8 or fewer years of school than among those with 9–11 years. The same pattern is true of mild cognitive impairment. These education differences are highly significant.

Table 12–4 presented information about the prevalence of cognitive impairment in the entire U.S. adult population. Table 12–5 presents comparable information about the U.S. population age 55 and older. As noted previously, cognitive impairment is likely to reflect different etiologies in younger versus older persons and the prevalence of cognitive impairment is strongly related to age. Therefore, it is important to focus attention on the prevalence and correlates of cognitive impairment among older adults.

Although the age range in Table 12–5 is much narrower than that in Table 12–4, large and statistically significant age differences are still observed. For severe cognitive impairment, regardless of the scoring method used, respondents in each successive age group exhibit much higher prevalences. The same pattern is true for mild cognitive impairment. More than 3% of persons 75–84 and 10% of those 85 and older suffer from severe cognitive impairment. At least 17% of those aged 75–84 and a quarter of those aged 85 and older suffer from mild cognitive impairment. Because of the large age differences observed, age will be retained as a control variable in all subsequent analyses.

As was the case for the entire adult population, there are no meaningful sex differences in the prevalence of either mild or severe cognitive impairment among persons aged 55 and older. Race/ethnicity differences observed among persons aged 55 and older are similar to those observed for all American adults. For severe cognitive impairment, regardless of the scoring method used, blacks have a higher prevalence than either whites or Hispanics. For mild cognitive impairment, the prevalences for older persons vary even more widely than for the total sample, with blacks ranking highest, whites ranking lowest, and Hispanics in an intermediate position. The difference between Hispanics and whites is not significant for severe cognitive impairment but is statistically significant for mild impairment.

Education differences in the prevalence of cognitive impairment for persons aged 55 and older also are similar to those observed for the entire U.S. adult population. Both severe and mild cognitive impairment are concentrated among persons with eight or fewer years of education. This pattern is especially strong for severe impairment, although the education differences are highly significant for both mild and severe cognitive impairment. Because of this, education is used as a control variable in all subsequent analyses.

Because of methodological differences across studies, these prevalence

Table 12-5 Prevalence of Cognitive Impairment by Age, Race/Ethnicity, and Education Among Those Aged 55 and Older

| | | Severe Cognitive Impairment | | | | Mild Cognitive Impairment in Those without Severe Impairment | | | | |
| | | Errors Only | | Errors and Refusals | | | Errors Only | | | Errors and Refusals | |
	N[a]	%	(SE)	%	(SE)	N	%	(SE)	N	%	(SE)
Total	8,208	1.77	(0.22)	2.73	(0.27)	7,899	9.70	(0.49)	7,735	12.01	(0.55)
Age:											
55–64	2,381	0.81	(0.22)	1.32	(0.28)	2,337	4.98	(0.53)	2,316	7.23	(0.63)
65–74	3,530	1.29	(0.32)	2.06	(0.41)	3,446	11.16	(0.91)	3,395	13.28	(0.98)
75–84	1,832	3.83	(0.80)	5.84	(0.97)	1,710	17.82	(1.62)	1,641	20.43	(1.73)
85 and older	465	10.14	(2.70)	14.07	(3.11)	406	25.45	(4.11)	383	30.88	(4.46)
Sex:											
Male	3,118	1.76	(0.33)	2.60	(0.40)	2,991	9.06	(0.73)	2,926	11.93	(0.83)
Female	5,090	1.77	(0.29)	2.83	(0.37)	4,908	10.19	(0.67)	4,809	12.08	(0.73)
Race/Ethnicity:											
Black	1,479	5.71	(1.34)	8.50	(1.60)	1,358	27.73	(2.65)	1,290	33.32	(2.84)
Hispanic	309	2.18	(1.40)	3.35	(1.72)	299	12.91	(3.24)	291	25.67	(4.24)
White/Other	6,420	1.39	(0.21)	2.17	(0.26)	6,242	7.98	(0.48)	6,154	9.69	(0.53)
Education:											
< 9 years	3,545	4.33	(0.57)	6.14	(0.67)	3,285	21.95	(1.19)	3,172	26.32	(1.27)
9–11 years	1,642	0.74	(0.32)	1.29	(0.42)	1,613	6.08	(0.88)	1,591	8.04	(1.01)
12 years	1,508	0.20	(0.16)	0.79	(0.31)	1,499	3.16	(0.61)	1,478	4.53	(0.73)
> 12 years	1,513	0.26	(0.18)	0.62	(0.28)	1,502	1.12	(0.37)	1,494	1.93	(0.48)

[a] Ns reflect some missing data for the demographic variables.

estimates are not entirely comparable to the results of previous research. Relevant methodological differences that are frequently observed across studies include differences in sampling designs, differences in the age ranges of study participants, and differences in the measurement of cognitive impairment. Despite these differences, the prevalences of both severe and mild cognitive impairment reported here are similar to those reported in previous studies. Particularly relevant is Mortimer et al.'s (1981) review of eight studies in which the prevalence of severe cognitive impairment ranged from 1.3% to 6.2% of persons aged 65 and older. The range for mild cognitive impairment was from 2.6% to 15.4%. Though our data in Table 12–5 are based on persons aged 55 and older, all four of our prevalence estimates fall within the ranges reported by Mortimer et al.

A detailed view was appropriate for the basic prevalence data (Tables 12–4 and 12–5). In subsequent tables, however, the scope of information provided will be simplified in two ways. First, all subsequent tables are restricted to persons aged 55 and older for reasons previously discussed. Second, in all subsequent tables, cognitive impairment is based on the "errors only" scoring method for the MMSE. Although prevalences are consistently higher when refusals are added to errors, relationships with demographic and other variables are not significantly affected by the scoring method used.

We have seen that there are significant age, race/ethnicity, and education differences in the prevalence of both severe and mild cognitive impairment. It is possible that age-related or race/ethnicity-related differences in educational attainment explain or account for age and race/ethnicity prevalence differences. Tables 12–6 and 12–7 provide information pertinent to this issue.

For both severe and mild cognitive impairment, age differences remain within each category of educational attainment (Table 12–6). That is, regardless of level of education, persons aged 75 and older are significantly more likely to exhibit severe and mild cognitive impairment than are younger persons. Education continues to have a significant role in the prevalence of cognitive impairment, however. Thus, these results suggest that both age and education are significant correlates of cognitive impairment.

The same pattern is true for race/ethnicity (Table 12–7). Blacks have higher rates of both severe and mild cognitive impairment than whites and Hispanics within each level of educational attainment. This difference also remains statistically significant within each level of education. Thus, both race/ethnicity and education are significant correlates of cognitive impairment.

In general, these results suggest that education accounts partially, but not totally, for observed age and race/ethnicity differences in cognitive impairment. These results should not be interpreted too literally, however. There may be qualitative differences in the educational experiences of

Table 12-6 Prevalence of Cognitive Impairment (Errors Only) by Education and Age, Among Those Aged 55 and Older

Education and Age	Severe Cognitive Impairment			Mild Cognitive Impairment in Those without Severe Impairment		
	N	%	(SE)[a]	N	%	(SE)[a]
< 9 years:						
Age 55–64	726	2.89	(0.83)	689	15.90	(1.84)
Age 65–74	1,531	2.50	(0.70)	1,467	21.74	(1.88)
Age 75–84	1,046	6.28	(1.37)	938	27.67	(2.61)
Age 85 and older	264	15.70	(4.25)	213	33.26	(5.99)
9–11 years:						
Age 55–64	565	0.48	(0.36)	560	4.19	(1.05)
Age 65–74	737	0.74	(0.54)	725	7.21	(1.64)
Age 75–84	270	1.58	(1.25)	261	9.54	(2.96)
Age 85 and older	80	1.13	(2.20)	77	14.00	(7.27)
12 years:						
Age 55–64	590	0.10	(0.14)	588	0.96	(0.44)
Age 65–74	637	0.06	(0.15)	634	4.07	(1.28)
Age 75–84	234	0.73	(0.94)	232	10.04	(3.33)
Age 85 and older	56	3.61	(5.27)	54	26.85	(12.75)
> 12 years:						
Age 55–64	521	0.00	(—)	521	0.66	(0.37)
Age 65–74	636	0.56	(0.49)	631	1.42	(0.77)
Age 75–84	300	0.41	(0.67)	297	1.14	(1.11)
Age 85 and older	68	2.72	(4.06)	65	10.08	(7.63)

[a]Standard error not calculated when prevalence is zero.

ethnic groups and groups of different ages that are not captured by a measure of "years of education." For example, a high school degree earned in 1935 may not be equivalent to a high school degree earned in 1980. Similarly, many black respondents aged 55 and older (especially those in the southern U.S.) attended segregated schools in which educational resources are known to have been limited. Moreover, persons in the lowest educational level range from those with no education at all through those completing eighth grade. Undoubtedly blacks and the very old are the groups most likely to be found at the lower end of that broad educational range.

Although caution must be applied to these findings, there also are reasons to give credence to these results—that is, to believe that education will only partially account for age and race/ethnicity differences in the prevalence of cognitive impairment. As noted previously, dementing illnesses, which characteristically develop in later life, are one major reason that older

Table 12-7 Prevalence of Cognitive Impairment (Errors Only) by Education and Race/Ethnicity, Among Those Aged 55 and Older

Education and Ethnicity	Severe Cognitive Impairment			Mild Cognitive Impairment in Those without Severe Impairment		
	N	%	(SE)[a]	N	%	(SE)[a]
< 9 years:						
Black	945	9.04	(2.15)	834	40.00	(3.85)
Hispanic	185	3.57	(2.30)	176	19.99	(5.05)
White/Other	2,415	3.57	(0.58)	2,275	19.14	(1.25)
9-11 years:						
Black	266	0.92	(1.22)	258	16.55	(4.78)
Hispanic	59	0.00	—	59	5.84	(5.01)
White/Other	1,317	0.75	(0.34)	1,296	5.11	(0.86)
12 years:						
Black	145	1.20	(1.80)	144	8.78	(4.71)
Hispanic	39	0.48	(1.85)	38	0.00	—
White/Other	1,324	0.15	(0.14)	1,317	2.96	(0.61)
> 12 years:						
Black	123	0.62	(1.52)	122	4.21	(3.91)
Hispanic	26	[0.00]	—	26	[0.00]	—
White/Other	1,364	0.25	(0.18)	1,354	1.03	(0.36)

Note. [ ] signifies small cell size of 25–29.
[a]Standard error not calculated when prevalence is zero.

adults exhibit elevated prevalence of cognitive impairment. Thus, one would expect robust age differences in the prevalence of cognitive impairment. Similarly, the higher rates of cognitive impairment observed among older blacks may in part reflect higher rates of multi-infarct dementia—a dementing illness for which hypertension, which is known to be most prevalent among blacks, may be a risk factor.

In an effort to better understand MMSE performance, we also explored the possibilities of education, race/ethnicity, and age differences on individual items of the MMSE. Those results indicated that the same items were easy and hard for all respondents, regardless of age, race, or educational attainment. For example, orientation to place was the easiest MMSE item and the subtraction and spelling tasks were the most difficult for all demographic subgroups. Moreover, for every item on the MMSE, the largest proportion of errors were made by the oldest respondents, blacks, and those with the lowest levels of education. Similar results were reported by Jorm et al. (1988). Thus, item analysis provides no evidence that specific items account for the observed age, race, and education differences in overall MMSE performance.

GEOGRAPHIC REGION

For severe cognitive impairment, prevalence estimates for the total samples aged 55 and older range from 1.87% for Los Angeles to 3.71% for Durham (Table 12–8a). Thus, there are substantial differences across sites, with

Table 12–8a Prevalence of Cognitive Impairment (Errors Only) by Age and Site, Among Those Aged 55 and Older (Weighted to Local Population Distribution)

Site and Age	Severe Cognitive Impairment			Mild Cognitive Impairment in Those without Severe Impairment		
	N	%	(SE)	N	%	(SE)
New Haven:						
All ages	2,936	2.03	(0.39)	2,860	7.38	(0.74)
55–64	436	1.18	(0.43)	429	2.65	(0.64)
65–74	1,574	0.85	(0.46)	1,561	7.84	(1.34)
75–84	749	4.14	(1.42)	718	17.08	(2.74)
85 and older	177	15.27	(5.35)	152	31.63	(7.52)
Baltimore:						
All ages	1,489	2.73	(0.50)	1,393	10.52	(0.95)
55–64	496	1.08	(0.46)	486	5.19	(0.99)
65–74	599	2.25	(0.77)	575	13.72	(1.80)
75–84	303	6.77	(1.99)	262	18.46	(3.17)
85 and older	91	14.40	(6.19)	70	23.21	(8.05)
St. Louis:						
All ages	1,186	2.91	(0.71)	1,061	13.10	(1.45)
55–64	435	0.49	(0.44)	424	8.98	(1.80)
65–74	360	2.50	(1.16)	334	13.85	(2.60)
75–84	278	6.53	(2.49)	229	20.20	(4.18)
85 and older	113	16.25	(7.48)	74	25.00	(9.60)
Durham:						
All ages	2,016	3.71	(0.55)	1,911	18.78	(1.15)
55–64	716	2.24	(0.62)	692	12.34	(1.40)
65–74	777	4.00	(0.98)	741	22.06	(2.11)
75–84	416	6.68	(1.85)	381	28.56	(3.46)
85 and older	107	7.78	(4.15)	97	34.57	(7.68)
Los Angeles:						
All ages	850	1.87	(0.55)	817	7.07	(1.05)
55–64	355	0.41	(0.36)	352	2.96	(0.97)
65–74	270	1.76	(0.95)	265	9.45	(2.15)
75–84	182	5.14	(2.26)	166	15.51	(3.80)
85 and older	43	13.04	(8.95)	34	11.10	(8.95)

Durham exhibiting a prevalence that is almost twice as high as that in Los Angeles. The site differences are statistically significant. Age is significantly related to severe cognitive impairment in all five sites. Interestingly, however, the differences across age groups are much smaller for Durham than for the other four sites. There is even greater variation in the prevalence of mild than severe cognitive impairment across the five sites. Los Angeles and New Haven have the lowest prevalences (7.07% and 7.38%, respectively). Durham is again highest with an overall prevalence of 18.78%. Again, the site differences are statistically significant. For all five sites, age is strongly associated with the prevalence of mild cognitive impairment (Table 12–8a).

Education is significantly and negatively associated with both severe and mild cognitive impairment in all five ECA sites, with the major threshold being eight or fewer versus nine or more years of schooling (Table 12–8b). Moreover, the site differences in the prevalence of cognitive impairment are not explained by age or education differences in sample composition across the five sites.

These results suggest that the prevalence of cognitive impairment may be related to geographic region. Caution must be used in making that conclusion, however, because the ECA sites, though geographically dispersed, do not represent geographic regions (for example, Durham does not adequately represent the entire southeastern U.S.). If there are, in fact, reliable differences in the prevalence of cognitive impairment across geographic regions, it is difficult to identify the causes of those differences. These results suggest that regional differences are not explained by age or level of education. Geographic differences may, in part, reflect racial or ethnic composition (for example, Durham has the largest proportion of blacks and the highest prevalence of cognitive impairment). Geographic differences also may, in part, be due to differences in urbanization or the quality of educational facilities. It is unlikely that geographic differences in the prevalence of cognitive impairment reflect comparable differences in the distribution of organic brain syndromes—previous studies do not suggest regional differences in the prevalence of dementia (Mortimer et al., 1981; Mortimer & Hutton, 1985). Thus, the factors underlying geographic differences in the prevalence of cognitive impairment are more likely to be cultural or social factors affecting cognitive status than etiologic factors related to dementia.

URBAN-RURAL RESIDENCE

Two ECA sites included both urban and rural residents: Durham and St. Louis. Rural residents from the Durham ECA area lived in four predominantly rural counties; most residents of those counties were farmers or in

Table 12–8b Prevalence of Cognitive Impairment (Errors Only)
by Education and Site, Among Those Aged 55 and Older
(Weighted to Local Population Distribution)

Site and Age	Severe Cognitive Impairment			Mild Cognitive Impairment in Those without Severe Impairment		
	N	%	(SE)[a]	N	%	(SE)[a]
New Haven:						
< 9 years	1,048	6.34	(1.31)	988	18.62	(2.16)
9–11 years	577	0.56	(0.47)	572	5.96	(1.51)
12 years	589	0.38	(0.35)	585	3.72	(1.08)
> 12 years	715	0.27	(0.27)	711	1.52	(0.63)
Baltimore:						
< 9 years	775	4.61	(0.92)	702	17.97	(1.72)
9–11 years	354	1.50	(0.73)	346	5.06	(1.33)
12 years	218	0.07	(0.20)	216	2.21	(1.08)
> 12 years	118	0.72	(0.88)	117	1.62	(1.31)
St. Louis:						
< 9 years	524	2.07	(0.94)	499	28.20	(2.90)
9–11 years	217	0.26	(0.48)	214	7.83	(2.53)
12 years	161	0.00	—	161	1.79	(1.30)
> 12 years	141	0.00	—	141	1.18	(1.14)
Durham:						
< 9 years	944	7.67	(1.18)	855	37.42	(2.24)
9–11 years	348	1.15	(0.76)	340	9.20	(2.06)
12 years	364	0.57	(0.47)	362	6.73	(1.56)
> 12 years	351	0.64	(0.53)	346	1.57	(0.84)
Los Angeles:						
< 9 years	276	3.32	(1.35)	263	17.93	(2.95)
9–11 years	156	0.30	(0.53)	151	7.57	(2.56)
12 years	185	0.08	(0.23)	184	1.84	(1.10)
> 12 years	200	0.07	(0.21)	199	0.18	(0.34)

[a]Standard error not calculated when prevalence is zero.

local retail or service trades. Rural residents from the St. Louis sample lived outside of St. Louis proper, but were less likely to be farmers and more likely to commute to the urban area for employment oppotunities. In addition, rural residents from the Durham area were about equally split between blacks and whites; all rural residents in the St. Louis sample were white. Because of these differences, Durham and St. Louis are examined separately.

Table 12–9 presents the prevalence of severe and mild cognitive impairment for urban and rural household residents aged 55 and older in the Durham and St. Louis samples. In Durham, urban–rural residence was not

Table 12-9 Prevalence of Cognitive Impairment (Errors Only) by Urban Versus Rural Household Residence, in Durham and St. Louis, Controlling on Age and Education, Aged 55 and Older (Weighted to Local Population)

| | | Percent with Cognitive Impairment in | | | | | | | |
| | | Durham | | | | | | St. Louis[c] | |
		N	Severe %	(SE)[d]	N	Mild[b] %[a]	(SE)	N	Mild %[a]	(SE)
Urban household residents		827	3.44	(0.75)	795	14.07	(1.46)	847	13.51	(1.60)
Rural household residents		1,033	3.40	(0.75)	994	22.83	(1.78)	69	4.69	(2.58)
Education										
< 9 years:	Urban	333	8.04	(1.90)	306	34.45	(3.46)	395	28.09	(3.31)
	Rural	572	6.56	(1.45)	485	38.94	(2.96)	38	6.78	(4.17)
9–11 years:	Urban	145	1.42	(1.19)	143	8.13	(2.77)	189	7.81	(2.62)
	Rural	181	0.52	(0.73)	179	9.68	(3.00)	8	—	—
12 years:	Urban	161	1.01	(0.84)	160	4.28	(1.71)	137	1.10	(1.10)
	Rural	188	0.00	—	188	9.15	(2.69)	14	—	—
> 12 years:	Urban	188	0.70	(0.69)	186	0.96	(0.81)	126	1.24	(1.23)
	Rural	142	0.00	—	142	2.00	(1.64)	9	—	—
Age										
55–64:	Urban	320	1.90	(0.80)	314	6.47	(1.46)	368	9.36	(1.95)
	Rural	363	2.35	(0.93)	352	8.63	(2.41)	24	—	—
65–74:	Urban	349	4.26	(1.40)	334	19.24	(2.79)	273	15.51	(2.96)
	Rural	393	3.28	(1.29)	381	24.51	(3.17)	23	—	—
75–84:	Urban	127	6.61	(2.86)	118	24.61	(5.13)	170	20.72	(4.73)
	Rural	231	5.63	(2.32)	217	30.00	(4.74)	16	—	—
85 and older:	Urban	31	5.55	(5.60)	29	[38.12]	(12.22)	36	20.22	(10.65)
	Rural	46	7.19	(5.66)	44	28.64	(10.29)	6	—	—

[a] [ ] signifies cell size of 25–29, and thus an unstable rate. — signifies cell size less than 25, and so no prevalence calculated.
[b] Based on those without severe impairment.
[c] Because no cases of severe cognitive impairment were found in rural St. Louis households, only mild disorder is shown.
[d] Standard error not calculated when prevalence is zero.

significantly related to either severe or mild cognitive impairment in the total household sample; that pattern also held true for the four levels of educational attainment and the four age categories.

Because none of the rural household residents in the St. Louis sample was categorized as severely cognitively impaired, no column for severe cognitive impairment appears for St. Louis in Table 12-9. The prevalence of severe cognitive impairment among urban household residents in St. Louis was 1.03%, suggesting that severe impairment is more characteristic of urban than rural residents in the St. Louis sample. The higher rate in the St. Louis urban population appears confirmed for mild cognitive impairment; the prevalence was significantly lower among rural than urban residents (4.69% versus 13.51%). This pattern holds true for the one level of educational attainment for which enough cases were available to test it.

Although the differences between urban and rural residents in the Durham sample were not significant, it is interesting to note that the pattern in the data suggests more mild cognitive impairment among rural residents— which is the opposite of the pattern observed among St. Louis respondents. This may reflect the fact that the rural area of Missouri surveyed was entirely white, while the rural counties around Durham had as high a proportion of blacks as did Durham itself. Overall, urban–rural residence does not appear to be a very potent correlate of cognitive status, and the limited data available in the ECA study suggest that the direction of the relationship may vary across geographic regions.

MARITAL STATUS

Married respondents have a substantially lower prevalence of severe cognitive impairment than persons who are widowed, divorced/separated, or who have never married (Table 12-10). This pattern falls just short of statistical significance ($p = .06$). The same pattern holds true within the four levels of educational attainment and three of the four age categories. Married individuals also have a (statistically significant) lower prevalence of mild cognitive impairment than do persons in other marital status categories. This pattern is found at all four levels of educational attainment, but in only the two younger age categories. Nonetheless, no statistical interaction between marital status and age for mild cognitive impairment was found.

Our data suggest that marital status may be related to cognitive status, with marriage being associated with a lower prevalence of impairment. The meaning of this relationship, however, is unclear. On the one hand, marriage may serve to protect individuals from cognitive decline—though the etiologic process that would generate this protection remains uncertain. Alternatively, the pattern observed in Table 12-10 may represent a consequence of cognitive impairment. That is, the onset of cognitive impairment

Table 12-10 Prevalence of Cognitive Impairment (Errors Only) by Marital Status, Controlling on Age and Education, Aged 55 and Older

Marital Status	Severe Cognitive Impairment			Mild Cognitive Impairment in Those without Severe Impairment		
	N	%	(SE)	N	%	(SE)
Married	3,607	0.98	(0.21)	3,540	7.04	(0.54)
Widowed	3,174	3.22	(0.58)	3,015	14.29	(1.16)
Divorced/Separated	879	2.56	(0.91)	837	13.99	(2.02)
Never married	595	2.34	(1.07)	554	11.57	(2.28)
Education						
< 9 years:						
Married	1,323	2.77	(0.63)	1,267	17.45	(1.49)
Widowed	1,621	6.13	(1.14)	1,482	25.49	(2.15)
Divorced/Separated	369	5.63	(2.29)	336	32.18	(4.78)
Never married	250	5.48	(2.66)	218	26.06	(5.27)
9–11 years:						
Married	735	0.40	(0.30)	732	5.21	(1.07)
Widowed	599	1.07	(0.73)	585	7.39	(1.87)
Divorced/Separated	215	1.67	(1.55)	209	9.51	(3.58)
Never married	102	1.23	(1.81)	96	5.78	(3.85)
12 years:						
Married	776	0.11	(0.14)	773	2.58	(0.66)
Widowed	498	0.30	(0.43)	496	4.49	(1.64)
Divorced/Separated	132	0.88	(1.24)	130	4.15	(2.65)
Never married	111	0.16	(0.62)	109	4.07	(3.05)
> 12 years:						
Married	773	0.17	(0.18)	768	0.71	(0.36)
Widowed	456	0.43	(0.56)	452	1.76	(1.13)
Divorced/Separated	163	0.57	(0.86)	162	2.56	(1.80)
Never married	132	0.31	(0.80)	131	1.64	(1.83)
Age						
55–64:						
Married	1,351	0.63	(0.22)	1,339	3.54	(0.52)
Widowed	489	0.98	(0.66)	476	6.90	(1.71)
Divorced/Separated	397	1.55	(0.93)	388	10.30	(2.30)
Never married	163	1.38	(1.32)	153	10.49	(3.50)
65–74:						
Married	1,682	0.93	(0.36)	1,656	9.74	(1.12)
Widowed	1,251	1.66	(0.69)	1,224	12.00	(1.76)
Divorced/Separated	340	2.28	(1.58)	326	19.14	(4.22)
Never married	266	1.63	(1.48)	249	13.25	(4.01)
75–84:						
Married	508	2.35	(0.99)	486	16.89	(2.48)
Widowed	1,082	4.23	(1.21)	1,011	19.26	(2.42)
Divorced/Separated	124	8.58	(4.80)	107	17.84	(6.87)
Never married	134	5.03	(3.39)	122	9.79	(4.73)
85 and older:						
Married	66	7.42	(5.36)	59	17.83	(8.13)
Widowed	352	11.80	(3.43)	304	28.25	(5.09)
Divorced/Separated	18	—	—	16	—	—
Never married	32	3.97	(6.49)	30	15.46	(12.26)

Note. — signifies cell size less than 25, and so no prevalence calculated.

may lead to marital dissolution. The fact that the relationship is equally strong for widowed as for divorced and separated persons, however, argues against viewing marital dissolution as a consequence of cognitive impairment.

CONSEQUENCES OF COGNITIVE IMPAIRMENT

Cognitive impairment has the potential to negatively affect several aspects of the individual's life, increasing use of specialty mental health and general medical services, financial problems, and institutionalization. Note that these are *assumed* consequences of cognitive impairment—given the fact that our data were collected at a single point in time, we cannot make clear inferences based on the timing of the presumed cause and consequence. Nonetheless, it is highly reasonable to view these factors as outcomes of cognitive impairment. It would make no sense, for example, to argue that health service use causes impairment—though it is possible that the two might be associated only because other factors (for example, alcohol abuse, cerebrovascular disease) led to both cognitive dysfunction and health service use. Financial problems were assumed to exist if there was either receipt of welfare or household income of less than $5,000 per year. Although it is possible that financial resources are a risk factor for cognitive impairment, it is more likely that cognitive impairment, with its associated loss of self-care capacity and the demands it poses for medical and social services, leads to financial problems. Finally, it is more reasonable to expect that cognitive impairment, and its associated lack of self-care capacity, leads to institutional placement than to believe that institutionalization leads to cognitive dysfunction. This is especially the case when the cognitive impairment is severe.

HEALTH SERVICE USE

Previous literature reveals a virtual absence of information about health service use and cognitive status in later life. In this section, four types of care are examined: outpatient and inpatient specialty mental health services (Table 12–11) and outpatient and inpatient general medical care (Table 12–12) by persons over 55 residing in households. Prior to examining those relationships, it is worth noting general differences in use of specialty mental health services and general medical care by comparing Tables 12–11 and 12–12. There are stark differences in rates of service use across the two health service sectors. In terms of outpatient services, only 6.19% of older Americans report one or more visits to a specialty mental health provider during a six-month interval, compared to 62.2% who report at

Table 12-11 Utilization of Mental Health Services and Cognitive Impairment (Errors Only) Controlling on Education and Age, Aged 55 and Older (Household Residents Weighted to National Demographic Distribution)

	Used Outpatient Services for Mental Health in Past 6 Months			Used Inpatient Services for Mental Health in Past 12 Months		
	N	%	(SE)[a]	N	%	(SE)[a]
Total household residents aged 55 or older	8,258	6.19	(0.40)	8,139	0.45	(0.11)
Cognitive Impairment						
No impairment	6,745	6.14	(0.42)	6,669	0.39	(0.11)
Mild impairment	1,204	7.32	(1.39)	1,100	1.12	(0.57)
Severe impairment	309	2.80	(2.05)	290	0.13	(0.48)
Education						
< 9 years:						
No impairment	2,379	6.28	(0.78)	2,336	0.55	(0.24)
Mild impairment	928	7.79	(1.63)	908	1.14	(0.65)
Severe impairment	260	2.74	(2.20)	244	0.00	—
9–11 years:						
No impairment	1,478	6.45	(0.94)	1,464	0.16	(0.15)
Mild impairment	143	9.11	(4.26)	142	1.54	(1.84)
Severe impairment	29	[0.00]	—	28	[1.15]	(5.20)
12 years:						
No impairment	1,413	5.73	(0.82)	1,401	0.66	(0.29)
Mild impairment	94	1.81	(2.62)	92	0.29	(1.08)
Severe impairment	9	—	—	8	—	—
> 12 years:						
No impairment	1,475	6.12	(0.84)	1,468	0.11	(0.12)
Mild impairment	39	0.00	—	38	1.01	(3.39)
Severe impairment	11	—	—	10	—	—
Age						
55–64:						
No impairment	2,159	7.95	(0.67)	2,146	0.41	(0.16)
Mild impairment	199	10.51	(3.31)	197	0.61	(0.84)
Severe impairment	44	1.02	(2.70)	41	0.00	—
65–74:						
No impairment	2,986	5.20	(0.68)	2,950	0.56	(0.23)
Mild impairment	468	5.42	(1.94)	464	0.70	(0.72)
Severe impairment	84	4.25	(5.10)	82	0.51	(1.84)
75–84:						
No impairment	1,328	2.60	(0.74)	1,310	0.00	—
Mild impairment	400	6.06	(2.39)	388	1.54	(1.26)
Severe impairment	122	3.69	(4.00)	116	0.00	—
85 and older:						
No impairment	272	2.37	(1.66)	263	0.00	(0.00)
Mild impairment	137	11.14	(5.89)	131	3.41	(3.51)
Severe impairment	59	1.39	(3.29)	51	0.00	—

Note. — signifies cell size below 25.
   [ ] signifies cell size of 25–29.
[a]Standard error not calculated when prevalence is zero.

Table 12–12 Utilization of General Health Services and Cognitive Impairment (Errors Only), Controlling on Age and Education, Aged 55 and Older (Household Residents Weighted to National Demographic Distribution)

	Used Outpatient Services in Past 6 Months			Used Inpatient Services in Past 12 Months		
	N	%	(SE)[a]	N	%	(SE)[a]
Total household residents aged 55 or older	8,258	62.20	(0.80)	8,148	15.90	(0.61)
Cognitive Impairment						
No impairment	6,745	62.52	(0.85)	6,676	14.84	(0.63)
Mild impairment	1,204	61.18	(2.61)	1,182	23.36	(2.29)
Severe impairment	309	51.60	(6.23)	290	30.81	(6.07)
Education						
< 9 years:						
No impairment	2,379	61.49	(1.57)	2,339	16.20	(1.20)
Mild impairment	928	61.69	(2.97)	910	22.38	(2.57)
Severe impairment	260	53.64	(6.71)	244	28.49	(6.36)
9–11 years:						
No impairment	1,478	62.90	(1.84)	1,464	14.73	(1.36)
Mild impairment	143	67.35	(6.94)	142	28.85	(6.75)
Severe impairment	29	[45.78]	(21.35)	28	[43.46]	(24.20)
12 years:						
No impairment	1,423	61.66	(1.72)	1,404	15.27	(1.27)
Mild impairment	94	51.44	(9.82)	92	27.10	(8.86)
Severe impairment	9	—	—	8	—	—
> 12 years:						
No impairment	1,475	64.27	(1.69)	1,469	12.92	(1.18)
Mild impairment	39	42.81	(16.41)	38	13.47	(11.61)
Severe impairment	11	—	—	10	—	—
Age						
55–64:						
No impairment	2,159	58.97	(1.21)	2,149	12.38	(0.81)
Mild impairment	199	55.55	(5.37)	197	19.21	(4.27)
Severe impairment	44	55.28	(13.32)	41	14.96	(10.14)
65–74:						
No impairment	2,986	65.02	(1.46)	2,952	15.41	(1.11)
Mild impairment	468	62.61	(4.15)	464	22.68	(3.61)
Severe impairment	84	53.39	(12.61)	82	33.27	(12.14)
75–84:						
No impairment	1,328	69.07	(2.14)	1,310	20.86	(1.90)
Mild impairment	400	66.56	(4.73)	389	25.22	(4.43)
Severe impairment	122	47.71	(10.60)	116	32.17	(10.39)
85 and older:						
No impairment	272	63.75	(5.25)	265	23.07	(4.69)
Mild impairment	137	52.52	(9.34)	132	33.18	(9.08)
Severe impairment	59	52.18	(14.03)	51	43.70	(15.52)

Note. — signifies cell size less than 25 and therefore no prevalence calculated.
[ ] signifies cell size of 25–29.

[a]Standard error not calculated for cells smaller than 25.

least one visit to a general medical provider. Similarly, for inpatient services, less than half of one percent of older adults have been admitted to inpatient psychiatric facilities in the past year, compared to 15.9% admitted to a general medical hospital. Clearly, specialty mental health services account for a very small percentage of all medical services used by older adults.

Table 12-11 provides information about the percentages of persons at three levels of cognitive status (no impairment, mild impairment, and severe impairment) who used outpatient specialty mental health services in the six months prior to interview and who used inpatient specialty mental health services in the year prior to interview. For outpatient care, there was a trend for persons with severe cognitive impairment to be least likely to use outpatient services ($p = .10$). This pattern held in the one educational level with sufficient cases to test it and in three of the four age categories. For use of inpatient services, the pattern was similar, but not identical: persons with severe cognitive impairment were the least likely to have received inpatient services, those with mild cognitive impairment were most likely to have received inpatient services, and those with no cognitive impairment were intermediate in rates of inpatient service use. Again, this trend fell just short of statistical significance ($p = .07$). The pattern for inpatient care applied to the one educational level with enough cases to test it and to all four age categories.

Persons with severe cognitive impairment are less likely to use outpatient general medical services than either those with mild impairment or no impairment (Table 12-12). This pattern is not quite statistically significant ($p = .08$). This pattern holds true for the two levels of education for which testing was possible and the four age categories, although differences in some categories are very small. The pattern for inpatient care is different: persons with severe cognitive impairment are the most likely to have been hospitalized during the past year, persons with no cognitive impairment are least likely to have been hospitalized, and those with mild impairment are intermediate. This difference is statistically significant and applies to the two testable levels of educational attainment and three of four age categories.

Overall, these results suggest that persons with severe cognitive impairment are relatively underserved in terms of outpatient health care in both the specialty mental health and general medical care sectors and in terms of inpatient use in the specialty sector. In light of the fact that there are no effective treatments for many forms of dementia, we perhaps should not expect elevated rates of health service use for the severely cognitively impaired. Nonetheless, dementias are debilitating diseases and regular medical management as well as monitoring of secondary conditions is needed. Therefore, we should not be content to observe decreased rates of service use among older adults with severe cognitive impairment. Higher usage of inpatient general medical care suggests that, to some extent, hospitalization may substitute for outpatient service use among the severely cognitively impaired.

FINANCIAL PROBLEMS

Cognitive status is significantly related to receipt of welfare assistance among adults aged 55 and older (Table 12–13). Persons with severe cognitive impairment are most likely to receive welfare, those with no impairment are least likely to receive welfare, and those with mild impairment are intermediate. This pattern holds true for the one testable level of education and three of four age categories. Moreover, receipt of welfare is related to both education and age. As might be expected, receipt of welfare is negatively related to education and positively correlated with age (regardless of cognitive status).

Similar patterns are observed for household income of less than $5,000 per year (Table 12–13), despite the low response rate for this item. Low income is more characteristic of persons with both severe and mild cognitive impairment than among those with no impairment. This pattern is statistically significant and applies to all testable categories of education and age. In addition, low income is related to both education and age, regardless of cognitive status. As expected, low income is associated with low education and with older age.

Overall, these findings suggest that both mild and, especially, severe cognitive impairment are associated with financial problems.

COMMUNITY VERSUS INSTITUTIONAL RESIDENCE

As noted previously, the prevalence of cognitive impairment is known to be high among institutional residents (for example, Butler & Lewis, 1977; Gottesman, 1977). Consequently, we expected that community versus institutional residence would be significantly related to cognitive status. As expected, there is a strong and significant relationship between cognitive status and place of residence (Table 12–14). More specifically, institutional residence is most common among persons with severe cognitive impairment, least prevalent among those with no impairment, and intermediate for persons with mild impairment. Indeed, those with severe cognitive impairment are more than 23 times as likely to be in an institutional facility as those with no impairment. A similar, but less dramatic pattern is characteristic of mild cognitive impairment. Persons with mild impairment are more than eight times as likely to reside in institutions as those with no cognitive impairment. This pattern holds for all levels of education for which tests are possible and all four age categories. In addition, it is not

Table 12–13 Financial Indicators by Age, Education, and Cognitive Impairment (Errors Only) Aged 55 and Older

	Receives Welfare			Household Income < $5,000[a]		
	N	%	(SE)	N	%	(SE)
Total aged 55 or more	7,974	12.33	(0.55)	5,253	14.32	(0.66)
Cognitive Impairment						
No impairment	6,564	11.47	(0.56)	4,579	12.39	(0.65)
Mild impairment	1,148	18.50	(2.11)	569	36.53	(3.47)
Severe impairment	262	24.25	(5.81)	105	36.09	(8.19)
Education						
9 years:						
No impairment	2,296	13.65	(1.12)	1,482	25.93	(1.71)
Mild impairment	890	19.12	(2.43)	441	39.73	(4.11)
Severe impairment	225	24.59	(6.18)	87	35.82	(8.75)
9–11 years:						
No impairment	1,437	13.69	(1.33)	1,007	15.28	(1.55)
Mild impairment	135	16.47	(5.57)	67	26.73	(8.28)
Severe impairment	21	—	—	12	—	—
12 years:						
No impairment	1,380	9.97	(1.07)	979	7.16	(1.00)
Mild impairment	86	14.07	(7.11)	47	28.06	(10.48)
Severe impairment	7	—	—	3	—	—
> 12 years:						
No impairment	1,451	8.54	(0.99)	1,111	2.98	(0.62)
Mild impairment	37	22.60	(14.47)	14	—	—
Severe impairment	9	—	—	3	—	—
Age						
55–64:						
No impairment	2,113	12.00	(0.81)	1,458	6.57	(0.67)
Mild impairment	192	24.28	(4.69)	87	25.00	(6.77)
Severe impairment	39	40.84	(14.17)	16	—	—
65–74:						
No impairment	2,910	11.01	(0.97)	2,152	15.75	(1.24)
Mild impairment	455	16.95	(3.27)	260	38.66	(5.43)
Severe impairment	73	28.53	(12.48)	33	34.16	(15.40)
75–84:						
No impairment	1,282	9.92	(1.41)	833	25.79	(2.44)
Mild impairment	379	15.28	(3.67)	174	42.99	(6.59)
Severe impairment	106	21.50	(9.30)	42	50.12	(14.27)
85 and older:						
No impairment	259	15.69	(4.09)	136	26.97	(6.44)
Mild impairment	122	19.65	(7.82)	48	32.27	(12.07)
Severe impairment	44	3.62	(5.97)	14	—	—

Note. — signifies cell size smaller than 25.

[a]Income not available for St. Louis sample.

Table 12-14 Institutionalization by Age, Education, and Cognitive Impairment (Errors Only) Aged 55 and Older

	Institutionalized		
	N	%	(SE)
Total aged 55 or more	8,261	1.21	(0.18)
Cognitive Impairment			
No impairment	6,747	0.58	(0.13)
Mild impairment	1,205	4.75	(0.14)
Severe impairment	309	13.55	(4.26)
Education			
< 9 years:			
No impairment	2,379	0.79	(0.29)
Mild impairment	928	3.68	(1.15)
Severe impairment	260	11.28	(4.26)
9–11 years:			
No impairment	1,479	0.58	(0.29)
Mild impairment	144	7.07	(3.79)
Severe impairment	29	[19.51]	(16.98)
12 years:			
No impairment	1,414	0.45	(0.24)
Mild impairment	94	8.83	(5.58)
Severe impairment	9	—	—
> 12 years:			
No impairment	1,475	0.46	(0.24)
Mild impairment	39	12.86	(11.10)
Severe impairment	11	—	—
Age			
55–64:			
No impairment	2,159	0.18	(0.11)
Mild impairment	199	2.21	(1.59)
Severe impairment	44	8.12	(7.32)
65–74:			
No impairment	2,988	0.48	(0.21)
Mild impairment	469	2.40	(1.31)
Severe impairment	84	6.13	(6.07)
75–84:			
No impairment	1,328	1.59	(0.58)
Mild impairment	400	6.62	(2.49)
Severe impairment	122	14.93	(7.56)
85 and older:			
No impairment	272	4.11	(2.17)
Mild impairment	137	16.97	(7.02)
Severe impairment	59	26.24	(12.36)

Note. — signifies cell size smaller than 25.
    [ ] signifies cell size between 25 and 29.

surprising that age is also related to institutional residence regardless of cognitive status, since physical health worsens with age.

In spite of the strong relationship between cognitive status and place of residence, it should be noted that the vast majority of persons suffering from severe cognitive impairment remain in the community. Thus, the major burden of providing care and supervision to severely cognitively impaired older adults falls on family members and other informal providers (George & Gwyther, 1986).

COGNITIVE IMPAIRMENT AND OTHER PSYCHIATRIC DISORDERS

Mental health professionals are appropriately concerned about patterns of psychiatric comorbidity. The extent to which specific psychiatric disorders tend to co-occur can have important implications for etiology, illness course, treatment decisions, and prognosis for recovery. Our examination of comorbidity will be limited to two disorders that have been examined in previous research: major depression and alcohol abuse/dependence.

Unfortunately, it is very difficult to examine the comorbidity of cognitive impairment in the context of epidemiologic surveys, including the ECA program. As described elsewhere in this volume, the DIS was used to obtain the information needed to assign diagnoses for specific psychiatric disorders. Some respondents who were evaluated as having severe cognitive impairment on the basis of their MMSE scores were not administered the remainder of the DIS because they were incapable of answering the questions. Consequently, estimates of comorbidity between cognitive impairment and DIS diagnoses are based on a nonrepresentative subset of respondents, a subset especially compromised with regard to severe cognitive impairment.

MAJOR DEPRESSION

A number of studies based on clinical samples have suggested that depressive disorder commonly accompanies cognitive impairment in general and the organic mental disorders of later life in particular (for example Kiloh, 1961; Weingartner et al., 1981). A number of recent community-based surveys, however, have failed to detect a significant relationship between cognitive status and depressive disorder (for example, Kay et al., 1985). Because of the continuing debate surrounding this issue, we examined the relationship between cognitive status and a DIS/DSM-III diagnosis of recent major depressive episode (see Table 12–15).

Prevalence estimates for the total sample suggest that both mild and

Table 12–15 Major Depressive Episode in Past Year by Age, Education, and Cognitive Impairment (Errors Only), Aged 55 and Older

	Major Depressive Episode in Past Year		
	N	%	(SE)[a]
Total aged 55 or more	8,116	1.33	(0.19)
Cognitive Impairment			
No impairment	6,651	1.22	(0.19)
Mild impairment	1,179	2.18	(0.79)
Severe impairment	286	2.54	(2.08)
Education			
< 9 years:			
No impairment	2,331	1.43	(0.39)
Mild impairment	908	1.88	(0.84)
Severe impairment	241	2.92	(2.39)
9–11 years:			
No impairment	1,455	1.06	(0.39)
Mild impairment	142	1.04	(1.51)
Severe impairment	27	[0.00]	—
12 years:			
No impairment	1,398	0.81	(0.32)
Mild impairment	91	8.07	(5.43)
Severe impairment	8	—	—
> 12 years:			
No impairment	1,467	1.52	(0.43)
Mild impairment	38	0.00	—
Severe impairment	10	—	—
Age			
55–64:			
No impairment	2,142	1.73	(0.32)
Mild impairment	197	3.91	(2.10)
Severe impairment	42	0.00	—
65–74:			
No impairment	2,941	0.83	(0.28)
Mild impairment	460	1.85	(1.17)
Severe impairment	81	0.00	—
75–84:			
No impairment	1,306	0.40	(0.29)
Mild impairment	391	1.25	(1.13)
Severe impairment	115	3.21	(3.92)
85 and older:			
No impairment	262	0.69	(0.93)
Mild impairment	131	1.69	(2.50)
Severe impairment	48	8.48	(9.07)

Note. — signifies cell size smaller than 25.
[ ] signifies cell size between 25 and 29.
[a]Standard error not calculated where prevalence is zero.

severe cognitive impairment are associated with slightly elevated prevalences of major depression. This trend, however, is not statistically significant. Moreover, the pattern does not hold up well within categories of age and educational attainment (though there are no significant interactions).

Overall, age is negatively related to having a major depressive episode. That is, the prevalence of major depression decreases across successively older age groups. Given that older age is associated with higher prevalence of cognitive impairment and lower prevalence of major depression, it is not surprising that we find little evidence of comorbidity. Thus, these findings support other recent epidemiologic studies. Perhaps the depressed older patients seen in many clinical studies view difficulty concentrating and slowed thoughts (which are symptoms of depression) as memory problems and report them as such to their clinicians. It also is possible, however, that comorbidity cannot be examined meaningfully in this kind of epidemiologic study for the methodological reasons noted above.

ALCOHOL ABUSE/DEPENDENCE

Previous clinical studies strongly suggest that chronic alcohol abuse or dependence is associated with dementia in later life (for example, Roth, 1981; Victor & Banker, 1978). The ECA data provide an opportunity to examine the association between alcohol abuse/dependence and cognitive impairment in the context of a large epidemiologic study. We examine the relationship between cognitive status and lifetime alcohol abuse/dependence (as compared to current/recent major depression) because the cognitive consequences of chronic alcohol use may be experienced after drinking has stopped. (We also would have liked to examine the relationship between cognitive status and lifetime drug abuse/dependence. However, the number of ECA respondents aged 55 and older who reported lifetime drug abuse/dependence was too small to permit meaningful analysis.)

Results indicate that, for the total sample of persons aged 55 and older, lifetime alcohol abuse/dependence is significantly related to both severe and mild cognitive impairment (see Table 12–16). The prevalence of alcohol abuse/dependence is about 1.5 times greater among persons with both mild and severe cognitive impairment than among persons with no impairment. Alcohol abuse/dependence is significantly negatively related to both education and age. Thus, both low education and younger age are associated with higher prevalence of alcohol abuse/dependence.

Cognitive status is not related to lifetime alcohol abuse/dependence in the same way across all levels of education and age (see Table 12–16). In terms of education, severe cognitive impairment is significantly associated with alcohol abuse/dependence only among those with eight or fewer years of education. In contrast, mild cognitive impairment is significantly related

Table 12–16 Alcohol Abuse/Dependence (Lifetime) by Age, Education, and Cognitive Impairment (Errors Only) Aged 55 and Older (Five-Site Data Weighted to National Demographic Distribution)

	Alcohol Abuse Dependence (Lifetime)		
	N	%	(SE)
Total aged 55 or more	8,058	7.87	(0.45)
Cognitive impairment			
No impairment	6,615	7.42	(0.46)
Mild impairment	1,167	11.46	(1.72)
Severe impairment	276	11.65	(4.31)
Education			
< 9 years:			
No impairment	2,316	8.62	(0.92)
Mild impairment	901	8.58	(1.73)
Severe impairment	233	12.71	(4.75)
9–11 years:			
No impairment	1,451	9.18	(1.11)
Mild impairment	138	24.79	(6.44)
Severe impairment	26	[6.25]	(12.67)
12 years:			
No impairment	1,387	5.15	(0.79)
Mild impairment	91	17.65	(7.60)
Severe impairment	8	—	—
> 12 years:			
No impairment	1,461	6.80	(0.89)
Mild impairment	37	11.43	(10.83)
Severe impairment	9	—	—
Age			
55–64:			
No impairment	2,131	9.14	(0.72)
Mild impairment	195	17.46	(4.12)
Severe impairment	42	26.38	(12.52)
65–74:			
No impairment	2,934	6.61	(0.77)
Mild impairment	459	13.46	(2.95)
Severe impairment	76	10.58	(8.34)
75–84:			
No impairment	1,293	4.32	(0.96)
Mild impairment	384	5.93	(2.41)
Severe impairment	112	8.76	(6.30)
85 and older:			
No impairment	257	0.82	(1.02)
Mild impairment	129	2.22	(2.84)
Severe impairment	46	0.00	(0.00)

Note. — signifies cell size less than 25.
    [ ] signifies cell size 25 and 29.

to alcohol abuse/dependence among all respondents except those with eight or fewer years of schooling. For the age groups, severe cognitive impairment is significantly related to alcohol abuse/dependence only for persons aged 55–64 and those aged 75–84. Mild cognitive impairment is significantly associated with alcohol problems for all the age groups except for respondents aged 75–84. This relative instability of results appears to reflect the small cell sizes in many of the comparisons. Overall, alcohol abuse/dependence appears to be significantly associated with both mild and severe cognitive impairment.

CONCLUSION

We will end this chapter by addressing, in general terms, two issues. First, we will comment on the limitations of using instruments such as the MMSE for measuring cognitive impairment in the context of epidemiologic surveys such as the ECA study. Second, we will summarize and put into broader perspective what the ECA experience has taught us about cognitive impairment in America.

Though the MMSE has been a useful tool for obtaining information about the cognitive status of American adults, there clearly are limits associated with use of the MMSE (or similar measures). The results reported in this chapter reflect those limitations—and though they have been previously noted, they merit reiteration. For our purposes, three major limitations were associated with use of the MMSE. First, as compared to diagnostic sections of the DIS, the MMSE is restricted to the measurement of current cognitive status. Because we were unable to obtain information about age of onset and symptom history, we also were unable to examine a variety of research questions for which information about onset and duration of symptoms is necessary. Second, given that some respondents who scored as severely cognitively impaired on the MMSE could not be administered the DIS, we were unable to examine comorbidity using data from the entire ECA sample. Third, though the results suggested that cognitive status is strongly related to race, education, and age, we were unable to distinguish the degree to which those factors serve as risk factors for cognitive impairment versus the degree to which low MMSE scores reflect educational deprivations or other factors related to age and race.

Identifying the limitations of a measurement tool is an important task. More important, however, is the question of whether anything can be done to improve the MMSE. Frankly, it appears that there are only modest prospects for overcoming those limitations. With regard to the focus on current cognitive status, very little can be done. Persons suffering from cognitive impairment simply cannot provide symptom histories or information about the onset and remission of symptoms. The only feasible altern-tive is for investigators to perform longitudinal studies so that cognitive status is monitored on a regular basis. Unfortunately, such studies are very expensive—and, for large cohorts, probably prohibitively expensive. There also appears to be little that could be done to enhance the study of co-morbidity of cognitive impairment in epidemiologic studies. It is not clear that clinical studies can disentangle cognitive decline from other psychiat-ric disorders, but clinical studies have a higher probabiity of success than do epidemiologic surveys.

The issue of test error, however, is one that merits increased attention and has the potential to be usefully addressed in both clinical and epidemi-ologic studies. Clinical studies can be used to identify "false positive" MMSE scores and the factors that generate false positives. Research by Anthony et al. (1982) serves as an excellent illustration of this approach. Issues of test error also can be addressed using epidemiologic data. For example, it would be very useful to carefully examine the degree to which self-care capacity is related to MMSE scores across age, race, and education groups. To the degree that severe cognitive impairment has similar implica-tions for self-care capacity across demographic subgroups, the less likely it is that MMSE scores reflect bias. Conversely, to the extent that severe cognitive impairment is differentially related to self-care capacity across subgroups, the more likely that bias is present. Jorm et al. (1988) recently used this approach to examine education as a possible source of bias in the MMSE. Their results indicated that cognitive impairment has the same relationship to self-care capacity among those with both high and low levels of educational attainment.

In previous research, the most commonly identified limitation of the MMSE is the fact that it measures cognitive status rather than organic brain syndromes or organic mental disorders—that is, that it is not a diag-nostic tool. Obviously, that limitation applied to the ECA data also—and, in an ideal world, we would have preferred the ability to report the preva-lence of specific organic brain syndromes or mental disorders. Nonetheless, we found this limitation of the MMSE to be less troublesome than those noted above. We believe that the epidemiology of cognitive impairment is itself an important issue.

In spite of the limitations of the MMSE, the results of this chapter provide important information about the prevalence, correlates, and conse-quences of cognitive impairment in America. Our results indicate that cognitive impairment constitutes an important component of the burden of mental illness in America. The burden of cognitive impairment is borne primarily by older Americans. The nature of that burden is evidenced not only by the relatively high prevalence of cognitive impairment among older adults, but also by its observed consequences in terms of increased hospitalizations, increased financial dependency, and increased likelihood of institutional placement.

As is true for many illnesses, cognitive impairment is found most commonly among those older persons who are socially and culturally disadvantaged—that is, among the very old, among members of racial and ethnic minorities, among the unmarried, and among those with low levels of education. Whether these associations represent risk factors in an etiological sense is unclear. Nonetheless, it is clear that cognitive impairment is most prevalent among those with the fewest resources—which heightens its public health significance.

The importance of cognitive impairment among older Americans also is heightened by comparing the prevalence of cognitive impairment with the prevalences of DSM-III/DIS disorders. As described in other chapters in this volume, most psychiatric disorders are less prevalent among older adults than among their younger peers. In contrast, cognitive impairment is relatively common in later life and is especially prevalent among the very old. Any discussion of psychiatric disorders in America cannot afford to neglect cognitive impairment because it is the major psychiatric burden experienced by our older citizens.

13 An Overview of Psychiatric Disorders in America

LEE N. ROBINS / BEN Z. LOCKE /
DARREL A. REGIER

The ECA study describes America's problems in the early 1980s with 30 of the major psychiatric disorders listed in the official nomenclature of the American Psychiatric Association at that time, the *Diagnostic and Statistical Manual (3rd ed.)* (1980). Now that each of the disorders investigated by the ECA has been discussed, it is time to look at the larger picture of psychiatric disorder as a whole in America. By persons with a psychiatric disorder we will be referring to persons with any of the disorders covered in earlier chapters except for three—generalized anxiety, because that disorder was studied in only three sites, bereavement, and mild cognitive impairment, because the latter two are not usually considered disorders by clinicians. The disorders covered include the most common and serious adult disorders, and account for the majority of persons thought of as psychiatrically ill or treated for psychiatric disorder.

This broad look at the whole group of psychiatric disorders taken together allows us to estimate how many Americans have experienced common psychiatric disorders in their lifetimes and in the current year, and how those affected differ from the rest of the population in their work and family lives and in their use of health services. Thus the ECA study provides a summary estimate of how great the social and personal costs of psychiatric disorder are, as well as specifying which parts of the population are most likely to be in need of care. We can also ask at what age disorders typically began and how long they usually lasted, whether the generations differ in their rates of disorder, whether men or women were more likely to develop psychiatric disorders and to recover from them, whether minority groups were at particularly high risk of disorder. Knowing which groups are particularly susceptible can help planners to target their mental health programs, as well as stimulating ideas about possible reasons for differential susceptibility.

After answering these questions about liabilities to psychiatric disorder taken as a whole, we will ask how specific disorders differ from each other. Which disorders are most common in the total population and in particular population groups? Which begin earliest and last longest? Which disorders occur together? For which disorders is treatment most likely to be sought? For this comparison, disorders will be grouped into 12 categories: 7 affective disorders are combined into 3—major depressive episode, manic episode, and dysthymia; the 2 forms of alcoholism, dependence and abuse, into one; the 11 types of drug abuse and dependence into one; schizophrenia and schizophreniform are combined, as are the 3 types of phobia. Also included are the single disorders, somatization, panic disorder, obsessive compulsive, and antisocial personality. Generalized anxiety, which was excluded from the summary measure of any psychiatric disorder, is included when feasible in these specific comparisons with other disorders.

This chapter will also comment briefly on what the ECA study results suggest about the way diagnoses are grouped into larger categories in the standard American nomenclature. Diagnoses are grouped because they are thought to have something in common. Sometimes the grouping is based on a presumed common underlying problem (for example, the anxiety disorders), or on clinical experience showing that two disorders frequently appear in the same persons at different times (for example, depression and mania, alcohol and drug dependence), or share common symptoms (depression and dysthymia). While a survey such as the ECA cannot offer the clinical experience that psychiatrists brought to the groupings used in the *Diagnostic and Statistical Manual*, it has the advantage of total coverage of affected persons, both those who do and those who do not come to treatment. Thus it can add a dimension of knowledge that even the most expert diagnosticians lack.

Finally, new insights growing out of the ECA experience about paths that future research should take will be discussed.

Psychiatric Disorder as a Whole

PREVALENCE

One or more of the psychiatric disorders described in this volume had been experienced at some time in their lives by 32% of American adults, and 20% had an active disorder, defined as a disorder for which criteria had been met at some time in the person's life and at least one symptom (or one episode) has been present in the year prior to interview. This estimate, that one in five Americans has an active psychiatric disorder, is considerably higher than the 10% to 15% estimated as the annual prevalence of psychiatric disorder by the President's Commission on Mental Health (1978). Indeed, the estimate by the President's Commission for the annual rate is lower than the ECA's estimate for disorder in the current month (15.4%) (Regier et al., 1988a). However, the President's Commission's estimate was based on a single prevalence study conducted in the city of Baltimore plus estimates of annual incidence from a variety of sources. The recognition of the inadequacy of that data base was a major reason for undertaking the ECA (Regier et al., 1978).

The figures of a 32% lifetime and 20% annual prevalence are the best current estimates of the prevalence of psychiatric disorder in America, and like all estimates, they cannot claim to be precisely correct. Factors that might contribute to errors in that estimate were reviewed in chapter 2. They include the fact that not all diagnoses in the official manual of the American Psychiatric Association were covered (though, as we shall see, there is enough co-occurrence of psychiatric disorders to make us believe that many with uncovered diagnoses will also have had a covered diagnosis and so will have been counted), the ambiguity of some of the criteria in the Manual, the dropping of a few diagnostic questions at the request of the government, dependence on what respondents are able and willing to tell an interviewer (and consequently possible concealment of some socially disapproved symptoms), nonrandom refusals to participate, and the fact that the five sites selected were not necessarily representative of the nation as a whole.

Despite these limitations, the ECA certainly provides better estimates than has any earlier study of psychiatric disorder in America because it brings together a large number of unprecedented features. The ECA is the first survey for which estimates are based on the newly specific diagnostic criteria of the American Psychiatric Association (subject to the limitations cited in chapter 2), and in which respondents had the time periods over which they were to report symptoms clearly defined to them. Questions were carefully designed to match each of the official criteria for the diagnoses selected, and to be combined by computer programs that summed those criteria in just the way specified by the diagnostic manual. All questions were spelled out in detail, so that interviews were reliable and equivalent across sites. The subjects were a large, randomly selected sample of the general population, including institutionalized persons as well as those in households. Interviewer comparability was achieved both by the fully articulated questions and by intensive two-week training programs and careful supervision throughout the field period. Interviewer error was minimized by independent editing of all interviews and a uniform data cleaning pro-

gram that detected impossible responses and inconsistent patterns of responses. Response rates (above 75% overall) were high enough to make it
likely that the sample is representative of the population in the areas
sampled. Estimates of rates in the localities sampled were further improved
by adjustment for sample design (including the fact that only one person
per household was interviewed, that larger proportions of the institutional
than household populations were surveyed, and that blacks and the elderly
were oversampled in some sites) and for nonresponse through refusal or
inability to locate the respondent. State-of-the-art standards for survey procedures were maintained through close collaboration among the NIMH
scientists who coordinated the project and all five sites and by seeking
expert advice throughout. Finally, estimates for the country as a whole
were developed by adjusting the demographic profile of the sampled areas
to that of the country as a whole, and evaluation of differences in prevalence between groups made allowance statistically for the increased variance attributable to weighting to the reference local and national
populations.

AGE OF ONSET

Psychiatric disorders typically began when sample members were young.
Of all those affected, the median age at the first symptom of their disor-
der(s) was 16. Since the average age of the U.S. population is 40, most of our
sample had many years ahead of them in which those without disorder
could develop one or more. However, even if we were to follow the sample
to their deaths, we would not expect the total with disorders to increase
greatly or the median age of first symptom to get very much higher. This
expectation is based on the fact that over 75% of our sample with any
disorder had experienced its first symptoms by age 24, and 90% by age 38.
The half of the sample over age 40 added relatively few late-life onsets. (An
exception, of course, was cognitive impairment, which increases in frequency after age 70, but for which we do not have age of onset.)

REMISSION AND DURATION

Since 32% have had a disorder, but only 20% have been active within the
year, 37.5% of those ever affected (12%/32%) must have recovered by
time of interview.
    Among those with a past but no active disorder, the median age of onset

was 19, indicating that later onset is associated with more recovery. The average age at experiencing the last symptom of a disorder from which they recovered was 30, with an average interval between the first and the last symptom experienced of 10.4 years. If the respondent had more than one disorder and recovered from all, this interval covered the time from the first symptom of the earliest to the last symptom of the latest disorder. Thus the affected individual typically has symptoms for a considerable interval before recovery takes place.

CORRELATES OF EVER HAVING A DISORDER

The association of group membership with psychiatric disorder is of interest both as a way of identifying persons likely to benefit from treatment or prevention activities and as a hint of possible causes or consequences of having a psychiatric disorder. Group memberships determined at birth, like race, sex, and age, can provide ideas about causal mechanisms, while memberships acquired after the typical age of onset, like marital status and job level, may either be evidence for the degree of impairment resulting from psychiatric illness or related to situations that cause disorders to persist or recur. It is not possible in a cross-sectional study like the ECA to be certain which of these explanations is correct. However, whether the association between a disorder and group membership indicates a cause or effect of the disorder, identifying groups with high rates of current disorder helps planners of mental health services to know where to direct their efforts.

GENDER

More men than women had had a psychiatric disorder over their lifetime (36% versus 30%), but men and women did not differ at all in the proportion with active disorder in the last year—20% of both had had symptoms in the current year (Table 13-1). One of the important results of the ECA has been to question the excess of mental disorder among women compared to men reported in earlier surveys (Hagnell, 1966; Leighton et al., 1963; Srole et al., 1964). As Helgason's work in Iceland (1964) shows, results by gender vary with the mix of disorders covered. The sexes had similar rates of psychoses in Iceland, while women had more neurotic disorders and men had ten times women's rate of substance abuse. The predominance of disorders in women in these early studies reflects the inclusion of illnesses then considered psychosomatic and less attention to substance abuse and antisocial personality than in the current study.

BIRTH COHORT

If birth cohorts had equal risks of mental disorder, and if mental disorder did not affect survival, one would expect to find increasing rates of lifetime disorder in each successively older cohort because each had more years in which to develop a disorder than the next oldest. In contrast, the ECA found the younger two cohorts (18–29 and 30–44) to have the highest lifetime rates of disorder (Table 13–1). Disorder had been experienced at some time by only 21% of those 65 or older, by 27% of those 45–64, but by 39% of those 30–44. Active disorder was also lower in those over 45.

The fact that older persons had rates of *active* disorder as low or lower than rates of younger people contradicts results of earlier surveys in America, which showed a positive correlation of current disorder with age (Leighton et al., 1963; Srole et al., 1964), but these studies had not systematically attempted to determine whether symptoms could be explained by physical illness rather than psychiatric disorder, as the ECA did, and of course, the older half of the sample has more physical illness. Our results about current

Table 13–1 Prevalence of Any Psychiatric Disorder in Particular Groups

| | | Prevalence of Any Disorder[a] in Percent (SE) | | |
	N	Lifetime Prevalence	Active Cases in Last Year	Remission[b]
Total	19,640	32 (0.48)	20 (0.41)	38
Gender:				
Men	8,419	36 (0.72)	20 (0.59)	44
Women	11,221	30 (0.65)***	20 (0.57)	33
Age:				
<30	4,872	37 (0.90)	25 (0.80)	32
30–44	4,650	39 (0.97)	23 (0.84)	41
45–64	4,194	27 (0.88)***	15 (0.69)***	44
65+	5,912	21 (1.10)***	13 (0.90)	38
Ethnicity:				
White	13,091	32 (0.53)	19 (0.44)	41
Black	4,697	38 (1.56)***	26 (1.40)***	32
Hispanic	1,606	33 (2.10)	20 (1.78)**	39
Education:				
Not complete high school	8,818	36 (0.86)	23 (0.76)	36
High school or more	10,565	30 (0.58)***	18 (0.48)***	40
Financial dependence:				
Yes	2,767	47 (1.67)	31 (1.55)	34
No	16,318	31 (0.50)***	18 (0.42)***	42

Table 13-1 continues

Table 13–1 continued

	N	Prevalence of Any Disorder[a] in Percent (SE)		
		Lifetime Prevalence	Active Cases in Last Year	Remission[b]
Occupational status of men 30–64:				
Total	3,452	35 (0.81)	17 (0.77)	51
Unemployed	774	48 (2.46)	29 (2.24)	40
Unskilled	599	40 (2.48)*	19 (2.00)*	53
Skilled or higher	2,061	30 (1.15)***	14 (0.86)*	53
Site:[c]				
Baltimore	3,586	41 (0.98)	27 (0.89)	34
Durham	4,123	35 (1.00)***	23 (0.88)	34
Los Angeles	3,503	33 (0.94)	18 (0.78)***	45
St. Louis	3,327	31 (1.12)	18 (0.92)	42
New Haven	5,101	28 (0.85)*	18 (0.37)	36
Rural/Urban:[c]				
Urban	4,694	34 (0.89)	21 (0.77)	38
Rural	2,107	32 (1.37)	20 (1.18)	38
Marital history:				
Married and never div/sep	9,216	24 (0.63)	13 (0.50)	46
Single and never cohabited for one year	3,424	33 (1.07)***	22 (0.95)***	33
Never divorced/separated	5,906	44 (0.99)***	27 (0.88)***	39
Unmarried and cohabited	986	52 (2.77)**	36 (2.66)**	31

[a]Negative cases who failed to answer questions in person about one-third or more of the specific diagnoses are considered uninformative and are not included in these analyses. See Appendix Table A–2 for explanation of sample sizes.

[b]Lifetime minus active (one-year) divided by lifetime: $(Lt - 1 Yr)/Lt$.

[c]Weighted to local populations, rather than the nation. The two sites for which rural/urban comparisons were made were Durham and St. Louis.

Significantly different from group just above:

*$p < .05$

**$p < .01$

***$p < .001$

illness are in keeping with results from studies of clinical populations, which note the dearth of older people in psychiatric treatment settings (Bahn, Chandler, & Lemkau, 1962; Sturt, Wykes, & Creer, 1982).

There are many possible explanations for the puzzling observation that older persons do not have higher *lifetime* rates of disorder than younger persons. We explored many of the possible artifacts that could account for this finding, such as the elderly attributing their symptoms to physical illness or dismissing their symptoms as trivial, or having mild cognitive impairment (which is not counted as a disorder in these analyses) that might have made them poor historians, or having a longer interval since last experiencing symptoms and so forgetting their occurrence. Yet the phenomenon persisted when first, symptoms attributed to physical illness were counted as psychiatric, second, symptoms originally assessed as trivial because no treatment had been sought and they were said not to have interfered much with activities were counted as positive, third, prevalences were compared by age only for those who made no more than one or two errors on the Mini-Mental State Examination, showing they did not have dementia. The fourth possibility, that the elderly forgot more past disorders because they occurred longer ago, may be a factor, since they have particularly low rates of current disorders (Table 13-1). We also considered whether the highly structured interview used in the ECA might have worked less well for older adults, but this explanation is unlikely because the same phenomenon has been found in samples interviewed in a more clinical fashion (Bland, Newman, & Orn, 1986; Klerman, 1988; Lavori et al., 1987). The most telling argument against believing that the finding was entirely a methodological artifact was that it did not apply equally to *all* elderly in the ECA, but chiefly to whites (Table 13-2). It is hard to imagine any artifacts explaining a low rate in the elderly that would apply uniquely to whites. In addition, a lower rate in the elderly was not found when the identical interview used in the ECA was given in cultures very different from the U.S., that is, in Puerto Rico, Seoul, and Taiwan (Canino et al., in press; Lee et al., 1984; Yeh et al., 1984).

Since artifacts do not seem to be the explanation, what might occasion

Table 13-2 Age, Sex, and Ethnicity and Lifetime Disorder

| | Percent Ever Experiencing a Disorder | |
	Men	Women
Whites:		
Under 45	41	35
45–64	28	24
65+	21	19
Blacks:		
Under 45	41	37
45–64	47***	33*
65+	39*	30
Hispanics:		
Under 45	42	28
45–64	33	32
65+	30	18

Significantly different from whites in this sex and age group:
*$p < .05$
***$p < .001$

the lower lifetime rate of disorder in older persons? One plausible explanation is that psychiatric disorder accounts for premature deaths, leaving behind psychiatrically healthy older survivors. Follow-up studies of psychiatric patients do show an elevated risk of death (Tsuang & Woolson, 1978). And deaths from psychiatric causes might play a relatively more important role among the more advantaged parts of a population, for whom competing physical causes of death were longer delayed. The second possibility is that white Americans have experienced a gradual increase in psychiatric illnesses beginning early in life over the past 50 years, an increase the elderly were born too early to have been affected by. There is evidence compatible with an increase of disorder affecting only younger persons in the steady rise in per capita alcohol consumption since the end of Prohibition in 1933 and in medical and legal problems with drug abuse since 1970. Rising rates of criminal offenses over the last 50 years are also consistent with increasing antisocial personality among the young, although they might also reflect effects of improved record-keeping or increasing population density. Increasing suicide rates in young men and decreasing rates in elderly men are also consistent with the young having an increased rate of major depression and substance abuse, the two disorders most closely associated with suicide (Robins & Kulbok, 1986). However, it is not clear that blacks would not have had similar experiences. In any case, comparing age distributions for specific diagnoses will show whether the disorders that seem to have increased—alcohol and drug absuse, antisocial personality, and depression—account for most of the relative increase in disorder among the young.

ETHNIC GROUP

Blacks had a higher rate of both lifetime (38%) and active (26%) disorder than did whites or Hispanics (Table 13-1). Hispanics fell between the other two groups, and did not differ significantly from either. Because, on average, blacks are younger and poorer than whites and receive less education, their higher rates might be attributable to their demographic characteristics rather than their ethnic membership. Their younger age was not the answer (Table 13-2). Black rates exceeded white rates only for men and women over 45 and the principal difference occurred in men in the 45-64 year age range.

As will be seen below, the higher rates for older blacks was largely attributable to their having more errors on the Mini-Mental State Examination used to diagnose current cognitive impairment. Scores on that test have been shown to be strongly correlated with education and social status (Anthony et al., 1982). The fact that many older blacks grew up in rural areas where their racially segregated schools were particularly inadequate, and that they dropped out of school earlier than whites, spent more time unemployed, and when employed typically held unskilled jobs is a likely explanation for their lower scores. However, as will be explained below, survey data cannot definitively answer questions about the degree to which poor education and subsequent low social status account for the cognitive impairment in older blacks.

EDUCATION AND SOCIOECONOMIC STATUS (SES)

If the ECA had gathered information about parents' education and occupation when the respondent was a child as measures of social status, SES could have been investigated as a possible cause of disorder, because it would have predated the onset of illness. Instead SES was measured by the respondents' own educational level, current income, and current occupation. The earliest of these measures is final educational level, which is set for a large proportion of Americans by age 18. However, as we noted above, the median age of first symptom is age 16. Therefore, even educational level often does not predate disease onset. Income and occupation were assessed at the time of interview, clearly subsequent to the onset of disorder, but because both are influenced by educational level and early occupational history, they often reflect premorbid characteristics as well as the effects of intercurrent physical and psychiatric illness. Thus, they may be both indicators of risk factors for psychiatric disorder and its consequence. Persons who failed to complete high school had a distinctly greater risk of disorder than those who were high school graduates (36% versus 30%) (Table 13-1).

An unequivocal measure of poverty is being on welfare or receiving disability payments from Social Security. For persons in this situation, rates of disorder are even higher than among those who failed to graduate from high school—almost half (47%) had a disorder at some time and almost one-third (31%) had active symptoms (Table 13-1). This high rate may in part reflect the fact that severe psychiatric disorder itself can be a disability qualifying for support.

Employment is an effective measure of social status only for those in the labor market, excluding young people still in school, older people who have retired, and women who work parttime or as housewives. To study employment, we limited our sample to people who could be expected to be in the labor market: men aged 30–64. Occupational level is a valid measure only for those in full-time employment. To look at its correlates with disorder, we looked only at employed men 30–64.

Men 30 to 64 had the same level of lifetime disorder (35%) as the whole sample of men, but less active disorder (17%) (Table 13–1). Highest rates of both lifetime (48%) and active (29%) disorder were found among those not working full-time. But men working in unskilled jobs also had more disorder both over their lifetime (40%) and actively (19%) than those in better jobs.

SITE DIFFERENCES

The highest rates of lifetime and active disorder were found in Baltimore (41% lifetime; 27% active), and the lowest rates in New Haven (28% lifetime; 18% active).

The differences between sites could not be explained by different proportions nonwhite. For both blacks and whites, Baltimore had the highest and New Haven had the lowest rates (Table 13–3). It is beyond the scope of this study to explain why the sites differed. For Baltimore, the explanation for its high rate may lie in the low socioeconomic status of the particular catchment areas selected. The particularly low rate in New Haven may be related to the fact that it is the site with the largest proportion of college graduates.

RURAL–URBAN RESIDENCE

Little difference was found between rural and urban settings in the two sites that had both, St. Louis and Durham (Table 13–1).

Table 13–3 Site and Ethnicity as Predictors of Lifetime Psychiatric Disorder

Site	Lifetime Prevalence[a] of Any Disorder (Percent)		
	Total	Whites	Blacks
Baltimore	41***	38*	46*
Durham	35	34	38
Los Angeles	33	32	33
St. Louis	31	31	35
New Haven	28	28	31

[a]Weighted to populations of catchment areas sampled in each site.
Significantly different from each other site:
*$p < .05$
***$p < .001$

MARITAL HISTORY

Rates of lifetime disorder were particularly high among those who had been separated or divorced (44%) or who had cohabited without ever marrying (52%)(Table 13-1). These groups also had higher rates than others of active disorder (27% and 36%, respectively). Those who married and never divorced or separated had the lowest rate of disorder (24% lifetime and 13% active), less even than single persons who never cohabited for a year.

As with unemployment and poverty, these strong relationships may be both a cause and effect of psychiatric disorder: psychiatric disorder clearly causes marital difficulties, and marital difficulties are stressful events than may cause or prolong disorder.

While we cannot disentangle cause from consequence for these correlates of active disorder, the best social indicators of psychiatric disorder are being divorced or separated or cohabiting, financial dependency, and, among men in the labor market, unemployment.

INSTITUTIONALIZATION

Long-term institutions care for the mentally ill, the profoundly mentally retarded, convicts, those with severe chronic physical illnesses or disabilities, and those in long-term treatment for substance abuse. If only because they include long-term psychiatric patients and substance abuse clients, one would expect that, taken as a whole, institutional residents would have higher rates of psychiatric disorder than household residents. And this was the case. Indeed, 65% of all institutionalized individuals had a history of psychiatric disorder, and 51% were active cases (Table 13-4). Although the institutionalized population's rate of disorder is very high, its inclusion in the sample had little impact on overall lifetime rates because so small a proportion of the population is institutionalized. However, including the institutionalized did reduce estimated rates of remission; rates of remission are somewhat higher in the household sample than in the total population (41% versus 38%).

We divided the institutionalized population into three groups: those in mental hospitals, those in jails or residential drug and alcohol treatment settings, and those in nursing homes and other chronic care facilities. Residents in all three types of institutions had high rates of active psychiatric disorder as compared with household residents. Surprisingly, rates of disorder did not differ significantly among the institutions. The fact that some patients in psychiatric hospitals did not meet criteria for an active disorder is probably explained by uncovered psychiatric diagnoses, cases whose poor insight into their conditions made their report of symptoms incomplete, and those in need of hospitalization despite not meeting cri-

Table 13–4 Psychiatric Disorder and Institutionalization

	N	Lifetime Prevalence %	Active (One-Year) %	Proportion of Affected in Remission %
Not institutionalized	18,059	32	19	41
Any institution:	1,581	65	51	22
Psychiatric hospital	174	78	73	6
Prison or residential alcohol/drug center	709	83	57	31
Nursing home or chronic hospital	698	57	46	19

teria for a diagnosis, perhaps because they had very serious symptoms such as a suicide attempt. Much institutional care flows to those with severe cognitive impairment (see chapter 12). Among those with other active disorders, only 1% were in institutions.

CORRELATES OF REMISSION

Overall, more than one-third (38%) of those who ever met criteria for one or more psychiatric disorders had no signs of their disorders in the current year, and so could be considered to be in remission.

Employed men 30–64 years of age had higher rates of remission than others (51%) (Table 13–1). Remission was least common, not surprisingly, in the very young (32%), whose disorders, having begun most recently, had had least time in which to remit. A similarly low rate of remission in the never married reflects their youth.

TREATMENT

To assess the amount of treatment received by the psychiatrically disordered, those *not* institutionalized were asked whether they had seen any professional about a mental health problem or a problem with drugs or alcohol in the six months before interview, and whether they had been hospitalized because of emotional or mental problems or substance abuse in the prior year. Treatment was broadly defined. The professionals seen were limited neither to psychiatrists nor to physicians, and hospitalization in a general hospital would have counted if the reason was a mental health problem.

Only 19% of household residents with an active disorder in the current year reported either inpatient treatment in the last year or outpatient treatment in the last six months (Table 13-5). Hospitalizations were reported by 2.4%. Clearly, there is a very large volume of untreated mental disorder in the population.

Treatment among those actively affected did not differ by age. But, affected women got more treatment than affected men (23% versus 14%), and the unmarried more than the married (20% versus 17%). Married men with little education who had active disorders were particularly unlikely to receive treatment—only 11% did (Table 13-6). Active disorder had the greatest likelihood of receiving treatment when it occurred in unmarried women who had completed high school, but even this affected group had had recent treatment in only 27% of cases.

We also found that a more than trivial proportion of those without an active disorder had been in treatment, 10% of those with a past disorder but no symptoms of that disorder in the past year and 4% of those who never had one of the covered disorders. Some of those with past disorders may have been seen in follow-up or prophylactically. Some of those who did not meet criteria for having ever had a disorder may have suffered from disorders we had not covered in our interview; others may have had disturbing symptoms of covered disorders but did not quite meet diagnostic criteria; and still others may have sought care for "problems of living," such as marital counseling.

Finally, in any clinical setting, one should expect some persons without a

Table 13-5 Household Residents Receiving Mental Health Services

Mental Health of Household Residents	N	Mental Health Services Received (%)		
		Inpatient (Last Year)	Out-Patient Only (Last Six Months)	Total
Active (one-year) cases	3,678	2.4	16.4[a]	18.7[a]
Cases in remission	2,220	0.5	9.7	10.1
No positive diagnosis	12,161	0.3	3.8	4.1

[a]Rises to 18.9% receiving outpatient care and to 21.3% receiving any mental health care if the group of active cases is limited to those with symptoms in the last six months.

Table 13–6 Mental Health Services if Active (One-Year) Disorder Among
Household Residents by Marital Status and Education

		Number with Active Disorder	Percent Treated as Inpatients (1 Yr.) or Outpatients (6 Mo.)
Men:			
Married	Not high school graduate	297	11
	High school graduate	306	13
Unmarried	Not high school graduate	393	17
	High school graduate	436	14
Women:			
Married	Not high school graduate	336	21
	High school graduate	441	22
Unmarried	Not high school graduate	767	22
	High school graduate	668	27

disorder because some of those self-referred or referred by a primary care physician to be screened for suspected mental disorder will be found not to have such a disorder.

Differences Between Specific Disorders

Thus far, this chapter has been concerned with psychiatric disorders in America without distinguishing type of disorder, in much the fashion of older surveys. This has given us an opportunity to estimate the total burden of disorder in the population, to discover that much disorder goes un-treated, and to correct some of the misperceptions from these older stud-ies—in particular, that women have more psychiatric disorder than men and that older people have more disorder than younger. It has also con-firmed the associations reported by previous studies between psychiatric disorder and poverty, low education, and disrupted marriages, while raising questions about whether such correlates of disorder should be interpreted as its cause or its consequences. But the great strength of the ECA is that it makes specific diagnoses. We now bring together the results from the earlier chapters to contrast and compare the various disorders with respect to their prevalence, their risk periods for onset, their correlates, their patterns of co-occurrence, and the frequency with which they come to treatment.

PREVALENCE

The most common disorders in America are phobia and alcohol abuse (Table 13-7). Fourteen percent of adults have had a phobia at some time in their lives, 9% within the current year, and 14% have abused alcohol at some time, 6% within the current year. The next most common lifetime disorder is generalized anxiety, found in 8.5%, followed in frequency by a history of major depressive episode or abuse of illicit drugs, approximately 6% each. Generalized anxiety and major depressive episodes had occurred in the last year in almost 4% of the population, drug abuse in less than 3%. Cognitive impairment was assessed only on a current basis, and was found

Table 13-7 Prevalence of Specific Disorders (Percent)

	Lifetime	Active (One-Year)
Phobia	14.3	8.8
Alcohol abuse/dependence	13.8	6.3
Generalized anxiety	8.5	3.8
Major depressive episode	6.4	3.7
Drug abuse/dependence	6.2	2.5
Cognitive impairment: mild or severe	a	5.0
Dysthymia	3.3	a
Antisocial personality	2.6	1.2
Obsessive compulsive	2.6	1.7
Panic	1.6	0.9
Schizophrenia or schizophreniform	1.5	1.0
Manic episode	0.8	0.6
Cognitive impairment: severe	a	0.9
Somatization	0.1	0.1

[a]Not ascertained.

to be the third most common active disorder when mild as well as severe cases were counted, but severe cognitive impairment was rare (about 1%).

The rarest of all the disorders reported here was somatization disorder, which occurred in only 1 per thousand. Anorexia nervosa was even less prevalent, and is not reported in this volume because only 11 cases were identified (see Appendix Table A–3).

REMISSION

The disorders most likely to remit, that is, to have no symptoms present in the last year although criteria had been met earlier, were alcohol and drug disorders, antisocial personality, and generalized anxiety. More than half the persons with a history of these disorders had been free of their symptoms for a year (Table 13–8). This high rate of remission for alcohol and drug disorders differs from results for clinical samples, where relapse rates are traditionally very high, but agrees with previous follow-up studies in the general population, which show high rates of instability in the reporting of

Table 13–8 Likelihood of Remission[a]

Disorder	Number Ever Affected	No Symptoms within One Year %
Drug abuse/dependence	1,316	59
Generalized anxiety	722	56
Alcohol abuse/dependence	2,630	54
Antisocial personality	628	53
Major depressive episode	1,258	42
Panic	304	42
Phobia	3,053	38
Schizophrenia	305	36
Obsessive compulsive	571	33
Manic episode	172	28
Somatization	67	8

[a]Omitted are dysthymia, for which active status is unknown, and cognitive impairment, for which past occurrence is unknown.

current problems between interviews a few years apart (Taylor & Helzer, 1983). The high recovery rate for antisocial personality may seem surprising, given that this is a personality disorder from Axis II, and personality disorders are supposed to be essentially lifelong. However, it is confirmed in earlier studies (Robins, 1966).

The disorders with the lowest recovery rates were somatization disorder (only 8% of those ever affected had been free of its symptoms for the last year) and mania (only 28% of those affected had been free of its symptoms for the last year). However, the numbers with somatization disorder and mania were small, and therefore, the estimates for their remission rates are not very stable.

Persons with episodes of major depression were in remission in less than half the cases (42%). The fact that the majority of lifetime cases of both mania and depressive episodes, the only disorders unequivocally discussed as episodic in DSM-III, reported an episode in the last year may seem surprising. Perhaps those with a serious past episode are misperceiving recent normal elation or sadness as a recurrence. It is also possible that some who recover forget their earlier episodes, and so are counted as never having been manic or depressed rather than in remission. However, recent follow-up studies of clinical samples with major depressive disorder have shown a much higher level of chronicity than was previously thought to be the case (Keller et al., 1986); similar prospective studies of community samples will be needed to learn whether chronicity is also the rule for affective disorders that do not come to treatment.

Schizophrenia, unlike manic and depressive episodes, is widely believed to be a chronic, unremitting illness. It should be emphasized that our definition of remission for schizophrenia refers only to the remission of what have been called the first-rank symptoms—hallucinations and delusions. We were not able to assess the persistence of more subtle residual symptoms of unusual ideas or diminished social and occupational effectiveness. Nonetheless, we found schizophrenia to be more chronic than most other disorders, with only 36% of those affected free of first-rank symptoms for at least a year.

AGE OF ONSET AND AGES AT RISK

Which disorders begin first? DSM-III sets maximum ages of onset for three disorders: age 15 for antisocial personality, age 30 for somatization disorder, and age 45 for schizophrenia. For all three, this upper limit is about double the age at which they typically begin: antisocial personality at 8, somatization at 15, and schizophrenia at 19 (Table 13-9). For other disorders there is no upper limit in the official diagnostic criteria. Yet three additional psychi-

Table 13-9 Onset, Risk Periods, and Duration of Disorders

	Number Who Recall Onset	Median Age of Onset	Age by Which 90% Had the First Symptom	Duration for Those in Remission	
				N	(Mean Yrs)
Antisocial personality	763	8	12	149	19.7
Phobia	2,645	10	48	646	15.4
Somatization	67	15	23	3	a
Drug abuse/dependence	1,575	18	27	458	2.7
Schizophrenia	346	19	35	76	5.4
Manic episode	156	19	37	44	5.9
Obsessive compulsive	777	20	50	138	6.4
Alcohol abuse/dependence	3,125	21	38	1,008	8.7
Panic	418	23	42	81	7.1
Depressive episode	1,536	25	52	439	6.4

[a]Cell size below 25. Too few to calculate.

atric disorders also typically begin before age 20: phobia at 10, drug abuse at 18, and manic episodes at 19. All the disorders covered by the ECA study began on average by the midtwenties. (Of course, this excludes cognitive impairment, for which we had no age of onset.)

The range of ages over which a disorder begins tells us what the risk period of new cases is. To exclude highly unusual cases, we defined the end of the risk period as the age by which 90% of those affected had had a first symptom or episode. We found no risk period, by this definition, extending past the early fifties, when it ended for depression and obsessive compulsive disorder (Table 13-9). The only other disorders whose risk periods extended past age 40 were phobia and panic. The period of risk for some disorders might have extended somewhat longer if the sample had been followed over time. However, since half were over 40 at interview and the great preponderance of the risk period is over by then, even follow-up to death would probably have resulted in only a modest lengthening of the risk periods.

Disorders varied in the length of their risk periods. Longest risks (measured by the interval between the 50th and 90th percentiles) were for phobia, obsessive compulsive disorder, and depression; shortest periods of risk were for antisocial personality, somatization, and drug abuse/dependence.

DURATION

The average duration of a disorder can be estimated for those in remission by subtracting the age of onset from the age at which the last symptom appeared. We do not attempt to estimate duration for those still active, because we do not know how long the disorder is likely to continue.

Among those who recovered from their disorders, the longest average duration was experienced by persons with antisocial personality (19.7 years) (Table 13-9). Thus, while antisocial personality has a high recovery rate, it is not a brief disorder and seems appropriately placed in DSM-III on Axis II among the early onset, long duration personality disorders. Other disorders with long durations are phobia and alcoholism (an average of 15.4 and 8.7 years respectively). Shortest durations were experienced by recovered drug abusers (2.7 years).

INSTITUTIONALIZATION

The relative frequency of disorders in institutions is quite different from that found in the general population. In the institutionalized sample, current cognitive impairment (mild or severe) leads all others, with 51% of the institutionalized population affected, more than ten times the rate among household residents (Table 13-10). Severe cognitive impairment was found in 24% of the institutional residents, 24 times the rate in households; mild cognitive disorders in 27%, 7 times the rate among household residents. Other disorders with rates in institutional residents at least three times that in the household population are schizophrenia (3% of the institutionalized), somatization disorder (2% of the institutionalized), drug abuse (9% of the institutionalized), and antisocial personality (5% of the institutionalized). While these disorders may well have occasioned institutionalization, disorders can also be more common in institutional populations than in household residents just because they tend to occur along with the disorders that occasion institutionalization. This probably explains why every disorder is more common in institutionalized than in household populations.

People with different types of disorder are handled in different kinds of institutions (Table 13-11). Of those institutionalized with cognitive impairment, whether mild or severe, 92% were in nursing homes and similar settings, while over 75% of those institutionalized with substance abuse or

Table 13-10 Active Psychiatric Disorder in Institutionalized Persons

	% Institutionalized Residents Affected (1,640)	% Household Residents Affected (18,198)
Cognitive impairment:		
Mild or severe	51	5
Severe	24	1
Phobia	13	9
Alcohol abuse/dependence	12	6
Depressive episode	10	4
Drug abuse/dependence	9	2
Generalized anxiety	6	4
Antisocial personality	5	1
Obsessive compulsive	5	2
Schizophrenia	3	1
Manic episode	2	1
Somatization	2	a
Panic	2	1

[a]Less than 0.5%.

antisocial personality were in prisons or residential substance abuse programs. Persons with schizophrenia and manic episodes, however, appear in substantial numbers in all three types of institutions, prisons, mental hospitals, and chronic care settings. It has been documented that the closing of many large mental hospitals has resulted in the scattering of persons who would have been their patients among a variety of institutions (Redick, 1974).

RISK FACTORS
FOR PREVALENCE OF SPECIFIC DISORDERS

We have noted above that taking all psychiatric disorders together, men have had more disorders over their lifetime than women, as have younger more than older persons, blacks more than whites, and the undereducated

Table 13-11 Types of Institutions in Which Institutionalized
Active Cases Were Found

Institutionalized with Active Disorder	Number in Any Institution	Percent Institutionalized in:		
		Prison	Psychiatric	Chronic Care
Somatization	22	13	15	72
Cognitive impairment				
Mild or severe	597	1	7	92
Severe	259	0	7	93
Schizophrenia	76	34	24	41
Antisocial personality	131	88	4	8
Drug abuse/dependence	243	85	10	5
Manic episode	27	42	26	32
Obsessive compulsive	86	50	31	19
Major depressive episode	145	40	13	47
Panic	38	45	36	18
Generalized anxiety	39	50	10	40
Alcohol abuse/dependence	182	78	11	11
Phobia	218	38	12	50
Any active disorder	1,640	24	8	68

more than the well-educated. We also noted that active disorder, again as a whole, is more common in those who are financially dependent, the unemployed, and those with low job status if employed. Disorder is also common in those divorced, separated, or cohabitating. We ask now whether these findings apply uniformly across all disorders or whether these correlates of mental disorder as a whole apply only to certain disorders.

To categorize a risk factor as substantial, we will require that persons with the risk factor have a prevalence of disorder that is at least twice that among persons without the risk factor, that is, a prevalence ratio of two or more. No risk factors for psychiatric disorder as a whole had a prevalence ratio this high because large prevalences limit their range. For example, men and women differ in their lifetime rates of any disorder by 6% (36% − 30%), but their prevalence ratio is only 1.2 (36%/30%). In contrast, men and women differ in their lifetime rates of antisocial personality by only 3.7% (4.5% −0.8%), but their prevalence ratio is 5.6 (4.5%/0.8%).

We report prevalence ratios of two or higher for both lifetime (L) and active (A) disorder in Table 13–12. There are more positive results for active than for lifetime disorders because the prevalence of an active disorder is always lower than the prevalence category of the same disorder on a lifetime basis.

Table 13–12   Demographic Correlates[a] of Lifetime and Active Diagnosis

	Sex		Age			Education	Ethnic	
	F Vs. M	M Vs. F	18–29 Vs. Next	30–44 Older	45–64 Group	<12 Years Vs. More	Black Vs.	Hispanic White
Antisocial		LA	LA	LA	LA	LA		
Drug abuse/ dependence		A	LA	LA	LA			
Manic episode			LA	LA	LA			
Schizophrenic				LA	LA			
Somatization	LA		b			LA	LA	
Alcohol abuse/ dependence		LA	A		A			
Obsessive compulsive	L		A	A				
Depressive episode	LA				LA			
Cognitive impairment, severe				b	b	A	A	c
Generalized anxiety	A							
Panic	A				A			
Phobia	A							
Dysthymia								

[a]Entries shown when prevalence ratios are greater than 2 for lifetime (L) or active (A) disorders. The prevalence ratio is the percent positive for the disorder in the first demographic category divided by the percent positive in the second demographic category.

[b]Prevalence ratio vs. next older is less than 0.5.

[c]Prevalence ratio is greater than 2 if mild as well as severe cognitive impairment included.

Those interested in the specific percentages on which these ratios are based will find them in earlier chapters covering the individual disorders.

GENDER

Although overall men had more lifetime disorder than women (Table 13-1), a sizeable male excess was found for only two disorders—alcohol abuse and antisocial personality—while women's lifetime rates substantially exceeded men's for three disorders—somatization disorder, obsessive compulsive disorder, and major depressive episode. The high overall rate for men despite an excess of fewer specific disorders is explained by the fact that alcohol abuse/dependence is so common a disorder and the male excess of it is so great. Men and women did not differ in their overall active disorder rates, and the distribution of gender dominance for specific disorders is reasonably even: four active disorders more common in women than in men, and three more common in men than women.

The higher ratio for lifetime than active obsessive compulsive disorder suggests that its remission is more common in women than in men.

AGE

We had found overall that the younger half of the age range had experienced more psychiatric disorder than their elders. Their high lifetime rates are largely explained by antisocial personality, drug disorders, and manic episodes (Table 13-12). For these three, there was a substantial increase in prevalence in each successively younger cohort. These three disorders may be increasing over time and their rates still rising. An alternative possibility is that all lead to premature death, and that the risk of excess deaths continues over the lifetime, so that each successively older cohort will have lost more cases by death. However, for two out of three of these disorders, drug disorders and antisocial personality, there is good objective evidence for a true increase in prevalence, as shown by rising demand for treatment for drug addiction and rising proportions of young people arrested.

Schizophrenia was substantially higher in those 30-44 than in those 45-64, who in turn suffered more cases of schizophrenia than did those over 65. The fact that the youngest cohort did not show a significant excess over the next oldest may be explained by the fact that more of its members are still in the age of major risk of a first schizophrenic episode, since the end of the risk period for schizophrenic onsets is age 35 (Table 13-9). For major depressive and panic episodes, the only substantial age difference is a low rate in the elderly. No substantial excess was found in younger people for five disorders: somatization, generalized anxiety, phobia, panic, and, of course, cognitive impairment. Somatization disorder was the one example of a disorder with twice the rate in those 30–44 than in those 18–29. Severe cognitive impairment was more common in each successively older cohort, but was more than twice as frequent in those 45–64 as in those 30–44, and more than twice as frequent in those over 65 as in those 45–64.

EDUCATION

The earlier observation that failure to complete high school is associated with a high lifetime rate of psychiatric disorder appears to depend on its relation to three disorders: somatization disorder, antisocial personality, and cognitive impairment. (Drug abuse and depression were actually somewhat higher in those who finished high school, but the excess was not substantial and so does not appear in Table 13–12).

Somatization disorder and antisocial personality are disorders with unusually early onsets, making it questionable that a lower rate of schooling was a cause rather than a consequence of these disorders. The association with cognitive impairment has been claimed by some to indicate that poor education is a contributing factor, and by others as showing that the Mini-Mental State Examination cannot distinguish reliably between dementia and low IQ or educational disadvantage (Anthony et al., 1982; Mortimer, 1988).

ETHNIC GROUP

Blacks older than 45 had a higher lifetime risk of disorder overall than older whites (Table 13–2). This was accounted for largely by their higher rate of cognitive impairment (whether severe alone or both mild and severe are counted). Somatization disorder was also more common in blacks, but was such a rare disorder that it made little contribution to the overall rate. Since both the disorders more common in blacks than whites are strongly associated with low educational level, it is likely that the low educational level of the older black population plays a major role in explaining their higher rate of disorder.

The disorders associated with criminality, drug and alcohol abuse and antisocial personality, were not higher in blacks than whites, despite the overrepresentation of blacks in prisons and jails. The chapter on antisocial personality shows that this is consistent with a somewhat different pattern of symptoms for blacks than whites who have these disorders, more use of weapons by blacks, and blacks' greater chance of being incarcerated given similar arrestable behavior.

CURRENT LIFE-STYLE AND ACTIVE DISORDERS

As noted above, given the early age of onset of most disorders (Table 13-9), current life situations of persons with active disorder are at least as likely to be evidence for the social costs of mental disorder as evidence for social situations that cause it. However, these social situations may have been instrumental in prolonging the symptoms of disorders or causing relapses, and thus explain why disorders are still active rather than in remission.

JOB STATUS

Among men 30-64, there were too few cases of somatization and cognitive impairment to compare those unemployed or holding lower-ranking jobs with those holding better ones. For other disorders, the unemployed had at least double the rate of the employed of every disorder except drug abuse (Table 13-13). Mania, schizophrenia, and panic disorder were particularly

Table 13-13 Active Disorders in Males 30-64 by Job Level and Employment

	Prevalence of Disorder When Job Is:			Not Employed Full-Time	
	Skilled or Higher (2,062) %	Unskilled (598) %	Prevalence Ratio[a]	(861) %	Prevalence Ratio[b]
Manic episode	0.2	0.5	2.5	1.4	4.7
Depressive episode	1.7	1.7	-	4.3	2.5
Drug abuse	1.3	1.8	-	1.5	-
Schizophrenia	0.4	1.2	3.0	2.7	4.5
Obsessive compulsive	1.0	0.7	-	2.7	3.0
Phobia	4.6	4.8	-	10.7	2.3
Panic	0.3	0.8	2.7	2.3	5.7
Antisocial personality	0.7	2.6	3.8	3.1	2.6
Alcohol abuse	8.1	14.7	-	19.6	2.1

[a]Prevalence of disorder in the unskilled divided by prevalence in these skilled if greater than 2. A dash indicates a prevalence ratio below 2.

[b]Prevalence of disorder in unemployed divided by prevalence in those employed if greater than 2. A dash indicates a prevalence ratio below 2.

overrepresented among the unemployed, with prevalences more than four times that in the employed. These same three disorders were also over-represented among unskilled workers, as compared with other employed men. Thus, these disorders may both keep men from working and make them ineligible for promotion when they work. In addition, antisocial personality was associated with low-status jobs, perhaps because it interfered with completing an education (Table 13–12). No disorder was significantly more common in those with higher- than lower-status jobs.

MARITAL STATUS

In early studies, it was frequently reported that schizophrenia and alcoholism were associated with never marrying. However, some previous studies of alcoholics have not found many bachelors and have questioned whether elderly alcoholics may not fail to report brief early marriages (Bailey, 1961). And the emptying of mental hospitals beginning in the 1950s has greatly increased the opportunities for schizophrenics to marry (Bland & Orn, 1978).

The only disorder in which a majority of the affected (61%) have never married is drug abuse (Table 13–14). Other disorders in which more than one-third of those affected are still single are schizophrenia (36%), manic episode (37%), alcohol abuse (39%), and antisocial personality (35%). Drug abuse, mania, and antisocial personality are the only disorders in which lifetime prevalence is substantially highest in those under 30 (Table 13–12), and thus the only disorders in which a large proportion are still so young that many of those single are likely to marry in the future. The other two disorders with considerable numbers single are the two traditionally believed to prevent marriage—alcoholism and schizophrenia, although most people with both disorders have married.

Much more dramatic than the association with not marrying is the association of psychiatric disorder with marital breakup. Rates of being currently separated or divorced were at least twice as high for those with almost any active disorder as for those without the disorder of interest. The exceptions were drug abuse and cognitive impairment. The only reason drug abusers did not have that high a rate is that few had married. Among drug abusers who had ever married, the rate of divorce or separation (36%) was three times that for those without disorder, higher than for all other disorders except schizophrenia. Although cognitive impairment occurred at an age at which many were already widowed, and so not at risk for divorce, their risk of divorce and separation was still somewhat higher than rates for those without psychiatric disorder (16% versus 10%).

The highest proportion currently divorced or separated (26%) was found among those with schizophrenia. While early release from hospitals has

Table 13-14 Marital Status of Those with Active Mental Disorders

	Number with Active Disorder	Divorced/ Separated %	Single %	Widowed %	Married %	Divorced/ Separated of Those Ever Married %
Schizophrenia	229	26	36	5	33	41
Depressive episode	812	22	26	8	44	30
Panic	196	22	22	6	51	28
Somatization	64	21	25	26	28	28
Generalized anxiety	359	20	25	5	49	27
Manic episode	112	20	37	5	39	31
Alcohol abuse/ dependence	1,018	18	39	3	40	30
Antisocial personality	295	18	35	2	44	28
Phobia	2,118	16	22	7	55	21
Obsessive compulsive	385	16	25	7	52	21
Drug abuse/dependence	602	14	61	1	24	36
Cognitive impairment: Mild or severe	2,039	12	16	27	45	14
Severe	421	12	23	37	28	16
None of the diagnoses	5,777	8	23	8	61	10

increased chances that persons with schizophrenia will marry, the fact that two-fifths (41%) of those with schizophrenia who had married were not married at interview indicates that these marriages are unstable and remarriage difficult.

Widowhood, which occurs usually late in life, has been thought nonetheless to be a risk factor for depression. However, when episodes of depression identified specifically with bereavement were not counted, widowhood was found to be related only to the two disorders positively associated with older age—somatization disorder and cognitive impairment, both chronic disorders. It looks, therefore, as though widowhood was not an important risk factor either for causing new disorder or causing the relapse or persistence of preexisting disorders.

CO-OCCURRENCE OF DISORDERS

So far, we have examined each specific disorder separately. We turn now to look at the degree to which multiple disorders occur when the diagnostic preemptions in DSM-III are not used. Looking at co-occurrence has both practical, theoretical, and nosological interest. Practically, individuals who have multiple psychiatric disorders are in need of multifaceted treatment. Physicians should be urged to note the full diagnostic picture, rather than treating only the disorder that occasioned treatment seeking, because the presence of other disorders may defeat the therapeutic efforts or increase risks of relapse of the treated disorder.

Co-occurrence also raises important theoretical questions about why certain disorders occur together at a rate well above chance—are they caused by the same factors, or does having one of these disorders itself increase the risk of having another? If one disorder can cause another, then the risk factors we have identified for a particular disorder may be spurious: they may actually only be risk factors for another disorder that caused that disorder.

Finally, co-occurrence across diagnostic groupings raises nosological questions about the way our diagnostic system is organized. Adult disorders in DSM-III are assorted into broader categories identified as the affective disorders, substance abuse, anxiety disorders, schizophrenia, somatoform, personality disorders, and organic mental disorders. The basis for grouping disorders without known etiology or pathophysiology is, according to DSM-III, "shared clinical features." Shared clinical features should increase the chance of co-occurrence, because the same feature could simultaneously contribute to making both diagnoses. One would, therefore, other things being equal, expect co-occurrence chiefly among disorders that belong to the same broad category in DSM-III.

When exclusion rules that prevent giving a diagnosis if certain other diagnoses are present were ignored, we found that 18% of the total population or 60% of those with at least one disorder had had at least two psychiatric disorders in their lifetimes. Disorders with the highest rates of comorbidity are somatization, antisocial personality, panic, and schizophrenia, all over 90% (Table 13–15).

Of greater interest than comorbidity over the lifetime is co-occurrence of disorders within the last year, because that indicates how often people suffer from multiple disorders simultaneously. We considered whether reported concurrent disorders might be an artifact, explained by a general tendency to admit or deny symptoms. Reporting style would be the most likely explanation for co-occurrence if disorders were paired randomly. But if there are strong associations only between certain pairs of disorders, cooccurrence cannot be explained by general reporting style.

Table 13–15 Multiple Diagnoses Over the Lifetime Among Those Positive
for at Least One

Common Diagnoses	Number with this Diagnosis	Percent with at Least One Other Diagnosis
Somatization disorder	67	100
Antisocial personality	628	93
Panic	304	91
Schizophrenia/schizophreniform	340	91
Dysthymia	703	86
Agoraphobia	1,281	84
Obsessive compulsive	571	79
Depressive episode	1,258	75
Drug abuse/dependence	1,316	75
Simple phobia	2,482	63
Alcohol abuse/dependence	2,630	52
Cognitive impairment (mild or severe)	2,160	38

A standard way of comparing the strength of co-occurrence between pairs of events is by comparing their odds ratios. The odds ratio (OR) for the co-occurrence of two disorders is the ratio of the frequency with which the two disorders are simultaneously present or absent to the frequency with which one or the other appears alone. The formula is:

$$\frac{(\text{both present}) \times (\text{both absent})}{(\text{only the first present}) \times (\text{only the second present})}$$

On average, the odds that a pair of disorders would be concurrently active in the ECA study was 2, indicating that having any one disorder approximately doubled the chances of having any second disorder. If there are many disorders with odds ratios well above this average, then response set is an unlikely explanation. We chose an odds ratio of 10, with a lower bound of its confidence limits of 4, as an indicator of a strong association between disorders.

Without generalized anxiety, which was studied in only 3 sites, and dysthymia, for which active status was not assessed, there are 11 disorders reported in this volume. Eleven disorders can be combined into 55 pairs of disorders whose co-occurrence can be evaluated. Twenty-three of these 55 pairs had odds ratios greater than 10 (Table 13–16), and 21 had in addition a lower bound of its confidence limits above 4. These many extremely high odds ratios make a strong argument that comorbidity is not an artifact of response style.

Of the 55 pairs, 50 are cases where the two members come from different DSM-III categories, and 5 are cases where both members belong to the same broad DSM-III category, affective disorders, anxiety disorders, or substance abuse. Four of the 5 within-category pairs (80%) have an odds ratio for co-occurrence of 10 or higher, as do 19 (38%) of the cross-category pairs (Table 13–16). This higher average comorbidity within than across categories can perhaps be seen as a kind of validation of the DSM-III categories. However, 3 pairs of disorders that do not belong to the same DSM-III category had odds ratios as high or higher than the highest within-category odds ratio (which was found for depressive and manic episodes, OR = 36, lower bound = 21). Somatization was equally or more strongly associated with both panic (OR = 82, lower bound = 22) and schizophrenia (OR = 38, lower bound = 17), and mania was more strongly related to schizophrenia (OR = 46, lower bound = 23).

Co-occurrence of disorders must mean shared symptoms, shared risk factors, or that one disorder causes the other. The only shared symptoms in DSM-III were cardiopulmonary symptoms in both somatization and panic disorders, fatigue in both somatization disorder and depressive episodes, physical restlessness in both depressive and manic episodes, and speeding, fighting, and arrests as a result of drinking in both alcohol abuse/dependence and antisocial personality. Shared risk factors are shown in Table 13–12. Drug abuse and antisocial personality were both most common in young men; depressive episodes and somatization disorder were predominantly female disorders; somatization and cognitive impairment (mild or severe) were both associated with being black and not finishing high school. If shared risk factors explained co-occurrence, then when the sample was limited to people with the shared risk factors, the correlation between the two disorders should disappear. (It should also disappear when the sample was limited to people without the shared risk factor, but in that group there would be so few cases that results would be unstable.) Using the results in Table 13–12 to learn which pairs with ORs of ten or higher shared risk factors, we measured their co-occurrence within high-risk groups. The superscripts next to the odds ratios in Table 13–16 show what risk factors were shared and the odds ratios for co-occurrence for persons in the high-risk group. The lowest odds ratio within a high-risk group was 4.8, and most remained above 10, showing that even within high-risk groups, co-occurrence was much greater than chance. While there is still the possibility that co-occurrence was explained by some other unmeasured common

Table 13–16 Large Comorbidities in the Year of Interview:
Odds Ratios (OR) of 10 or Higher

Within Broad DSM-III Categories

	OR		OR
Affective		*Substance*	
Depression & mania	36	Drug & alcohol	14[f]
Anxiety			
Panic & obsessive compulsive	19		
Panic & phobia	11		

Across DSM-III Categories

Somatoform & Anxiety		*Affective & Anxiety*	
Somatization & panic	82[b]	Depression & panic	25[b]
Somatization & phobia	28[b]	Mania & panic	19
Somatization & ob-comp	23	Mania & ob-comp	15[d]
		Dep & ob-comp	10[e]
Schizophrenia & Affective			
Schizophrenia & mania	46	*Affective & Somatoform*	
Schizophrenia & depression	14	Depression & somatoform	22[b]
		Mania & somatoform	17
Schizophrenia & Somatoform			
Schizophrenia & somatization	38	*Personality & Affective*	
		Antisocial & mania	12[a]
Schizophrenia & Anxiety			
Schizophrenia & panic	35	*Somatoform & Organic*	
Schizophrenia & ob-comp	15	Somat & cognitive impairment*	10[g]
Schizophrenia & phobia	10		
Personality & Substance Abuse			
Antisocial & alcohol	29[f]		
Antisocial & drug	12[f]		

[a-g]Odds ratios controlling for demographic correlates of both active disorders.

	Odds Ratio in This Subgroup	
	Above 10	4 to 10
Demographic Correlates of Both Disorders		
Age < 30	a	d
Female	b	e
Male < 30	c	f
Blacks < 12 years education	d	g

*This OR is for mild and severe cognitive impairment combined; it would drop to 7 for severe cognitive impairment. Its lower confidence limit is below 4. All other ORs shown have lower confidence limits above 4 and all but 9 have lower limits above 10.

risk factor, it would have to be something *not* highly correlated with the shared demographic factors.

Since neither shared symptoms nor shared risk factors explained the strong co-occurrence between disorders, the most likely explanation for co-occurrence is that having one disorder puts the affected person at risk of developing other disorders. Such secondary cases are well recognized in clinical practice (Robins & Guze, 1972). Hypotheses as to which is typically the primary disorder and which typically the secondary one can be based on their typical ages of onset (Table 13-9). However, ages of onset may be different when there is comorbidity than when there is not, and this issue requires further investigation.

TREATMENT OF SPECIFIC DISORDERS

We noted earlier (Table 13-5) that only about one in five persons with an active disorder had had any mental health care in the last year. We now investigate which disorders are most likely to be brought to professional attention.

Each respondent affected at any time in his life was asked whether the symptoms of his particular disorder had ever been discussed with a doctor. Disorders varied greatly in the frequency with which a physician had been told about their symptoms (Table 13-17). All who had somatization disorder had told a doctor about some of those symptoms, as had more than half of those with panic or depressive episodes. Symptoms of schizophrenia had been discussed with a doctor in almost half the cases. Least likely to be brought to medical attention were drug abuse, alcohol abuse, antisocial behavior, and memory problems associated with cognitive impairment, all reported to physicians in less than one in five cases, and phobia had been brought to a doctor's attention only slightly more often than that. Note that the most common disorders were the ones least likely to be brought to a physician.

The fact that a particular disorder was mentioned to a doctor did not necessarily mean that the doctor undertook to treat it. Symptoms may have come up during a general check-up or while being treated for a physical problem or a different mental disorder. Similarly, the fact that a disorder was not discussed with a doctor did not necessarily mean that a physician had not been seen about another mental health problem. For example, many alcoholics saw doctors for other mental health purposes without discussing their drinking.

Residents of households were asked whether they had received services for a mental or emotional problem in the last six months, and whether they had had a hospitalization because of a mental health problem in the last

Table 13-17 How Many Ever Mentioned Their Symptoms to a Doctor

Positive for:	Number with a Lifetime Diagnosis	Percent Who Told Doctor of Symptoms
Somatization	67	100
Panic	425	73
Depressive episode	1,244	61
Schizophrenia	309	47
Obsessive compulsive	571	34
Manic episode	156	22
Phobia	2,645	22
Drug abuse	1,316	18
Alcohol abuse	2,620	15
Antisocial personality	628	11
Cognitive impairment:		
Mild or severe	1,224	6
Severe	244	11

year. (Since institutionalized persons often received care within their institution, these questions did not apply to them.) When persons with more than one disorder had been treated, it was not clear whether all disorders had been treated. Therefore, to compare the likelihood of particular disorders coming to treatment, we looked at persons with only one disorder active in the last year. If they received treatment for a mental health problem, whether from psychiatrists, primary care physicians, psychologists, or social workers, it was likely that this was the disorder being treated, although they could have been treated for symptoms of disorders for which they did not meet diagnostic criteria.

When we limited the sample to those with only one disorder (Table 13-18), treatment was even rarer (13%) than it was for the total affected sample (19%). This probably illustrates a well-recognized phenomenon called "Berkson's bias," which notes that persons with multiple diagnoses are more likely to appear for treatment than persons with a single diagnosis (Berkson, 1946).

The frequency of treatment varied markedly across diagnoses. Not surprisingly, the disorders most likely to have received recent care were those

Table 13–18 Treatment for Active One-Year Disorders in Persons with No Other Active Disorder (Household Sample)

	Percent with Any Mental Health Care[a]					
	Both Sexes		Males		Females	
	N	%	N	%	N	%
None of these disorders	14,077	5	5,971	4	8,106	6
Any single disorder	4,385	13	1,836	10	2,549	16
Specific single disorders:						
Somatization	22	67[c]	b	—	b	—
Panic	38	47	b	—	30	50
Schizophrenia	49	40	21	29[c]	28	50[c]
Depression	300	36	68	29	232	37
Mania	17	34[c]	b	—	b	—
Obsessive compulsive	107	20	42	11	65	25
Phobia	1,291	12	378	18	913	21
Alcohol	520	10	439	9	81	14
Drugs	233	10	160	11	73	7
Cognitive deficit (mild or severe)	1,733	5[d]	707	6	1,026	5
Antisocial personality	83	4	67	3	b	—

[a]Outpatient in last six months or inpatient in last year.
[b]Ns too small to calculate.
[c]Based on N less than 30.
[d]Results same for severe.

which respondents had most often *ever* mentioned to a physician. The active disorder most commonly receiving treatment was somatization disorder (two-thirds of a very small number of cases) and next most commonly treated (one-third to one-half of active cases) were panic, schizophrenia, depression, and mania. Persons with phobia, alcoholism, drug abuse, cognitive deficit, and antisocial personality had lowest rates of receiving any treatment.

Studies of patient loads in psychiatric clinics and other outpatient treatment settings often find that depression and anxiety are the most common disorders seen, a quite different picture from ECA findings in the general population, where alcoholism and phobia were the most common disorders. Our treatment results show how such different findings can occur. Depression and panic disorder are much more likely to be brought to the attention of clinicians than are alcoholism and phobia, probably in part because they are more limited to women, who seek care more readily, and partly because they are more widely recognized by the public as a mental health problem.

Conclusion

The ECA study was initiated to improve our knowledge about the frequency of psychiatric disorder in the community, in particular the frequency of the major specific disorders, and to identify underserved portions of the population. It was initiated because the President's Commission on Mental Health found that such information was sadly lacking, and consequently that empirically based planning was not possible.

This volume shows that the ECA's goals have largely been met. For the first time, with reasonable accuracy, the frequency of the major specific psychiatric disorders in the nation have been estimated, both on a lifetime and active basis. Those parts of the population with unusual burdens of mental illness have been identified, and the parts of the affected population who are underserved have been noted. The ECA study has also been able to achieve many subsidiary goals that were not entirely visualized at its beginning. It has been able to learn which disorders tend to co-occur in the same people, the age at which each disorder typically begins, the age at which the risk of beginning each disorder is essentially past, how often remission or recovery from each disorder occurred, and what the interval is between the first and last symptom when termination occurs.

These results not only provide estimates on which to base policy decisions, but they also provide key information with which to estimate whether and how policy has been successful. A successful policy is one that reduces the burden of mental illness. This reduction can come in several ways. It can come through earlier and more adequate treatment of those already ill. Shortening the duration of illness through early recognition and rapid treatment will cause the prevalence rate to drop. If this approach, now being used in the NIMH D/ART Program (Regier et al., 1988b), is successful, we should find earlier remissions and growing proportions of lifetime cases in remission.

But early treatment does not change the proportion who ever develop the disorder. Primary prevention can do so by reducing risk factors, by preventing symptoms, or by treating symptoms early before diagnostic criteria are met. The ECA not only provides the baseline data against which the success of treatment or prevention can be measured, but it can help in discovering how success in prevention was achieved. Because the ECA provides counts of the symptoms of a disorder even among persons who did not meet diagnostic criteria, a reduction in the proportion with any of these symptoms can be detected. Because it provides baseline data for calculating how many of those with any symptom went on to meet diagnostic criteria, future studies may be able to show that new programs were able to reduce the probability of progression from first symptom to illness. Information provided by the ECA about when the risk period for onset of a specific disorder ends can indicate by what age we can be reasonably sure that lifetime rates of disorders have been reduced by prevention, rather than possibly only delayed.

In addition to providing these baseline data against which the success of future programs can be measured, results of the ECA study suggest some directions that should be considered for future programs. It has shown, for example, that comorbidity occurs in more than half of those with any psychiatric disorder, but that when affected persons seek care, they often do not report symptoms of the secondary disorder to their doctors, whether they see a general medical physician or a psychiatrist. These results should encourage caretakers to carry out comprehensive evaulations of mental health status for each new patient, rather than focusing solely on the disorder that led to the consultation. Often they will find additional disorders that need treatment.

The ECA study also showed that only a minority of persons with psychiatric disability see mental health professionals or ask for care for their mental health problems from general medical physicians. Yet they have a substantial need for care, as shown by a marked level of impairment in ability to work and be self-supporting and in interpersonal relationships, as shown by their high level of disrupted marriages. If professionals in the general medical sector and social agencies are alerted to the association of mental disorder with work and marital problems, they can serve as detection, early treatment, and referral sources for those in need. To reach those with psychiatric disorders who are not in contact with medical and social agencies, a three-pronged educational program may be needed to (1) teach the public how to recognize these disorders, (2) inform them that many can be effectively treated, and (3) improve access to care. The NIMH-sponsored program now under way for the affective disorders, the D/ART program, may need to be extended to other disorders in the future.

The ECA has identified both treatable disorders that receive little care, particularly phobias and substance abuse, and population segments that are most unlikely to seek care, particularly married men. These findings underscore disorders for which educational outreach programs are indicated and the populations to which they most need to be addressed.

The ECA study also showed that institutionalized populations have enormous burdens of psychiatric disorder, even when they are in institutions not designated as mental health facilities. Institutions of all kinds need substantial mental health resources if they are to care for their residents adequately. Of particular concern with respect to public policy is the finding that people with schizophrenia are now being cared for in a variety of institutions, including nursing homes and prisons, where their disorders are unlikely to be recognized and treated. The burden of demented patients in nursing homes was also underscored by ECA results.

In addition to suggesting such practical policy considerations, the ECA results have overturned some erroneous views of the nature of psychiatric disorder in the community. Based on earlier studies, it was thought that women were particularly liable to psychiatric illness and that vulnerability increased with age. The stereotypic person with psychiatric disorder was a middle-aged anxious or depressed woman. The ECA has shown that disorders in men are as common as or slightly more common than in women and that most disorders begin in early adult life, with recovery from them in middle age the rule rather than the exception. The most common disorders of all are phobias and alcoholism rather than anxiety and depression. It was thought that minority groups must have high rates of antisocial personality and substance abuse because they have high rates of arrest and incarceration. The high arrest and incarceration rate among minority groups has been shown not to be explained by an excess of these disorders (see chapter 11). Of course, not all our previous beliefs were erroneous. The ECA confirmed the association of being female with the depressive disorders and the anxiety disorders, of being male with substance abuse and antisocial personality, of being elderly with cognitive impairment, of being young with drug abuse. It confirmed the fact that many persons with schizophrenia and alcoholism never marry, although it overthrows the stereotype that *most* do not.

In addition to revealing the prevalence and correlates of disorders described in the psychiatric nomenclature, ECA results can also affect the psychiatric nomenclature itself. This was not its original goal. Indeed, the ECA attempted to take the 1980 nomenclature as a given and operationalize it, in order to assess disorders based on that nomenclature. Nonetheless, its results have revealed difficulties with the official nomenclature, some of which have already been taken into account in the revision of the Diagnostic and Statistical Manual (American Psychiatric Association, 1987). One finding of importance to that revision was the discovery of how common was the occurrence of multiple disorders, and that the official exclusion criteria ruling out one disorder in the presence of another often did not reflect the most common comorbidities (Boyd et al., 1984). Further use of these results to modify the official nomenclature can be expected.

An important product of any major research effort like the ECA study should be to clarify the important next steps in research needed to answer remaining questions. The ECA was essentially a cross-sectional study of prevalence, although it provided two follow-up interviews, at six months and one year. Analysis of the first year's data in the current volume has demonstrated that a one-year follow-up of an adult population was both too brief and too late to teach us much about the incidence of new disorders, because most disorders begin in late adolescence and early adulthood. In a population with an average age of 40, few new disorders can be expected in a one-year period. Studies of incidence will require long-term follow-ups of the younger segments of the population.

The ECA was not designed to be a study of the causes of disorders, although it did identify many of their correlates. It showed that the study of causes would require information about respondents dating back to the first school years because the "adult" disorders often have their first symptoms in childhood or adolescence. The only variables in the ECA that could unequivocably be viewed as predictors of disorder were those demographic characteristics already determined at birth—sex, year of birth, ethnicity. Even a low level of education was as plausibly a product of disorder as its cause. Future psychiatric surveys interested in psychosocial causes of disorder can enrich the range of early causal variables to be studied by asking more about childhood experiences, including place of rearing, intactness of the family in which the respondent was reared, and that family's social status. To explore the question of whether later events were more likely causes or consequences of disorder, dates of school leaving, first marriage, first parenthood, and first divorce or separation should be obtained so that it can be determined whether they preceded or followed the onset of illness. To assess possible biological causes in addition will require seeking access to early medical records.

The ECA survey depended on personal retrospective reporting of symptoms in response to standardized questions. Retrospection was essential to making diagnoses and learning something about the course of psychiatric disorders, but it is nonetheless subject to error. The ECA's study of prevalence can serve as a guide to the needed design for what would be a reasonable next step in causal studies, a prospective longitudinal study that overcomes the weaknesses of long-term retrospective reporting. The ECA results make clear that such a prospective study should begin in childhood and should follow its subjects to about age 35, when the great majority of disorders that will ever occur will have appeared. Unlike earlier prospective studies that have studied risk factors for particular disorders such as schizophrenia or depression, it should encompass the whole range of child and adult psychiatric disorders because these disorders are closely linked, and one may be a risk factor for another. It should incorporate multiple assessment points to keep the intervals over which retrospective accounts are collected reasonably brief, and it should add validating information from parents, schools, and medical records.

The ECA fulfilled the goals set for it, and like all thoroughly satisfactory research projects, it has clarified what the next research goals might be and how they are to be accomplished.

References Cited

Adler, M., Anthony, J.C., Balster, R., et al. (1987). Scientific perspectives on cocaine abuse. *Pharmacologist, 29,* 20–24.

Agras, S., Sylvester, D., & Oliveau, D. (1969). The epidemiology of common fears and phobias. *Comprehensive Psychiatry, 10,* 151–156.

Akiskal, H.S. (1981). Subaffective disorders: Dysthymic, cyclothymic, and bipolar II disorders in the "borderline" realm. *Psychiatric Clinics of North America, 4,* 25–46.

Allebeck, P., & Wistedt, B. (1986). Mortality in schizophrenia. *Archives of General Psychiatry, 43,* 650–653.

American Psychiatric Association, Committee on Nomenclature and Statistics. (1952). *Diagnostic and statistical manual: Mental disorders.* Washington, DC: American Psychiatric Association Mental Hospital Service.

American Psychiatric Association. (1980). *Diagnostic and statistical manual of mental disorders* (3rd ed., DSM-III). Washington DC: Author.

———. (1987). *Diagnostic and statistical manual of mental disorders* (3rd ed. rev., DSM-III revised). Washington, DC: Author.

Ananth, J. (1985). Pharmacotherapy of obsessive-compulsive disorder. In M. Mavissakalian, S.M. Turner, & L. Michelson (Eds.), *Obsessive-compulsive disorder.* New York: Plenum Press.

Angst, J., & Dobler-Mikola, A. (1983). Anxiety states, panic and phobia in a young general population. In *World psychiatry proceedings, Vienna.* New York: Plenum.

———. (1984). The Zurich study: III. Diagnosis of depression. *European Archives of Psychiatric and Neurological Science, 234,* 30–37.

Angst, J., Dobler-Mikola A., & Scheidegger P. (1985). The Zurich study: V. Anxiety and phobia in young adults. *European Archives of Psychiatric and Neurological Sciences, 235,* 171–178.

Anthony, J.C. (1979). The effect of federal drug law on the incidence of drug abuse. *Journal of Health Politics, Policy and Law, 4,* 87–108.

———. (1983). The regulation of dangerous psychoactive drugs. In J.P. Morgan & D.V. Kagan (Eds.), *Society and medication: Conflicting signals for prescribers and patients.* (pp. 163–180). Lexington: DC Heath.

———. (1988a). *Models for substance abuse risk estimation.* Invited paper presented at the

1988 annual meeting of the Committee on Problems of Drug Dependence, North Falmouth, MA.

——— . (1988b). *DIS operational definitions for DSM-III drug abuse-dependence diagnoses* (Tech. Rep.). Baltimore, MD: The Johns Hopkins University, Department of Mental Hygiene.

Anthony, J.C., Folstein, M., Romanoski, A.J., et al. (1985). Comparison of lay Diagnostic Interview Schedule and a standardized psychiatric diagnosis. *Archives of General Psychiatry, 42,* 667–675.

Anthony, J.C., LeResche, L., Niaz, U., von Korff, M.R., & Folstein, M.F. (1982). Limits of the "Mini-Mental State" as a screening test for dementia and delirium among hospital patients. *Psychological Medicine, 12,* 397–408.

Anthony, J.C., & Petronis, K.R. (Forthcoming). Epidemiologic evidence on suspected causal associations between cocaine use and psychiatric disturbances. In C. Schade & S. Schober (Eds.), *Epidemiology of cocaine use and abuse.* Rockville, MD: National Institution on Drug Abuse.

Anthony, J.C., Tien, A.Y., & Petronis, K.R. 1989. Epidemiologic evidence on cocaine use and panic attacks. *The American Journal of Epidemiology, 129,* 543–549.

Ashok, R., & Sheehan, D.V. (1987). Medical evaluation of panic attacks. *Journal of Clinical Psychiatry, 48,* 309–313.

Auden, W.H. (1946). *The age of anxiety.* New York: Random House.

Babigian, H.M. (1985). Schizophrenia: Epidemiology. In H.I. Kaplan & B.J. Sadock (Eds.), *Comprehensive textbook of psychiatry, Vol. 1* (4th ed.). Baltimore, MD: Williams & Wilkins.

Baer, L., & Minichiello W.E. (1986). Behavior therapy for obsessive-compulsive disorder. In M.A. Jenike, L. Baer, & W.E. Minichiello (Eds.), *Obsessive compulsive disorders: Theory and management.* Littleton, MA: PSG Publishing.

Bahn, A.K., Chandler, C.A., & Lemkau, P.V. (1962). Diagnostic characteristics of adult outpatients of psychiatric clinics as related to type and outcome of services. *Milbank Memorial Fund Quarterly, 15,* 407–442.

Bailey, M. (1961). Alcoholism and marriage. *Quarterly Journal of Studies on Alcohol, 22,* 81–97.

Balter, M.B., Levine, J., & Manheimer, D.I. (1974). Cross-national study of the extent of anti-anxiety/sedative drug use. *New England Journal of Medicine, 290,* 769–774.

Barabas, G. (1988). Tourette's syndrome: An overview. *Psychiatric Annals, 18,* 395–398.

Barsky, A.J., & Klerman, G.L. (1983). Overview: Hypochondriasis, bodily complaints and somatic styles. *American Journal of Psychiatry, 140,* 273–283.

Bebbington, P., Hurry, J., Tennant, C., Sturt, E., & Wing, J.K. (1981). Epidemiology of mental disorders in Camberwell. *Psychological Medicine, 11,* 561–579.

Behar, D., Rapoport, J.L., Berg, C.J., et al. (1984). Computerized tomography and neuropsychological test measures in adolescents with obsessive-compulsive disorder. *American Journal of Psychiatry, 141,* 363–369.

Berkman, L.F. (1986). The association between educational attainment and mental status examinations: Of etiologic significance for senile dementias or not? *Journal of Chronic Disease, 39,* 171–174.

Berkson, J. (1946). Limitations of the application of fourfold table analysis to hospital data. *Biometric Bulletin, 2,* 47–53.

Black, A. (1974). The natural history of obsessional neurosis. In H. Beech (Ed.), *Obsessional states.* London: Methuen.

Black, D.W., & Winokur, G. (1988). Age, mortality and chronic schizophrenia. *Schizophrenia Research, 1,* 267–272.

Blacker, K.H. (1966). Obsessive-compulsive phenomena and catatonic states: A continuum. A five year case study of a chronic catatonic patient. *Psychiatry, 29,* 185.

Bland, R.C., Newman, S.C., & Orn, H. (1986). Recurrent and nonrecurrent depression. *Archives of General Psychiatry, 43,* 1085–1089.

Bland, R.C., & Orn, H. (1978). 14-year outcome in early schizophrenia. *Acta Psychiatrica Scandinavica, 58,* 327–338.

Blazer, D., Crowell, B.A., & George, L.K. (1987). Alcohol abuse and dependence in the rural south. *Archives of General Psychiatry, 44,* 736–747.

Blazer, D.G., George, L.K., Landerman, R., Pennybacker, M., Melville, M.L., Woodbury, M., Manton, K.G., Jordan, K., & Locke, B.Z. (1985). Psychiatric disorders: A rural/urban comparison. *Archives of General Psychiatry, 42,* 651–656.

Blazer, D.G., Hughes, D.C., & George, L.K. (1987a). The epidemiology of depression in an elderly community population. *The Gerontologist, 27,* 281–287.

———. (1987b). Stressful life events in the onset of a generalized anxiety syndrome. *American Journal of Psychiatry, 144,* 1178–1183.

Blazer, D., & Williams, C.D. (1980). Epidemiology of dysphoria and depression in an elderly population. *American Journal of Psychiatry, 137,* 439–444.

Boyd, J.H., Burke, J.D., Gruenberg, E.M., et al. (1984). Exclusion criteria of DSM-III: A study of co-occurrence of hierarchy-free syndromes. *Archives of General Psychiatry, 41,* 983–989.

Boyd, J.H., & Weissman, M.M. (1981). Epidemiology of affective disorders: A re-examination and future directions. *Archives of General Psychiatry, 38,* 1039–1046.

Braiker, H.B. (1982). The diagnosis and treatment of alcoholism in women. In *Special population issues.* Alcohol and Health Monograph No. 4. Publication No. (ADM) 82-1193, pp. 111–139. National Institute on Alcoholism and Alcohol Abuse. Rockville, MD.

Brecher, E.M., & the Editors of Consumer Reports. (1972). *Licit and illicit drugs.* Boston: Little, Brown.

Breslau, N. (1985). Depressive symptoms, major depression and generalized anxiety. A comparison of self-reports on the CES-D and results from diagnostic interviews. *Psychiatry Research, 15,* 219–229.

Breslau, N., & Davis, G.C. (1985). DSM-III generalized anxiety disorder: An empirical investigation of more stringent criteria. *Psychiatry Research, 15,* 231.

Briscoe, C.W., & Smith, J.B. (1973). Depression and marital turmoil. *Archives of General Psychiatry, 28,* 811–817.

Briscoe, C.W., Smith, J.B., Robins, E., Marten, S., & Gaskin, F. (1973). Divorce and psychiatric disease. *Archives of General Psychiatry, 29,* 119–125.

Brown, G.W., & Harris, T. (1978). *Social origins of depression: A study of psychiatric disorders in women.* London: Tavistock Publications.

Bruce, M.L., Kim, K., Leaf, P., & Jacobs, S. (in press). Depressive episodes and dysphoria resulting from conjugal bereavement in a prospective community sample. *American Journal of Psychiatry.*

Burke, J.D., Jr. (1986). Diagnostic categorization by the Diagnostic Interview Schedule (DIS): A comparison with other methods of assessment. In J. Barrett & R.M. Rose (Eds.), *Mental disorders in the community.* New York: Guilford Press.

Burnam, M.A., Hough, R.L., Escobar, J.I., Karno, M., Timbers, D.M., Telles, C.A., & Locke, B.Z. (1987a). Six-month prevalence of specific psychiatric disorders among Mexican-Americans and non-Hispanic whites in Los Angeles. *Archives of General Psychiatry, 44,* 687–694.

Burnam, M.A., Hough, R.L., Marvin, K., Escobar, J.I., & Telles, C.A. (1987b). Acculturation and lifetime prevalence of psychiatric disorders among Mexican Americans in Los Angeles. *Journal of Health and Social Behavior, 28,* 89–102.

Butler, R.N., & Lewis, M.I. (1977). *Aging and mental health* (2nd ed.). St. Louis: C.V. Mosby.

Canino, G.J., Bird, H., Shrout, P., Rubio-Stipec, M., Geil, K.P., & Bravo, M. (in press). The prevalence of alcohol abuse and/or dependence in Puerto Rico, In J.E. Helzer & G.J. Canino (Eds.), *Alcoholism in North America, Europe and Asia: A coordinated analysis of population data from ten regions.* New York: Oxford University Press.

Canino, G.L., Bird, H.R., Shrout, P.E., Rubio-Stipec, M., Bravo, M., Martinez, R., Sesman, G., & Guevara, L.M. (1987). Prevalence of specific psychiatric disorders in Puerto Rico. *Archives of General Psychiatry, 44,* 727–735.

Christie, K.A., Burke, J.D., Jr., Regier, D.A., Rae, D.S., Boyd, J.H., & Locke, B.Z. (1988). Epidemiologic evidence for early onset of mental disorders and higher risk of drug abuse in young adults. *American Journal of Psychiatry, 145,* 971–975.

Clark, W.B., & Cahalan, D. (1976). Changes in problem drinking over a four-year span. *Addictive Behaviors, 1,* 251–259.

Clayton, P.J. (1987). Anxious depression: A reemerging subtype of depression. In A. Racagni & E. Smeraldi (Eds.), *Anxious depression: assessment and treatment* (pp. 1–5). New York: Raven Press.

Clayton, R.R. (1984). *Cocaine use in the United States: In a blizzard or just being snowed?* Paper presented at a technical review on Patterns of Cocaine Use in the United States (pp. 37–39), Bethesda, MD, July 11–13.

Cleckley, H. (1955). *The mask of sanity.* St. Louis: Mosby.

Cloninger, C.R., & Guze, S.B. (1970). Psychiatric illness and female criminality: The role of sociopathy and hysteria in antisocial women. *American Journal of Psychiatry, 127,* 303–311.

Cloninger, C.R., & Guze, S.B. (1973). Psychiatric illness in the families of female criminals: A study of 288 first-degree relatives. *British Journal of Psychiatry, 122,* 697–703.

Cohen, M.E., Robins, E., Purtell, J.J., Altmann, M.W., & Reid, D.E. (1953). Excessive surgery in hysteria. *Journal of the American Medical Association, 151,* 977–986.

Commission on Chronic Illness. (1957). *Chronic illness in a large city* (Vol. 4). Cambridge, MA: Harvard University Press.

Cooper, J.E., Kendell, R.E., Gurland, B.J., Sharpe, L., Copeland, J.R.M., & Simon, R. (1972). *Psychiatric diagnosis in New York and London.* London: Oxford University Press.

Cornoni-Huntley, J.C., Foley, D.J., White, L.R., Suzman, R., Berkman, L.F., Evans, D.A., & Wallace, R.B. (1985). Epidemiology of disability in the oldest old: Methodologic issues and preliminary findings. *Milbank Memorial Fund Quarterly, 63,* 350–376.

Coryell, W. (1981a). Diagnosis-specific mortality: Primary unipolar depression and Briquet's syndrome (somatization disorder). *Archives of General Psychiatry, 38,* 939–942.

———. (1981b). Obsessive-compulsive disorder and primary unipolar depression. Comparisons of background, family history, course and mortality. *Journal of Nervous and Mental Disorders, 169,* 220–224.

Crowe, R.R. (1974). An adoptive study of antisocial personality. *Archives of General Psychiatry, 31,* 785–791.

Crowell, B.A., George, L.K., Blazer D., & Landerman, R. (1986). Psychosocial risk factors and urban/rural differences in the prevalence of major depression. *British Journal of Psychiatry, 149,* 307–314.

Cummings, J.L., & Frankel, M. (1985). Gilles de la Tourette syndrome and the neurological basis of obsessions and compulsions. *Biological Psychiatry, 20,* 1117–1126.

Davies, D.L. (1976). Definition issues in alcoholism. In R.E. Tarter & A.A. Sugarman (Eds.), *Alcoholism: Interdisciplinary approaches to an enduring problem.* Reading, MA: Addison-Wesley.

Dean, C., Surtees, P.G., & Sashidharian, S.P. (1983). Comparison of research diagnostic systems in an Edinburgh community sample. *British Journal of Psychiatry, 142,* 247–256.

Dohrenwend, B.P. (1989). "The problem of validity in field studies of psychological disorders" revisited. In L. Robins & J. Barrett (Eds.), *The validity of psychiatric diagnosis.* New York: Raven Press.

Dohrenwend, B.P., & Dohrenwend, B.S. (1969). *Social status and psychological disorder: A causal inquiry.* New York: John Wiley.

Dohrenwend, B.P., Shrout, P.E., Egin, G., & Mendelsohn, F.S. (1980). Nonspecific psychological distress and other dimensions of psychopathology: Measures for use in the general population. *Archives of General Psychiatry, 37,* 1229–1236.

Eaton, W.W. (1986). *The sociology of mental disorders* (2nd ed.). New York: Praeger.

Eaton, W.W., & Bohrnstedt, G. (1989). Latent variable models with dichotomous outcomes: Analyses of data from the NIMH Epidemiologic Catchment Area program. *Sociological Methods and Research,* special issue *(18).*

Eaton, W.W., & Kessler, L.G. (Eds.). (1985). *Epidemiologic field methods in psychiatry: The NIMH Epidemiologic Catchment Area program.* Orlando, FL: Academic Press.

Eaton, W.W., & Ritter, C.R. (1988). Distinguishing anxiety and depression with field survey data. *Psychological Medicine, 18,* 155–166.

Eaton, W.W., Weissman, M., Anthony, J.C., Robins, L.N., & Karno, M. (1985). Problems in the definition and measurement of prevalence and incidence of psychiatric disorders. In W.W. Eaton & L.G. Kessler (Eds.), *Epidemiologic field methods in psychiatry: The NIMH Epidemiologic Catchment Area program.* Orlando, FL: Academic Press.

Edwards, G., & Gross, M.M. (1976). Alcohol dependence: Provisional description of a clinical syndrome. *British Medical Journal, 1,* 1058–1061.

Edwards, G., Gross, M.M., Keller, M., Moser, J., & Room, R. (1977). *Alcohol-related disabilities.* (Offset Publication Number 32). Geneva: World Health Organization.

Egeland, J.A., Gerhard, D.S., Pauls, D.L., et al. (1987). Bipolar affective disorder linked to DNA markers on chromosome 11. *Nature, 325,* 783–787.

Endicott, J., & Spitzer, R.L. (1978). A diagnostic interview: The Schedule for Affective Disorders and Schizophrenia. *Archives of General Psychiatry, 35,* 837–844.

Escobar, J.I., Rubio-Stipec, M., Canino, G., & Karno, M. (1989). Somatic Symptom Index (SSI). A new and abridged somatization construct: Prevalence and epidemiological correlates in two large community samples. *Journal of Nervous and Mental Disease, 177,* 140–146.

Escobar, J.I., Burnam, M.A., Karno, M., Forsythe, A., & Golding, J.M. (1987a). Somatization in the community. *Archives of General Psychiatry, 44,* 713–718.

Escobar, J.I., Golding, J.M., Hough, R.L., & Karno, M., Burnam, M.A., & Wells, K.B. (1987b). Somatization in the community: Relationship to disability and use of services. *American Journal of Public Health, 77,* 837–840.

Faris, R.E.L., & Dunham, H.W. (1939). *Mental disorders in urban areas: An ecological study of schizophrenia and other psychoses.* Chicago: University of Chicago Press.

Feighner, J.P., Robins, E., Guze, S.B., Woodruff, R.A., Winokur, G., & Munoz, R. (1972). Diagnostic criteria for use in psychiatric research. *Archives of General Psychiatry, 26,* 57–63.

Feldman, A.R., Kessler, L., Myers, M.H., & Naughton, M.D. (1986). The prevalence of cancer: Estimates based on the Connecticut tumor registry. *New England Journal of Medicine, 315,* 1394–1397.

Fillenbaum, G.G., George, L.K., & Blazer, D.G. (1988a). Scoring non-response on the Mini-Mental State Examination. *Psychological Medicine, 18,* 1021–1025.

Fillenbaum, G.G., Hughes, D.C., Heyman, A., George, L.K., & Blazer, D.G. (1988b). Relationships of health and demographic characteristics to Mini-Mental State Examination score among community residents. *Psychological Medicine, 18,* 719–726.

Filstead, W.J., Goby, M.J., & Bradley, N.J. (1976). Critical elements in the diagnosis of alcoholism: A national survey of physicians. *Journal of the American Medical Association, 236,* 2767–2769.

Fishburne, P.M., Abelson, H.I., & Cisin, I. (1979). *National survey on drug abuse: Main findings 1979.* Washington, DC: National Institute On Drug Abuse.

Foa, E.B., & Steketee, G. (1984). Behavioral treatment of obsessive-compulsive ritualizers. In T.R. Insel (Ed.), *Obsessive-compulsive disorder.* Washington, DC: American Psychiatric Press.

Foa, E.B., Steketee, G.S., & Ozarow, B.J. (1985). Behavior therapy with obsessive-compulsives: From theory to treatment. In M. Mavissakalian, S.M. Turner, & L. Michelson (Eds.), *Obsessive-compulsive disorder.* New York: Plenum Press.

Folstein, M., Anthony, J.C., Parhad, I., Duffy, B., & Gruenberg, E.M. (1985). The meaning of cognitive impairment in the elderly. *Journal of the American Geriatrics Society, 33,* 228–235.

Folstein, M.F., Folstein, S.E., & McHugh, P.R. (1975). Mini-Mental State: A practical method for grading the cognitive status of patients for the clinician. *Journal of Psychiatric Research, 12,* 189–198.

Frances, A. (1979). Lecture at APA regional conferences on DSM-III. Unpublished manuscript.

Freud, S. (1979). *On psychopathology: Inhibitions, symptoms and anxiety.* (A. Richards, Ed.). Harmondsworth, Eng.: Penguin Books.

George, L.K., & Gwyther, L.P. (1986). Caregiver well-being: A multidimensional examination of family caregivers of demented adults. *The Gerontologist, 34,* 253–259.

George, L.K., Hughes, D.C., & Blazer, D.G. (1986). Urban/rural differences in the prevalence of anxiety disorders. *American Journal of Social Psychiatry, 6,* 249–258.

German, P.S., Shapiro, S., & Skinner, E.A. (1985). Mental health of the elderly: Use of health and mental health services. *Journal of the American Geriatrics Society, 33,* 246–252.

Gershon, E.S., Hamovitt, J.H., Guroff, J.J., et al. (1982). A family study of schizoaffective, bipolar I, bipolar II, unipolar, and normal control probands. *Archives of General Psychiatry, 39,* 1157–1167.

Gittleson, N.L. (1966) The fate of obsessions in depressive psychosis. *British Journal of Psychiatry, 112,* 705–708.

Goldberg, D. (1977). WHO consultation: Report on the research methodology appropriate for the current research program of the Department of Biometry and Epidemiology of the National Institute of Mental Health (Dec 3–21, 1977). Washington, DC: Pan American Health Organization, Unpublished mimeo.

Goldin, L.R. & Gershon, E.S. (1988). The genetic epidemiology of major depressive illness. In A.J. Frances & R.E. Hales (Eds.), *Psychiatry update: Vol. 7* (pp. 149–168). Washington, DC: American Psychiatric Press.

Goldstein, P. (forthcoming). Frequency of cocaine use and violence: A comparison between men and women. In C. Schade & S. Schober (Eds.), *Epidemiology of cocaine use and abuse.* National Institute on Drug Abuse Research Monograph. Rockville, MD: National Institute on Drug Abuse.

Goodwin, D.W., & Guze, S.B. (1979/1984). *Psychiatric Diagnosis* (2nd and 3rd eds.). New York: Oxford University Press.

Goodwin, D.W., Guze, S.B., Robins, E. (1969). Follow-up studies in obsessional neurosis. *Archives of General Psychiatry, 20,* 182–187.

Gottesman, L. (1977). Clinical psychology and aging: A role model. In D. Gentry (Ed.), *Geropsychology.* Cambridge, MA: Ballinger.

Green, R.C., & Pitman, R.K. (1986). Tourette syndrome and obsessive-compulsive disorder. In M.A. Jenike, L. Baer, & W.E. Minichiello (Eds.), *Obsessive-compulsive disorders: Theory and management.* Littleton, MA: PSG Publishing.

Greenberg, E.D. (1981). Obsessive-compulsive neurosis and season of birth. *Biological Psychiatry, 16,* 513–516.

Gunderson, J.G., & Mosher, L.R. (1975). The cost of schizophrenia. *American Journal of Psychiatry, 132,* 901–906.

Guze, S.B. (1964). Conversion symptoms in criminals. *American Journal of Psychiatry, 121,* 580–583.

Guze, S.B., Goodwin, D.W., & Crane, J.B. (1969). Criminality and psychiatric disorders. *Archives of General Psychiatry, 20,* 583–591.

Guze, S.B., & Perley, M.J. (1963). Observations on the natural history of hysteria. *American Journal of Psychiatry, 119,* 960–965.

Guze, S.B., Woodruff, R.A., & Clayton, P.J. (1971a). A study of conversion symptoms in psychiatric outpatients. *American Journal of Psychiatry, 128,* 643–646.

——— . (1971b). Hysteria and antisocial behavior: Further evidence of an association. *American Journal of Psychiatry, 127,* 957–960.

Hagnell, O. (1966). *A prospective study of the incidence of mental disorder.* Lund, Sweden: Berlingska Boktryckeriet.

Hagnell, O., Lanke, J., Rorsman, B., & Ojesjo, L. (1982). Are we entering an age of melancholy? *Psychological Medicine, 12,* 279–289.

Hall, W., Goldstein, G., Andrews, G., et al. (1985). Estimating the economic costs of schizophrenia. *Schizophrenia Bulletin, 11,* 598–611.

Hare, R.D. (1983). Diagnosis of antisocial personality disorder in two prison populations. *American Journal of Psychiatry, 140* (7), 887–890.

Hare E.H., Price, J.S., & Slater, E.T. (1972). Fertility in obsessional neurosis. *British Journal of Psychiatry, 121,* 197–205.

Harris, M.J., & Jeste, D.V. (1988). Late-onset schizophrenia: An overview. *Schizophrenia Bulletin, 14*(1), 39–55.

Hasday, J.D., & Karch, F.E. (1981). Benzodiazepine prescribing in a family medicine center. *Journal of the American Medical Association, 246,* 1321–1325.

Helgason, T. (1964). *Epidemiology of mental disorders in Iceland.* Copenhagen: Munksgaard.

Helzer, J.E., Robins, L.N., Croughan, J.L., & Welner, A. (1981). Renard diagnostic interview: Its reliability and procedural validity with physicians and lay interviewers. *Archives of General Psychiatry, 38,* 393–398.

Helzer, J.E., Stoltzman, R., Farmer, A., Brockington, I.F., Plesons, D., Singerman, B., & Works, J. (1985). Comparing the DIS with a DIS/DSM-III based physician reevaluation. In W.W. Eaton & L.G. Kessler (Eds.), *Epidemiologic field methods in psychiatry: The NIMH Epidemiologic Catchment Area program* (pp. 285–308). Orlando, FL: Academic Press.

Henderson, S. (1977). The social network, support and neurosis: The function of attachment in adult life. *British Journal of Psychiatry, 131,* 185–191.

Henderson, S., Duncan-Jones, P., Byrne, D.G., Scott, R., & Adcock, S. (1979). Psychiatric disorder in Canberra: A standardized study of prevalence. *Acta Psychiatrica Scandinavica, 60,* 355–374.

Henderson, A.S., & Jorm, A.F. (1987). Is case-ascertainment of Alzheimer's disease in field studies practicable? (Editorial). *Psychological Medicine, 17,* 549–555.

Hesselbrock, M.N., Meyer, R.E., & Keener, J.J. (1985). Psychopathology in hospitalized alcoholics. *Archives of General Psychiatry, 42,* 1050–1055.

Hirschfeld, R.M.A., & Cross, C.K. (1982). Epidemiology of affective disorders. *Archives of General Psychiatry, 39,* 35–46.

Hollingshead, A.B., & Redlich, F.C. (1958). *Social class and mental illness.* New York: John Wiley.

Holzer, C.E., III, Spitznagel, E., Jordan, K.B., Timbers, D.M., Kessler, L.G., & Anthony, J.C. (1985). Sampling the household population. In W.W. Eaton & L.G. Kessler (Eds.), *Epidemiologic methods in psychiatry: The NIMH Epidemiologic Catchment Area program* (pp. 23–48). Orlando, FL: Academic Press.

Huizinga, D., & Elliott, D.S. (1983). A preliminary examination of the reliability and validity of the National Youth Survey (Project Report No. 27). Boulder, CO: Behavioral Research Institute.

Hunt, L.G. (1979). Incidence and prevalence of drug use and abuse. In R.I. Dupont, A. Goldstein, & J. O'Donnell (Eds.), *Handbook on drug abuse* (pp. 395–403). Washington, DC: National Institute on Drug Abuse.

Ingram, I.M. (1961). Obsessional illness in mental hospital patients. *Journal of Mental Science, 107,* 382–402.

Insel, T.R. (1984). Obsessive-compulsive disorder: The clinical picture. In T.R. Insel (Ed.), *Obsessive-compulsive disorder.* Washington, DC: American Psychiatric Press.

Insel, T.R., Gillin, J.C., Moore, A., et al. (1982). The sleep of patients with obsessive-compulsive disorder. *Archives of General Psychiatry, 39,* 1372–1377.

Insel, T.R., & Mueller, E.A. (1984). The psychopharmacologic treatment of obsessive-compulsive disorder. In T.R. Insel (Ed.), *Obsessive-compulsive disorder.* Washington, DC: American Psychiatric Press.

Institute of Medicine (IOM), Division of Health Sciences Policy. (1987). *Causes and consequences of alcohol problems: An agenda for research.* Washington, DC: National Academy Press.

Institute of Medicine Committee on Health Care for Homeless People. (1988). *Homelessness, health and human needs,* pp. 2–4. Washington, DC: National Academy Press.

Jablensky, A. (1986). Epidemiology of schizophrenia: A European perspective. *Schizophrenia Bulletin, 12,* 52–73.

Jellinek, E.M. (1959). Estimating the prevalence of alcoholism: Modified values in the Jellinek formula and an alternative approach. *Quarterly Journal of Studies on Alcohol, 20,* 261–269.

Jenike, M.A. (1986). Somatic treatments. In M.A. Jenike, L. Baer, & W.E. Minichiello (Eds.), *Obsessive-compulsive disorders: Theory and management.* Littleton, MA: PSG Publishing.

Jenike, M.A., Baer, L., & Minichiello, W.E. (Eds.). (1986). *Obsessive-compulsive disorders: Theory and management.* Littleton, MA: PSG Publishing.

Johnson, B.D. (1977). The race, class, and irreversibility hypotheses: myths and research about heroin. In J.D. Rittenhouse (Ed.), *The epidemiology of heroin and other narcotics.* National Institute on Drug Abuse Research Monograph 16 (pp. 51–57). Rockville, MD: National Institute on Drug Abuse.

Joint Commission on Mental Illness and Health. (1961). *Action for mental health.* New York: Basic Books.

Jorm, A.F., Scott, R., Henderson, A.S., & Kay, D.W.K. (1988). Educational level differences on the Mini-Mental State: The role of test bias. *Psychological Medicine, 18,* 727–731.

Kahn, R.L., Goldfarb, A.I., Pollack, M., & Peck, A. (1960). Brief objective measures for the determination of mental status in the aged. *American Journal of Psychiatry, 117,* 326–328.

Kandel, D.B. (1978). Homophily, selection, and socialization in adolescent friendship. *American Journal of Sociology, 84,* 427–436.

Karno, M., Golding, J.M., Sorenson, S.B., & Burnam, M.A. (1988). The epidemiology of obsessive-compulsive disorder in five U.S. communities. *Archives of General Psychiatry, 45,* 1094–1099.

Karno, M., Hough, R.L., Burnam, A., Escobar, J.I., Timbers, D.M., Santana, F., & Boyd, J.H. (1987). Lifetime prevalence of specific psychiatric disorders among Mexican Americans and non-Hispanic Whites in Los Angeles. *Archives of General Psychiatry, 44,* 695–701.

Kay, D.W.K., Henderson, A.S., Scott, R., Wilson, J., Richwood, D., & Grayson, D.A. (1985). Dementia and depression among the elderly living in the Hobart community: The effect of the diagnostic criteria on the prevalence rates. *Psychological Medicine, 15,* 771–788.

Keith, S.J., & Schooler, N.R. (1989). Treatment of schizophreniform illness. In B. Karasu & A.J. Frances (Eds.), *Treatment of psychiatric disorders* Washington, DC: American Psychiatric Association Press.

Keller, M.B., Lavori, P.W., Klerman, G.L., Andreasen, N.C., Endicott, J., Coryell, W., Fawcett, J., Rice, J.P., & Hirschfeld, R.M.A. (1986). Low levels and lack of predictors of somatotherapy and psychotherapy received by depressed patients. *Archives of General Psychiatry, 43,* 458–466.

Keller, M.B., & Shapiro, R.W. (1982). "Double depression": Superimposition of acute depressive episodes on chronic depressive disorders. *American Journal of Psychiatry, 139,* 438–442.

Kellner, R. (1965). Neurosis in general practice. *British Journal of Clinical Practice, 19,* 681–682.

Kellner, R. (1975). Psychotherapy in psychosomatic disorders: A survey of controlled studies. *Archives of General Psychiatry, 32,* 1021–1030.

———. (1985). Functional somatic symptoms in hypochondriasis. *Archives of General Psychiatry, 42,* 821–833.

Kendell, R.E. (1975). *The role of diagnosis in psychiatry.* London: Blackwell Scientific Publications.

Kenyon, F.E. (1964). Hypochondriasis: A clinical study. *British Journal of Psychiatry, 110,* 478–488.

Kessel, W.I.N. (1960). Psychiatric morbidity in a London general practice. *British Journal of Preventive and Social Medicine, 14,* 16–22.

Keyl, P. & Eaton, W.W. (1989). Risk factors for the onset of panic attacks and panic disorder.

Kiloh, L.G. (1961). Pseudo-dementia. *Acta Psychiatrica Scandinavica, 37,* 336–351.

Kirmayer, L.J. (1984). Culture, affect and somatization. *Transcultural Psychiatry Research Review, 21,* 159–188.

Kish, L. (1965). *Survey sampling.* New York: John Wiley.

Kittner, S.J., White, L.R. Farmer, M.E., Wolz, M., Kaplan, E., Moes, E., Brody, J.A., & Feinleib, M. (1986). Methodological issues in screening for dementia: The problem of education adjustment. *Journal of Chronic Disease, 39,* 163–170.

Kleinbaum, D.G., Kupper, L.L., & Morgenstern, H. (1982). *Epidemiologic research: Principles and quantitative methods.* Belmont, CA: Wadsworth.

Kleinman, A. (1982). Neurasthenia and depression: A study of somatization in China. *Culture, Medicine and Psychiatry, 6,* 117–190.

Klerman, G.L. (1988). The current age of youthful melancholia: Evidence for increase in depression among adolescents and young adults. *British Journal of Psychiatry, 152,* 4–14.

Klerman, G.L., Lavori, P.W., Rice, J., et al. (1985). Birth cohort trends in rates of major depressive disorder among relatives of patients with affective disorder. *Archives of General Psychiatry, 42,* 689–693.

Klerman, G.L., & Weissman, M.M. (1980). Depressions among women: Their nature and causes. In M. Guttentag, S. Salasin, & D. Belle, (Eds.), *The mental health of women* (pp. 57–92). New York: Academic Press.

Klorman, R., Strauss, J., & Kokes, R. (1977). Premorbid adjustment in schizophrenia: Concepts, measures, and implications. Part IV. Some biological approaches to research on premorbid functioning in schizophrenia. *Schizophrenia Bulletin, 3,* 226–239.

Kraepelin, E. (1921). *Manic-depressive insanity and paranoia.* Edinburgh: E. & S. Livingstone.

Kramer, M. (1969). Cross-national study of diagnosis of the mental disorders: Origin of the problem. *American Journal of Psychiatry,* 125 (Suppl. I-II).

————. (1977). Epidemiology, biostatistics and mental health planning. In R.R. Monroe, G.D. Klee, & E.B. Brody (Eds.), *Psychiatric research report 22. Psychiatric epidemiology and mental health planning* (pp. 1–63). Washington, DC: American Psychiatric Association.

————. (1980). The rising pandemic of mental disorders and associated chronic diseases and disabilities. *Acta Psychiatrica Scandinavica* (Supplementum 285), *62,* 382–396.

Kramer, M., German, P.S., Anthony, J.C., Von Korff, M., & Skinner, E.A. (1985). Patterns of mental disorders among the elderly residents of eastern Baltimore. *Journal of the American Geriatrics Society, 33,* 236–245.

Kringlen, E. (1965). Obsessional neurotics: A long-term follow-up. *British Journal of Psychiatry, 111,* 709–722.

Landerman, R., Pennybacker, M., Melville, M.L., Woodbury, M., Manton, K.G. Jordan, K., & Locke, B.Z. (1985). Psychiatric disorders: A rural/urban comparison. *Archives of General Psychiatry, 42,* 651–656.

Langner, T.S., & Michael, S. (1963). *Life Stress and mental health: The Midtown Manhattan study.* New York: Free Press.

Last, J.M. (1983). *A dictionary of epidemiology.* New York: Oxford University Press.

Lavori, P.W., Klerman, G.L., Keller, M.B., Reich, T., Rice, J., & Endicott, J. (1987). Age-period-cohort analysis of secular trends in onset of major depression: Findings in siblings of patients with major affective disorder. *Journal of Psychiatry Research, 21,* 23–35.

Leaf, P.J., German, P., Spitznagel, E. George, L., Landsverk, J., & Windle, C. (1985a). The institutional population. In W.W. Eaton & L.G. Kessler (Eds.), *Epidemiologic field methods in psychiatry: The NIMH Epidemiologic Catchment Area program* (pp. 49–66). Orlando, FL: Academic Press.

Leaf, P.J., Livingston, M.M., Tischler, G.L., Weissman, M.M., Holzer, C.E., III, & Myers, J.K. (1985b). Contact with health professionals for the treatment of psychiatric and emotional problems. *Medical Care, 23,* 1322–1337.

Leaf, P.J., Bruce, M.L., Tischler, G.L., Freeman, D.H., Weissman, M.M., & Myers, J.K. (1988). Factors affecting the utilization of specialty and general medical mental health services. *Medical Care, 26,* 9–26.

Lee, C.K., Kwak, Y.S., Rhee, H., Kim, Y.S., Han, J.H., Choi, J.O., & Lee, Y.H. (1984). DIS lifetime prevalence in Korea. (Unpublished manuscript).

Leighton, D.C., Harding, J.S., Macklin, D.B., MacMillan, A.M., & Leighton, A.H. (1963). *The character of danger: Psychiatric symptoms in selected communities.* New York: Basic Books.

Lewis, A.J. (1936). Problems of obsessional illness. *Proceedings of the Royal Society of Medicine, 29,* 325–326.

———. (1957). Obsessional illness. *Acta Neuropsiquiatrica Argentina, 3,* 323–325.

Lewis, C.E., Croughan, J.L., Whitman, B.Y., & Miller, J.P. (1983a). Association of alcoholism and antisocial personality in a narcotic-dependent population. The Lexington addicts. *Psychiatry Research, 10,* 31–46.

Lewis, C.E., Rice, J., & Helzer, J.E. (1983b). Diagnostic interactions: Alcoholism and antisocial personality. *Journal of Nervous and Mental Disease, 171,* 105–113.

Lin, E.H.B., Carter, W.B., & Kleinman, A.M. (1985). An exploration of somatization among Asian refugees and immigrants in primary care. *American Journal of Public Health, 75,* 1080–1084.

Lo, W.H. (1967). A follow-up study of obsessional neurotics in Hong Kong Chinese. *British Journal of Psychiatry, 113,* 823–832.

Maddux, J.F., & Desmond, D.P. (1975). Reliability and validity of information from chronic heroin users. *Journal of Psychiatry Research, 12,* 87–95.

Manderscheid, R.W., & Barrett, S.A. (Eds.). (1987). *Mental health, United States.* (p. 79). (DHHS Publication No. (ADM) 87-1518). Washington, DC: U.S. Government Printing Office.

Marks, I.M. (1987). *Fears, phobias, and rituals: Panic, anxiety, and their disorders.* New York: Oxford University Press.

Mavreas, V.G., Beis, A., Mouyias, A., Rigoni, F., & Lyketsos, G.C. (1986). Prevalence of psychiatric disorders in Athens: A community study. *Social Psychiatry, 21,* 172–181.

Mayou, R. (1976). The nature of bodily symptoms. *British Journal of Psychiatry, 129,* 55–69.

————. (1978). Chest pain in the cardiac clinic. *Journal of Psychosomatic Research, 17,* 353–357.

McKeon, J., Roa, B., & Mann, A. (1984). Life events and personality traits in obsessive-compulsive neurosis. *British Journal of Psychiatry, 144,* 185–189.

Merikangas, K.R., & Weissman, M.M. (1987). Epidemiology of anxiety disorders in adulthood. In R. Michaels & J.O. Cavenar (Eds.), *Psychiatry* (Vol. 3, chap. 14). Philadelphia: Lippincott.

Millon, T. (1981). *Disorders of personality. DSM-III, Axis II,* (p. 181). New York: John Wiley.

Morris, J.N. (1964). *Uses of epidemiology* (2nd ed.). Baltimore: Williams & Wilkins.

Mortimer, J.A. (1988). Do psychosocial risk factors contribute to Alzheimer's disease? In A.S. Henderson & J.H. Henderson (Eds.), *Etiology of dementia of Alzheimer's type.* Chichester: John Wiley.

Mortimer, J.A., & Hutton, J.T. (1985). Epidemiology and etiology of Alzheimer's disease. In J.T. Hutton & A.D. Kenney (Eds.), *Senile dementia of the Alzheimer's type* (Vol. 18). New York: Alan R. Liss.

Mortimer, J.A., Schuman, L.M., & French, L.R. (1981). Epidemiology of dementing illness. In J.A. Mortimer & L.M. Schuman (Eds.), *The epidemiology of dementia.* New York: Oxford University Press.

Murphy, J.M. (1980). Continuities in community-based psychiatric disorders. *Archives of General Psychiatry, 37,* 1215–1223.

Murphy, J.M., Sobol, A.M., Neff, R.K., Olivier, D.C., & Leighton, A.H. (1984). Stability of prevalence—depression and anxiety disorders. *Archives of General Psychiatry, 41,* 990–997.

Musto, D.F. (1973). *The American disease: Origins of narcotic control.* New Haven: Yale University Press.

Myers, J.K., Weissman, M.M., Tischler, G.I., Holzer, C.E., Leaf, P.J., Orvaschel, H ., Anthony, J.C., Boyd, J.H., Burke, J.D., Kramer, M., & Stoltzman, R. (1984). Six-month prevalence of psychiatric disorders in three communities. *Archives of General Psychiatry, 41,* 959–967.

Nam, C.B., & Powers, M.G. (1965). Variations in socioeconomic structure by race, residence, and life cycle. *American Sociological Review, 30,* 97–103.

National Center for Health Statistics. (1978): *Plan and operation of the Health and Nutrition Examination Survey, United States, 1971-1973.* (Vital and Health Statistics, Series 1, No. 10a, DHEW Publication No. (PHS) 79-1310, Public Health Service). Washington, DC: U.S. Government Printing Office.

————. (1979). *The national nursing home survey: 1977 summary for the United States.* (Vital and Health Statistics, Series 13, No. 43). Washington, DC: U.S. Government Printing Office.

National Institute of Alcoholism and Alcohol Abuse (NIAAA). (1985). *U.S. alcohol epidemiological data reference manual,* Vol. 1. Washington, DC: Author.

National Institute on Drug Abuse (NIDA). (1989). *National household survey on drug abuse. 1988 population estimates.* (DHHS Publication No. ADM 89-1636). Rockville, MD: Author.

Nemiah, J.C. (1984). Foreword. In T.R. Insel (Ed.), *Obsessive-compulsive disorder*. Washington, DC: American Psychiatric Press.

———. (1985). Obsessive-compulsive disorder (obsessive-compulsive neurosis). In H.I. Kaplan & B.J. Sadock (Eds.), *Comprehensive textbook of psychiatry*. (4th ed.). Baltimore: Williams and Wilkins.

Newcomb, M.D., & Bentler, P.M. (1985). The impact of high school substance use on choice of young adult living environment and career directions. *Journal of Drug Education, 2,* 253–261.

O'Donnell, J.A., Voss, H.L., Clayton, R.R. Slatin, G.T., & Room, R.G.W. (1976). *Young Men and Drugs*. (NIDA Research Monograph No. 5). Rockville, MD: National Institute on Drug Abuse.

O'Malley, P.M., Johnston, L.D., & Bachman, J.A. (1985). Cocaine use among American adolescents and young adults. In N.J. Kozel & E.H. Adams (Eds.), *Cocaine use in America: Epidemiologic and clinical perspectives*. (NIDA Research Monograph No. 61 (pp. 50–75). Rockville MD: National Institute on Drug Abuse.

Parry, H.J. (1979). Sample surveys of drug abuse. In R.I. Dupont, A. Goldstein, & J. O'Donnell (Eds.), *Handbook on drug abuse*, (pp. 381–394). National Institute on Drug Abuse. Washington DC.

Perley, M.J., & Guze, S.B. (1962). Hysteria: The stability and usefulness of clinical criteria. *New England Journal of Medicine, 266,* 421–426.

Pfeiffer, E. (1975). A short portable mental status questionnaire for the assessment of organic brain deficit in elderly patients. *Journal of the American Geriatrics Society, 23,* 433–441.

Pilowski, I. (1970). Primary and secondary hypochondriasis. *Acta Psychiatrica Scandinavica, 46,* 273–285.

Plum, F. (1979). Dementia: An approaching epidemic. *Nature, 279,* 372–373.

Polich, J.M., & Kaelber, C.T. (1985). Sample survey and the epidemiology of alcoholism. In M.A. Schuckit & A.E. Slaby (Eds.), *Alcohol patterns and problems*. (Series in Psychosocial Epidemiology, Vol. 5). New Brunswick, NJ: Rutgers University Press.

Pollit, J. (1957). Natural history of obsessional states. *British Medical Journal, 1,* 194–198.

President's Commission on Mental Health. (1978). *Report to the President from the President's Commission on Mental Health* (Stock No. 040-000-00390-8, Vol. 1). Washington, DC: U.S. Government Printing Office.

Price, R.A., Kidd, K.K., Pauls, D.L., et al. (1985). Multiple threshold models for the affective disorders: The Yale-NIMH collaborative family study. *Journal of Psychiatric Research, 19,* 533–546.

Purtell, J.J., Robins, E., & Cohen, M.E. (1951). Observations on clinical aspects of hysteria. *Journal of the American Medical Association, 146,* 902–909.

Racagni, G., & Smeraldi, E. (Eds.). (1987). *Anxious depression: assessment and treatment*. New York: Raven Press.

Rasmussen, S.A., & Tsuang, M.T. (1984). Epidemiology of obsessive-compulsive disorder: A review. *Journal of Clinical Psychiatry, 45,* 450–457.

———, M.T. (1986). Epidemiology and clinical features of obsessive- compulsive disorder. In M.A. Jenike, L. Baer, & W.E. Minichiello (Eds.), *Obsessive-compulsive disorders*. Littleton, MA: PSG Publishing.

Ray, O.S. (1983). *Drugs, society and human behavior* (3rd ed.). St. Louis: C.V. Mosby.

Redick, R.W. (1974). Patterns in use of nursing homes by the aged mentally ill (Statistical Note 107). Rockville, MD: Division of Biometry and Epidemiology, National Institute of Mental Health.

Redick, R.W., Manderscheid, R.W., Witkin, M.J., & Rosenstein, M.J. (1983). *National Institute of Mental Health: A history of the US national reporting program for mental health statistics, 1840-1983.* (DHHS Publication No. ADM 83-1296). Washington, DC: U.S. Government Printing Office.

Regier, D.A., Boyd, J.H., Rae, D.S., Burke, J.D., Locke, B.Z., Myers, J.K., Kramer, M., Robins, L.N., George, L.K., & Karno, M. (1988a). One month prevalence of mental disorders in the U.S.—based on the five Epidemiologic Catchment Area sites. *Archives of General Psychiatry, 45,* 977-986.

Regier, D.A., Hirschfeld, R.M.A., Goodwin, F.K., Burke, J.D., Lazar, J.B., & Judd, L.L. (1988b). The NIMH Depression Awareness Recognition and Treatment (D/ART) program: Structure, aims and scientific basis. *American Journal of Psychiatry, 145,* 1351-1357.

Regier, D.A., Goldberg, I.D., & Taube, C.A. (1978). The de facto US mental health services system: A public health perspective. *Archives of General Psychiatry, 35,* 685-693.

Regier, D.A., Myers, J.K., Kramer, M., et al. (1984). The NIMH epidemiologic catchment area program. *Archives of General Psychiatry, 41,* 934-941.

Regier, D.A., & Burke, J.D. (1989). Epidemiology—Quantitative and experimental methods in psychiatry. In H.I. Kaplan & B.J. Sadock (Eds.), *Comprehensive textbook of psychiatry.* (5th ed. pp. 308-326). New York: Williams & Wilkins.

Rice, J., Reich, T., Andreasen, N.C., et al. (1984). Sex-related differences in depression: Familial evidence. *Journal of Affective Disorders, 71,* 199-210.

Ricks, D.F., & Berry, J.C. (1973). Family and symptom patterns that precede schizophrenia. In M. Roff & D.F., Ricks (Eds.), *Life history research in psychopathology.* Minneapolis: University of Minnesota Press.

Robins, E. Sociopathy. (1977). In *International encyclopedia of psychiatry, psychology, psychoanalysis, and neurology.* New York: Aesculapius Publishers.

Robins, E., Gentry, K.A. Munoz, R.A., & Marte, S. (1977). A contrast of the three more common illnesses with the ten less common in a study and 18-month follow-up of 314 psychiatric emergency room patients. *Archives of General Psychiatry, 34,* 269-281.

Robins, E., & Guze, S.B. (1972). Classification of affective disorders: The primary—secondary, the endogenous–reactive, and the neurotic–psychotic concepts. In T.A. Williams, M.M. Katz, & J.A. Shields, Jr. (Eds.), *Recent advances in the psychobiology of the depressive illnesses.* Washington, DC: U.S. Government Printing Office.

Robins, E., Purtell, J.J., & Cohen, M.E. (1952). "Hysteria" in men. *New England Journal of Medicine, 246,* 677-685.

Robins, L.N. (1966). *Deviant children grown up: A sociological and psychiatric study of sociopathic personality.* Baltimore: Williams & Wilkins.

———. (1978). Sturdy childhood predictors of adult outcomes: Replications from longitudinal studies. *Psychological Medicine, 8,* 611-622.

———. (1982). The diagnosis of alcoholism after DSM-II. In E.M. Pattison & E. Kaufman (Eds.), *Encyclopedic handbook of alcoholism.* New York: Gardner Press.

———. (1985). Epidemiology: Reflections on testing the validity of psychiatric interviews. *Archives of General Psychiatry, 42,* 918–924.

———. (1989). Diagnostic grammar and assessment. In L. Robins & J. Barrett (Eds.), *The validity of diagnosis.* New York: Raven Press.

Robins, L.N., Davis, D.H., & Nunco, D.N. (1974). How permanent was Vietnam drug addiction? *American Journal of Public Health, 64* (Suppl.), 38–43.

Robins, L.N., Helzer, J.E., Croughan, J., & Ratcliff, K. (1981a). National Institute of Mental Health Diagnostic Interview Schedule: Its history, characteristics, and validity. *Archives of General Psychiatry, 38,* 381–389.

Robins, L.N., Helzer, J.E., Croughan, J., Williams, J.B.W., & Spitzer, R.L. (1981b). *NIMH Diagnostic Interview Schedule: Version III* (May 1981). Rockville, MD: National Institute of Mental Health.

Robins, L.N., Helzer, J.E., Ratcliff, K.S., & Seyfried, W. (1982). Validity of the Diagnostic Interview Schedule, Version II: DSM-III diagnoses. *Psychological Medicine, 12,* 855–870.

Robins, L.N., & Kulbok, P.A. (1986). Methodological strategies in suicide. In J. Mann & M. Stanley (Eds.), Psychology of suicidal behavior. *Annals of the New York Academy of Sciences, 487,* 1–15.

Robins, L.N., & Murphy, G.E. (1967). Drug use in a normal population of young Negro men. *American Journal of Public Health, 57,* 1580–1596.

Robins, L.N., Orvaschel, H., Anthony, J., Blazer, D., Burnam, A., & Burke, J. (1985). The Diagnostic Interview Schedule. In W.W. Eaton & L.G. Kessler (Eds.), *Epidemiologic methods in psychiatry: The NIMH Epidemiologic Catchment Area Program.* Orlando, FL: Academic Press.

Robins, L.N., & Przybeck, T. (1985). Age of onset of drug use: A factor in drug and other disorders. In C.L. Jones & R.J. Battjes (Eds.), *Etiology of drug abuse: Implications for prevention* (pp. 178–192). (DHHS Publication No. ADM 85-1335). Washington, DC: U.S. Government Printing Office.

Rocca, W.A., Amaducci, L.A., & Schoenberg, B.S. (1986). Epidemiology of clinically diagnosed Alzheimer's disease. *Annals of Neurology, 19,* 415–424.

Rohan, W.P. (1982). The concept of alcoholism: Assumptions and issues. In E.M. Pattison & E. Kaufman (Eds.), *Encyclopedic handbook of alcoholism.* New York: Gardner Press.

Roth, M. (1981). The diagnosis of dementia in late and middle life. In J.A. Mortimer & L.M. Schuman (Eds.), *The epidemiology of dementia.* New York: Oxford University Press.

Rounsaville, B.J. (forthcoming). Patterns of use and psychiatric consequences in treated and untreated cocaine users. In C. Schade & S. Schober (Eds.), *Epidemiology of cocaine use and abuse.* National Institute on Drug Abuse Research Monograph. Rockville MD: National Institute on Drug Abuse.

Roy, A. (1986). Depression, attempted suicide, and suicide in patients with chronic schizophrenia. *Psychiatric Clinics of North America, 9,* 193–206.

Rudin, E. (1953). Beitrag zur Frage der Zwangskrankheit insbesondere ihrere Hereditaren beziechungen. *Archive Für Psychiatrie und Nervenkrankheiten, 191,* 14–54.

Rutter, M., & Madge, N. (1976). *Cycles of disadvantage.* London: Heinemann.

Salzman, L., & Thaler, F.H. (1981). Obsessive-compulsive disorders: A review of the literature. *American Journal of Psychiatry, 138,* 286–296.

Schneider, K. (1959). *Clinical psychopathology.* (M. W. Hamilton, Trans.). New York: Grune & Stratton.

Schulsinger, F. (1972). Psychopathy: Heredity and environment. In M. Roff, L.N. Robins, & M. Pollack (Eds.), *Life history research in psychopathology.* Minneapolis: University of Minnesota Press.

Schwab, J.J., Bell, R.A., Warheit, G.J., & Schwab, R.B. (1979). *Social order and mental health.* New York: Brunner/Mazel.

Shapiro, S., Skinner, E.A., Kessler, L.G., et al. (1984). Utilization of health and mental health services: Three Epidemiologic Catchment Area sites. *Archives of General Psychiatry, 41,* 971–978.

Somervell, P.D., Leaf, P.J., Weissman, M.M., Blazer, D.G., & Bruce, M.L. (1989). The prevalence of major depression in black and white adults in five United States communities. *American Journal of Epidemiology, 130,* 725–735.

Spalt, L. (1980). Hysteria and antisocial personality. *Journal of Nervous and Mental Disease, 168,* 456–464.

Spitzer, R.L., Endicott, J., & Robins, E. (1978). Research Diagnostic Criteria: Rationale and reliability. *Archives of General Psychiatry, 35,* 773–782.

Srole, L., Langner, T.S., Michael, S.T., Opler, M., & Rennie, T. (1962). *Mental health in the metropolis: the Midtown Manhattan Study.* New York: McGraw-Hill.

Strauss, J.S., & Carpenter, Jr., W.T. (1981). *Schizophrenia.* New York: Plenum Press.

Sturt, E., Wykes, T., & Creer, C. (1982). Demographic characteristics of the sample. In J.K. Wing, C. Creer, E. Sturt, & T. Wykes, *Long-term community care: Experience in a London borough.* Psychological Medicine (Monograph Suppl 2).

Surtees, P.G., Sashidharan, S.P., & Dean, C. (1986). Affective disorder amongst women in the general population: A longitudinal study. *British Journal of Psychiatry, 148,* 176–186.

Swartz, M.S., Blazer, D.G., George, L.K., & Landerman, R. (1986a). Somatization disorder in a community population. *American Journal of Psychiatry, 143,* 1403–1408.

Swartz, M.S., Blazer, D.G., Woodbury, M., George, L.K., & Landerman, R. (1986b). Somatization disorder in a U.S. southern community: Use of a new procedure for analysis of medical classification. *Psychological Medicine, 16,* 595–609.

Swartz, M.S., Hughes, D., Blazer, D.G., & George, L.K. (1987). Somatization disorder in the community: A study of diagnostic concordance among three diagnostic systems. *Journal of Nervous and Mental Disorder, 175,* 26–33.

Swartz, M.S., Landerman, R., Blazer, D.G., & George, L.K. (1989). Somatization symptoms in the community: A rural/urban comparison. *Psychosomatics, 30,* 44–53.

Taylor, J.R., & Helzer, J.E. (1983). The natural history of alcoholism. In B. Kissen & H. Begleiter (Eds.), *The biology of alcoholism, Vol. 6.* New York: Plenum Press.

Templer, D.I. (1972). The obsessive-compulsive neurosis: Review of research findings. *Comprehensive Psychiatry, 13,* 375–383.

Terry C.E., & Pellens, M. (1928). *The opium problem.* New York: Bureau of Social Hygiene.

Tsuang, M.T., & Woolson, R.F. (1978). Excess mortality in schizophrenia and affective disorders. *Archives of General Psychiatry, 35,* 1181–1185.

Uhlenhuth, E.G., Balter, M.B., Mellinger, G.D., et al. (1983). Symptom checklist syndromes in the general population: Correlations with psychotherapeutic drug use. *Archives of General Psychiatry, 40,* 1167–1173.

U.S. Department of Health & Human Services, Office on Smoking and Health. (1988). *The health consequences of smoking: Nicotine addiction. A report of the Surgeon General.* (DHHS Publication No. [PHS] CDC 88-8406). Washington DC: U.S. Government Printing Office.

Vaillant, G.E. (1983). *The natural history of alcoholism.* Cambridge, MA: Harvard University Press.

Victor, M., & Banker, B.Q. (1978). Alcohol and dementia. In R. Katzman, R.D. Terry, & K.L. Bick (Eds.), *Alzheimer's disease: Senile dementia and related disorders.* New York: Raven Press.

Videbech, T. (1975). The psychopathology of anancastic endogenous depression. *Acta Psychiatrica Scandinavica, 52,* 336–373.

Von Korff, M.R., & Anthony, J.C. (1982). The NIMH Diagnostic Interview Schedule modified to record current mental status. *Journal of Affective Disorders, 4,* 365–371.

Von Korff, M., & Eaton, W.W. (1989). Epidemiologic findings on panic. In R. Baker (Ed.), *Panic disorder.* New York: John Wiley.

Von Korff, M., Eaton, W.W., & Keyl, P. (1985). The epidemiology of panic attacks and panic disorder: Results of three community surveys. *American Journal of Epidemiology, 122,* 970–981.

Warheit, G.J., & Auth, J.B. (1985). Epidemiology of alcohol abuse in adulthood. In J.O. Cavenar (Ed.), *Psychiatry* (Vol. 3, chap. 18). Philadelphia, Lippincott.

Warheit, G.J., Bell, R.A., Schwab, J.J., & Buhl, J.M. (1986). An epidemiologic assessment of mental health problems in the southeastern United States. In M.M. Weissman, J.K. Myers, & C.E. Ross (Eds.), *Community surveys of psychiatric disorders* (pp. 191–208). New Brunswick, NJ: Rutgers University Press.

Washton, A.M., & Gold, M.S. (1986). Crack [Letter to the editor]. *Journal of the American Medical Association, 256* (6), 711.

Wattis, J.P. (1983). Alcohol and old people. *British Journal of Psychiatry, 143,* 306–307.

Weingartner, H., Cohen, R.M., Murphy, D.L., Martello, J., & Gerdt, C. (1981). Cognitive process in depression. *Archives of General Psychiatry, 38,* 42–47.

Weissman, M.M. (1985). The epidemiology of anxiety disorders: Rates, risks, and family patterns. In. A.H. Tuma & J.D. Maser (Eds.), *Anxiety and the anxiety disorders.* Hillsdale, NJ: Lawrence Erlbaum.

———. (1988). The epidemiology of panic disorder and agoraphobia. In A. Frances & R. Hales (Eds.), *Review of psychiatry, Vol. 7.* Washington, DC: American Psychiatric Press.

Weissman, M.M., Gershon, E.S., Kidd, K.K., et al. (1984). Psychiatric disorder in relatives of probands with affective disorders: The Yale-NIMH collaborative family study. *Archives of General Psychiatry, 41,* 13–21.

Weissman, M.M., & Klerman, G.L. (1982). Sex differences and the epidemiology of depression. In F.G. Guggenheim & C.C. Nadelson, *Major psychiatric disorders: Overviews and selected readings* (pp. 95–114). New York: Elsevier Science Publishing.

———. (1985). Gender and depression. *Trends in Neurosciences, 8,* 416–420.

Weissman, M.M., Leaf, P.J., Holzer, C.E. III, Myers, J.K., & Tischler, G.L. (1984). The epidemiology of depression: An update on sex differences in rates. *Journal of Affective Disorders, 7,* 179–188.

Weissman, M.M., & Myers, J.K. (1978). Affective disorders in a United States community: The use of Research Diagnostic Criteria in an epidemiological survey. *Archives of General Psychiatry, 35,* 1304–1311.

Weissman, M.M., Myers, J.K., & Harding, P.S. (1978). Psychiatric disorders in a U.S. urban community: 1975–1976. *American Journal of Psychiatry, 135,* 459–462.

Weissman, M.M., Myers, J.K., Tischler, G.L., Holzer, C.E., Leaf, P.J., Orvaschel, H., & Brody, J.A. (1985). Psychiatric disorders (DSM-III) and cognitive impairment in the elderly in a U.S. urban community. *Acta Psychiatrica Scandinavica, 71,* 366–379.

Weissman, M.M., & Paykel, E.S. (1974). *The depressed woman: A study of social relationships,* Chicago, IL: University of Chicago Press.

Welner, A., Marten, S., Wochnick, E., et al. (1979). Psychiatric disorders among professional women. *Archives of General Psychiatry, 36,* 169–173.

Wilcox, A.J., & Horney, L.F. (1984). Accuracy of spontaneous abortion recall. *American Journal of Epidemiology, 120,* 727–733.

Wilsnack, S.C. (1982). Prevention of alcohol problems in women. In *Special population issues,* Alcohol and Health Monograph No. 4 (pp. 77–108). Publication No. ADM 82-1193). Washington, DC: U.S. Government Printing Office.

Wing, J.H., Nixon, J., Mann, S.A., & Leff, J.P. (1977). Reliability of the PSE (9th ed) used in a population survey. *Psychological Medicine, 7,* 505–516.

Winokur, G., Clayton, P.J., & Reich, T. (1969). *Manic-depressive illness.* St. Louis, MO: C.V. Mosby.

Winokur, G., & Tsuang, M. (1975). The Iowa 500: Suicide in mania, depression and schizophrenia. *American Journal of Psychiatry, 132,* 650–651.

Wittchen, H-U. (1987). Chronic difficulties and life events in the long-term course of affective and anxiety disorders. In M.C. Angermeyer (Ed.), *From social class to social stress.* Berlin: Springer-Verlag.

Wittchen, H-U., Semler, G., & Von Zerssen, D. (1985). A comparison of two diagnostic methods: Clinical ICD diagnosis v. DSM-III and Research Diagnosis Criteria using the Diagnostic Interview Schedule (Version 2). *Archives of General Psychiatry, 42,* 677–684.

Woodruff, R.A., Robins, L.N., Winokur, G. et al. (1971). Manic-depressive illness and social achievement. *Acta Psychiatrica Scandinavica, 47,* 237–249.

World Health Organization (WHO). (1987). Draft text submitted to the second Expert Committee on the Tenth Revision of the International Classification of Diseases (Chap 5). Geneva: WHO.

Yamaguchi, K., & Kandel, D.B. (1985). On the resolution of role incompatibility: Life event history analysis of family roles and marijuana use. *American Journal of Sociology, 90*, 1284–1325.

Yeh, E-K., Hwu, H-G., & Chang, L-Y. (1984). Prevalence of mental disorders in Taipei City by Chinese modified Diagnostic Interview Schedule: A preliminary report. *Bulletin of Chinese Society of Neurology & Psychiatry, 10*, 88–103.

Yolles, S.F., & Kramer, M. (1969). Vital statistics. In L. Bellak & L. Loeb (Eds.), *The schizophrenia syndrome.* New York: Grune & Stratton.

Zahn, T.P., Insel, T.R., & Murphy, D.L. (1984). Psychophysiological changes during pharmacological treatment of patients with obsessive-compulsive disorder. *British Journal of Psychiatry, 145*, 39–44.

APPENDIX A
Demographic Tables

Table A–1a Total Number of Persons in Basic Subsamples in the ECA (Sex and Race by Age and Site)

		Males				Females			
	Total	White	Black	Hispanic	Unknown	White	Black	Hispanic	Unknown
Overall	20,862[a]	5,927	1,988	824	151	8,053	2,974	796	148
Age:									
18–29	4,949	1,363	681	342	53	1,387	815	276	32
30–44	4,736	1,335	508	280	30	1,488	809	250	36
45–64	4,396	1,299	372	138	23	1,718	661	154	31
65+	6,753	1,928	426	64	34	3,457	688	112	44
Unknown	28[a]	2	1	0	11	3	1	4	5
Site:									
New Haven	5,372[a]	1,970	237	48	27	2,745	286	35	23
Baltimore	4,034	1,056	525	13	0	1,563	861	16	0
St. Louis	3,498	970	489	11	0	1,228	792	8	0
Durham	4,423	1,148	659	11	0	1,645	954	6	0
Los Angeles	3,535	783	78	741	124	872	81	731	125

[a]One case unknown for sex, race, and age.

Table A–1b Total Number of Persons in Standard Subsamples by Age, Sex, and Ethnicity

		Total	Males			Females		
			White	Black	Hispanic	White	Black	Hispanic
Age	*Last School Year Completed*							
18–29	<8th	190	20	14	69	8	9	68
	8	127	47	23	14	19	14	9
	9–11	1,252	258	296	122	210	273	71
	12	1,436	379	166	65	475	277	62
	13–15	1,148	323	126	61	385	184	47
	16+	726	316	43	10	278	52	17
30–44	<8th	336	36	29	95	32	34	107
	8	140	28	28	8	44	23	8
	9–11	904	177	152	68	223	226	51
	12	1,225	268	124	43	474	263	46
	13–15	1,006	322	106	43	319	171	27
	16+	1,056	477	57	22	385	88	10
45–64	<8th	706	161	119	46	147	156	72
	8	429	115	43	10	175	72	11
	9–11	999	265	89	37	365	205	33
	12	1,093	302	49	23	558	123	27
	13–15	551	177	23	13	265	55	7
	16+	470	238	16	7	173	27	3
65+	<8th	1,801	401	240	37	714	328	67
	8	1,261	372	45	6	707	108	13
	9–11	1,155	370	42	5	618	95	13
	12	997	299	26	8	596	51	8
	13–15	589	187	18	6	349	22	4
	16+	433	182	7	0	216	24	2
	Residence							
18–29	Household	4,367	1,201	434	254	1,364	787	270
	Nursing home	14	9	1	0	0	2	0
	Prison	482	113	226	84	13	17	5
	Psych. hosp.	86	40	20	4	10	9	1
30–44	Household	4,406	1,243	387	246	1,452	784	240
	Nursing home	30	10	5	0	10	1	1
	Prison	192	41	85	28	8	12	9
	Psych. hosp.	108	41	31	6	18	12	0
45–64	Household	4,088	1,198	315	121	1,628	627	152
	Nursing home	182	52	30	5	61	28	1
	Prison	42	14	14	12	1	0	0
	Psych. hosp.	84	35	13	0	28	7	1
65+	Household	5,704	1,705	361	52	2,837	605	95
	Nursing home	990	198	58	11	607	70	17
	Prison	3	1	1	1	0	0	0
	Psych. hosp.	56	24	6	5	13	13	0

Table A-1b continues

Table A-1b continued

Age		Total	Males White	Black	Hispanic	Females White	Black	Hispanic
18–29	Number in Household							
	1	622	250	91	14	178	65	15
	2	1,170	361	89	58	420	174	49
	3	1,020	259	69	56	349	203	73
	4	798	194	81	62	250	151	49
	5+	741	134	103	64	162	189	84
30–44	1	696	260	101	32	202	78	9
	2	852	285	72	17	286	135	45
	3	802	192	60	34	301	172	36
	4	1,076	319	75	59	385	172	57
	5+	971	186	79	104	275	226	93
45–64	1	997	250	98	17	410	183	29
	2	1,622	529	88	35	702	201	46
	3	680	196	51	23	283	89	32
	4	403	123	36	16	140	67	18
	5+	374	100	42	30	87	86	26
65+	1	2,373	379	137	10	1,473	309	53
	2	2,394	1,056	130	24	981	166	27
	3	501	175	45	8	209	51	10
	4	181	48	15	3	75	37	3
	5+	225	46	31	7	96	42	2
	Urban/Rural (Durham and St. Louis)							
18–29	Rural	369	105	64	2	115	83	0
	Urban	1,263	353	171	6	414	315	4
30–44	Rural	432	114	69	0	135	114	0
	Urban	1,248	359	159	5	370	352	3
45–64	Rural	604	149	78	0	237	139	1
	Urban	1,190	363	120	2	458	244	3
65+	Rural	752	158	90	0	335	169	0
	Urban	1,067	230	156	0	438	241	2
	Unemployed 6 Mo. in Last 5 Yr. When Not Out of Labor Market							
	(St. Louis, Durham Los Angeles)							
18–29		622	135	115	68	99	158	32
30–44		393	74	68	55	83	80	25
45–64		217	58	32	11	45	53	15
65+		80	13	20	1	20	25	1
	Currently Working Full-time							
18–29		2,443	867	262	184	707	291	114
30–44		3,012	1,093	296	200	801	483	108
45–64		2,088	836	155	88	696	249	47
65+		308	181	22	3	83	16	2

Table A-1b continues

Table A–1b continued

		Males			Females		
	Total	White	Black	Hispanic	White	Black	Hispanic
Age	*Occupation of Current Full-time Workers*						
18–29 Mngmt/Prof	497	205	32	20	189	33	12
Tech/Sale	851	204	56	36	371	134	46
Service	296	60	44	24	83	62	19
Farm/Forest	33	17	6	9	1	0	0
Skilled Lab	295	199	43	27	12	7	6
Laborers	440	173	76	65	42	51	30
30–44 Mngmt/Prof	964	439	51	32	306	104	14
Tech/Sale	811	208	61	20	316	168	31
Service	316	63	34	19	72	106	19
Farm/Forest	25	14	1	6	4	0	0
Skilled Lab	337	212	43	43	23	7	7
Laborers	531	150	104	77	71	91	37
45–64 Mngmt/Prof	496	252	18	14	169	31	7
Tech/Sale	580	180	13	11	310	45	17
Service	316	62	31	12	88	117	6
Farm/Forest	35	21	6	2	5	1	0
Skilled Lab	255	171	24	22	22	8	4
Laborers	389	148	61	25	93	46	13
65+ Mngmt/Prof	88	62	4	0	21	1	1
Tech/Sale	84	43	3	1	32	4	0
Service	49	21	4	0	16	8	0
Farm/Forest	14	11	1	1	1	0	0
Skilled Lab	29	23	2	0	4	0	0
Laborers	43	20	8	1	9	3	1
Nam & Powers Job Status Percentile (Current Full-time Workers)							
18–29 0–20	346	76	48	51	71	61	36
21–40	570	174	78	52	147	92	23
41–60	673	225	70	49	214	78	34
61–80	563	245	38	22	193	44	15
81–100	260	138	23	7	73	12	5
30–44 0–20	304	45	29	32	68	91	38
21–40	601	148	85	58	143	134	30
41–60	675	224	67	53	194	113	18
61–80	923	406	75	44	267	105	14
81–100	481	263	38	10	120	33	8
45–64 0–20	327	47	39	16	103	106	13
21–40	451	147	42	22	166	63	9
41–60	486	181	39	23	192	36	11
61–80	588	328	26	19	164	33	13
81–100	219	131	7	6	62	10	1
65+ 0–20	45	15	6	1	17	5	1
21–40	63	32	6	0	16	7	1
41–60	69	38	5	1	22	3	0
61–80	94	65	3	1	24	1	0
81–100	36	30	2	0	4	0	0

Table A-1b continues

Table A–1b continued

		Males			Females		
	Total	White	Black	Hispanic	White	Black	Hispanic
Age	*Annual Personal Income of Current Full-time Workers*						
18–29 Less than 5,000	268	78	23	17	93	30	23
5,000–9,999	518	116	59	55	158	90	35
10,000–14,999	516	168	43	52	175	56	18
15,000–19,999	269	131	23	20	72	10	10
20,000–24,999	157	79	17	17	29	3	11
25,000–34,999	111	76	8	8	17	2	1
35,000–49,999	21	13	2	1	4	0	0
50,000 or more	11	9	0	1	1	0	0
30–44 Less than 5,000	137	16	9	15	58	28	10
5,000–9,999	365	45	23	23	145	94	33
10,000–14,999	537	126	61	41	177	104	26
15,000–19,999	441	184	45	41	118	40	7
20,000–24,999	339	176	36	25	65	25	11
25,000–34,999	288	170	16	18	61	11	3
35,000–49,999	140	95	7	7	26	1	0
50,000 or more	75	59	2	5	6	0	1
45–64 Less than 5,000	86	8	4	3	40	26	5
5,000–9,999	284	36	25	5	146	54	17
10,000–14,999	355	96	23	19	166	35	12
15,000–19,999	280	123	27	16	89	21	3
20,000–24,999	193	121	7	15	42	8	0
25,000–34,999	181	121	11	11	30	4	1
35,000–49,999	72	55	1	5	9	1	0
50,000 or more	70	62	1	2	3	1	0
65 + Less than 5,000	25	9	5	0	5	5	1
5,000–9,999	58	24	5	0	24	4	1
10,000–14,999	59	32	3	0	22	2	0
15,000–19,999	33	24	3	1	5	0	0
20,000–24,999	25	22	0	0	3	0	0
25,000–34,999	17	11	0	1	4	0	0
35,000–49,999	13	12	1	0	0	0	0
50,000 or more	19	17	1	0	1	0	0
Financial Dependence							
18–29	664	83	49	25	131	311	59
30–44	605	90	64	38	129	226	51
45–64	759	226	101	28	176	183	38
65 +	830	210	97	24	284	153	46

Table A–1b continues

Table A–1b continued

		Total	Males White	Males Black	Males Hispanic	Females White	Females Black	Females Hispanic
Age	Marital History							
18–29	Married, no div/sep	1,174	324	82	91	460	106	97
	Never married	2,225	704	375	148	493	385	83
	Div/Sep once	451	97	43	23	166	85	29
	Div/Sep more	420	83	38	17	148	96	30
	Cohabit, never married	649	142	137	62	115	139	37
30–44	Married, no div/sep	1,788	593	126	141	639	163	107
	Never married	556	169	79	25	138	116	21
	Div/Sep once	992	249	107	46	339	187	51
	Div/Sep more	1,092	226	137	54	319	283	57
	Cohabit, never married	269	81	52	14	43	57	14
45–64	Married, no div/sep	2,253	703	134	63	994	269	70
	Never married	348	129	40	13	110	39	10
	Div/Sep once	889	225	97	35	330	151	40
	Div/Sep more	804	210	85	24	259	182	30
	Cohabit, never married	50	13	12	2	9	11	3
65+	Married, no div/sep	4,621	1,384	216	39	2,450	423	63
	Never married	483	127	29	1	274	43	5
	Div/Sep once	884	226	84	16	395	126	23
	Div/Sep more	543	134	83	6	209	84	17
	Cohabit, never married	22	6	7	1	2	3	2
	Current Marital Status							
18–29	Married	1,563	414	118	114	618	159	120
	Widowed	14	4	1	0	2	6	1
	Sep/Div	468	86	44	17	154	122	35
	Never married	2,874	846	512	210	608	524	120
30–44	Married	2,555	823	221	192	890	263	140
	Widowed	74	3	2	1	34	29	4
	Sep/Div	1,243	242	147	48	373	341	71
	Never married	825	250	131	39	181	173	35
45–64	Married	2,416	868	171	87	967	224	77
	Widowed	668	68	42	5	346	178	22
	Sep/Div	862	202	103	30	270	200	41
	Never married	398	142	52	15	119	50	13
65+	Married	2,405	1,230	175	40	795	124	21
	Widowed	3,110	389	126	13	2,056	430	60
	Sep/Div	532	125	82	8	202	79	22
	Never married	505	133	36	2	276	46	7

Table A–1b continues

Table A–1b continued

Age	Total	Males			Females		
		White	Black	Hispanic	White	Black	Hispanic
	Outpatient Mental Health Services in Last 6 Mo. (Household Residents)						
18–29	412	116	44	19	138	63	20
30–44	561	142	34	26	244	80	26
45–64	420	111	28	16	173	68	18
65 +	341	67	24	0	188	55	4
	Inpatient Mental Health Services in Last Year (Household Residents)						
18–29	132	58	27	11	17	15	1
30–44	122	47	25	8	23	14	4
45–64	131	46	20	6	43	13	0
65 +	84	34	7	0	32	11	0

Table A–2 ECA Sample Sizes for Analyses of Correlates
of Psychiatric Disorder as a Whole

	Unweighted Sample Size
Total ECA Sample	20,862
Less those for whom fewer than 8 diagnoses were personally assessed and no diagnosis personally assessed was found positive	− 1,222
Psychiatric diagnosis as a whole assessed	19,640
Number of those assessed diagnostically for whom data on specific correlates available	
A. Based on whole sample:	
Sex, type of residence, site	19,640
Age: 12 unknown	19,628
Marital status: 108 unknown	19,532
Marital history: 222 unknown	19,418
Ethnicity: 246 unknown	19,394
Education: 257 unknown	19,383
Financial dependency: 555 unknown	19,085
B. Based on subsamples:	
Treatment (household sample)	18,059
Rural/urban (households in 2 sites only)	6,801
Employment (males 30–64 in households, 28 unknown)	3,452
Occupation (employed males 30–64, 19 unknown)	2,660

Table A-3 Number of Cases with Specific Diagnoses

	Diagnoses by Personal Interview			
	Positive			
	Lifetime	One-Year	Negative	Not Assessed[b]
Any diagnosis	7,026	4,536	12,614	1,235
Cognitive impairment:				
Mild or severe	—[a]	2,160	17,678	156
Severe	—[a]	516	19,322	156
Somatization	67	64	19,500	427
Phobia	3,053	2,120	16,461	480
Panic disorder	304	196	19,197	493
Depressive episode	1,258	812	18,239	497
Dysthymia	703	—[a]	18,792	497
Manic episode	172	113	19,298	524
Obsessive compulsive	571	386	18,856	567
Schizophreniform	35	21	19,389	570
Schizophrenia	305	229	19,122	567
Drug abuse/dependence	1,316	602	18,088	590
Anorexia nervosa	11[c]	—[a]	19,383	600
Alcohol abuse/dependence	2,630	1,018	16,747	617
Antisocial personality	628	295	18,740	626
Generalized anxiety	722	360	7,954	2,578[d]

[a]Not assessed.
[b]Except for generalized anxiety, varies from 0.8% to 3% of subjects.
[c]Not treated separately in this volume because of small numbers, but included in "any diagnosis" and count of number of diagnoses.
[d]Assessed in only three sites.

Table A-4 Wave 2 Numbers for Ethnic Group, Sex, and Age in Sites Assessing
Generalized Anxiety (Used for Tables 8-4 and 8-5)

	Durham	St. Louis	Los Angeles
Total	3,422	2,683	2,432
Males			
Total	1,390	1,101	1,141
White:	893	738	623
< 30	154	209	164
30–44	228	219	237
45–64	258	181	138
65+	253	129	84
Black:	497	363	51
< 30	107	120	18
30–44	110	118	21
45–64	115	55	9
65+	165	70	3
Hispanic:	a	a	467
< 30	—	—	152
30–44	—	—	194
45–64	—	—	89
65+	—	—	32
Females			
Total	2,032	1,582	1,291
White:	1,276	934	710
< 30	162	236	149
30–44	236	229	264
45–64	233	155	330
65+	527	235	142
Black:	756	648	63
< 30	125	185	16
30–44	165	229	27
45–64	180	135	12
65+	286	99	8
Hispanic:	a	a	518
< 30	—	—	115
30–44	—	—	182
45–64	—	—	105
65+	—	—	76

[a]Too few to report.

APPENDIX B
The Interview Used
in the ECA

Follow-up questions (i.e., those asked only if previous
answers made them appropriate) are marked ‡. As explained
in Chapter Two, each positive answer to a symptom question
was followed by a standard set of "probe" questions designed
to assess clinical importance and to rule out physical causes.
These follow-up probes have been omitted below to save space,
as have standard follow-up questions about the ages at which
symptoms occurred the first and last times, and a few other
probes.

DEMOGRAPHICS

RECORD SEX AS OBSERVED.

How old were you on your last birthday?

What is your birthdate?

What is the highest grade in school or year of college
that you completed?

‡Did you get a high school diploma or pass a high
school equivalency test?

‡What is the highest degree that you have?

Are you currently enrolled in school or college?

When was the last time you worked for pay?

‡What kind of business or industry (is/was) this?

‡What kind of work (are/did) you do(ing)?

Would you please look at this card and give me the
letter of the group that best describes your racial
background?

Are you now receiving any unemployment compensation?

Are you receiving any disability payments or
disability benefits from Social Security, the
Veterans Administration, the State of [   ], or
from any other source?

Are you receiving any Social Security benefits other
than disability payments?

Are you receiving any welfare payments from the State
of [   ] such as AFDC or general assistance?

Would you please look at this card and tell me which
letter represents your household's total income before
taxes for the past year, including salaries, wages,
social security, welfare, and any other income?

About how much of this total household income was
earned or brought in by you personally?

Did you ever serve in the armed forces of the
United States?

‡When did you serve?

Are you presently married or are you widowed,
separated, divorced, or have you never been married?

‡Are you currently living with your (husband/wife)?

‡Are you currently living with someone as though you
were married?

‡How many times have you been legally married?

‡(So you've never been/How many times have you been)
divorced?

‡(Other than when you separated just before a divorce,)
Have you and your (husband(s)/wife/wives) ever
separated for a few days or longer because of not
getting along?

‡Have you (ever) lived with someone for at least a year as
though you were married?

‡Did you and the person(s) you lived with ever separate
for a few days or longer because of not getting along?

How many children have you had, not counting any who
are yours by adoption or who were born dead?

Have you ever acted as a parent for children who
were not your own natural children?

‡Have you ever tried for a year or more to get (someone)
pregnant without being able to?

HEALTH SERVICES

When you want help with or care for a health problem, where do you usually go?

‡IF PHYSICIAN: Is this a doctor at a clinic or hospital, or does he have his own office?

‡IF HOSPITAL: Where in the hospital do you usually go? Is it to the emergency room, an outpatient clinic, a walk-in clinic?

Now I'd like to ask you some questions about your use of health services in the past six months. Not counting any care you may have received while you were a bed patient in a hospital or nursing home, how many times altogether did you receive care or treatment from a health professional in an office, clinic or emergency room in the past six months, that is since (DATE)?

‡Were all of these visits to the same place?

‡Where did you go (most often)?

‡How many visits did you make to this place?

‡During these visits, did you and the health professional talk about any problems you had with your emotions or nerves that might have been connected to or in addition to the reason for your visit? (PAUSE) How about problems with alcohol or drugs?

‡How about the visits you made to other places? Did you and the health professionals talk about any problems you had with your emotions or nerves, alcohol or drugs?

‡Were these problems the main reason for making (any of these/this) visit(s)?

Now I'm going to read you a list of different kinds of places and people where someone might get help for problems with emotions, nerves, drugs, alcohol, or their mental health. Have you ever gone to:

... A friend or relative for help with any of these problems?

... A minister, priest or rabbi for help with any of these problems

... A psychiatrist or other mental health specialist at a health plan or family clinic for help with any of these problems?

Did you ever go to a psychiatrist, psychologist,
social worker or counselor in private practice for
help with problems with your emotions, nerves,
drugs, alcohol, or your mental health?

Have you ever talked to a medical doctor in
private practice (except for a psychiatrist) or to
any medical person at a health plan or at a
primary care clinic about problems like that?

Have you ever gone to a mental health center?

... A psychiatric outpatient clinic at a general
hospital or university hospital?

... An outpatient clinic in a psychiatric
hospital?

... An outpatient clinic in a Veterans
Administration Hospital, for problems with
emotions, nerves, alcohol, or mental health?

... A drug clinic?

... An alcohol clinic?

Have you ever gone to a hospital emergency room
for problems with emotions, nerves, drugs, alcohol
mental health?

... A family service, child counseling, or social
service agency?

... Someone at a self-help group like Alcoholics
Anonymous, etc.?

... A community program like a crisis center or
hotline?

... A spiritualist, herbalist, natural therapist
or reader for problems with emotions, nerves,
drugs, alcohol, or mental health?

... Anyone else?

‡You mentioned that you went to (NAME TYPES OF PLACES
VISITED) for problems with your emotions, mental
health, drugs, or alcohol. Have you been to (this/any of
these) place(s) in the last six months? What was the
name of the place you went (most often)?

‡How many visits to this particular (place/person) did
you make in the last six months?

‡REPEAT FOR VISITS TO OTHER SETTINGS

How many different times in the last 12 months (that
is, since DATE) did you stay at least one night in a
hospital, nursing home, or other medical care facility
because of your physical health?

‡How many of these admissions were to a hospital?

‡What hospital did you go to the last time you were admitted?

‡How many nights did you stay in the hospital?

‡REPEAT FOR OTHER HOSPITALIZATIONS

Have you ever been admitted to a hospital or other treatment
program where you stayed overnight because of family or
personal problems, a mental or emotional problem, trouble
with your nerves, or a problem with drugs or alcohol?

‡How many times have you ever been admitted to a state
psychiatric hospital?

‡How many times have you ever been admitted to a
private psychiatric hospital?

‡How many times have you ever been admitted to a
community mental health center?

‡How many times have you ever been admitted to a VA
hospital because of family or personal problems, a
mental or emotional problem, trouble with your nerves,
or a problem with drugs or alcohol?

‡How many times have you ever been admitted to a
general hospital because of family or personal
problems, a mental or emotional problem, trouble with
your nerves, or a problem with drugs or alcohol?

‡How many times have you ever stayed overnight or
longer in an alcohol treatment unit?

How many times have you ever stayed overnight or
longer in a drug treatment unit?

Have you ever stayed overnight or longer any place
else because of family or personal problems, a mental
or emotional problem, trouble with your nerves, or a
problem with drugs or alcohol? IF YES: How many
times?

‡You have told me that you were admitted to (TYPES OF
PLACES). Were you admitted to any of these places in
the past year? What was the name of the place you
were admitted to most recently?

‡How many nights did you stay there?

‡REPEAT FOR OTHER ADMISSIONS

PSYCHIATRIC DISORDERS

SOMATIZATION DISORDER

Now I am going to ask you about health problems that might have occurred at any time in your life. Have you ever had a lot of trouble with abdominal or belly pain (not counting times when you were menstruating)?

Have you ever had a lot of trouble with back pain?

Have you ever had pain in the joints:

Have you ever had pains in your arms or legs other than in the joints?

Have you ever had chest pains?

Have you ever had a lot of troubles with headaches?

FOR WOMEN ONLY: Have you ever had a lot of trouble with excessively painful menstrual periods?

Have you ever had pain when you urinate, (that is, pass your water)?

Have you ever been completely unable to urinate (or pass water) for 24 hours or longer, other than after (childbirth or) surgery?

Have you ever had burning pain in your mouth or around your private parts?

Have you ever had pain anywhere else, other than in the places we've already talked about?

Have you ever had a lot of trouble with vomiting (when you were not pregnant)?

ASK ONLY IF FEMALE: During any pregnancy did you have vomiting all through the pregnancy?

   ‡A. Were you ever hospitalized during a pregnancy because of vomiting?

Have you ever had a lot of trouble with nausea-- feeling sick to your stomach but not actually vomiting?

Have there ever been times when you have had a lot of trouble with loose bowels or diarrhea?

Have you ever had a lot of trouble with excessive gas or bloating of your stomach or abdomen?

Have you found there were any foods that you couldn't eat because they made you ill?

Have you ever been blind in one or both eyes where you couldn't see anything at all for a few seconds or more?

Has your vision ever become blurred for some period, when it wasn't just due to needing glasses or changing glasses?

Have you ever been deaf where you completely lost your hearing for a period of time?

Have you ever had trouble walking?

Have you ever been paralyzed--that is, completely unable to move a part of your body for at least a few minutes?

Was there ever a time when you lost your voice for 30 minutes or more and couldn't speak above a whisper?

Have you ever had a seizure or convulsion of any kind since you were 12 where you were unconscious but your body jerked?

Have you ever had fainting or falling out spells where you felt weak or dizzy and then passed out?

Have you ever had been unconscious for any (other) reason?

Have you ever had a period of amnesia--that is, a period of several hours or days where you couldn't remember anything afterwards about what happened during that time?

Have you ever had any (other) problems which seemed strange, like double vision or unusual spells?

Have you ever gotten short of breath when you had not been exerting yourself?

Have you ever been bothered by palpitations, that is, your heart beating so hard that you could feel it pounding in your chest?

> ‡A. Has that happened only when you were exerting yourself or at other times too?

Have you ever been bothered by dizziness?

Have you ever been bothered by periods of weakness, that is, when you could not lift or move things you could normally lift or move?

Have you ever been bothered by a feeling that there was a lump in your throat?

‡A. Was that only when you felt like crying?

Has your physical health been pretty good or have you
been sickly for the majority of your life?

WOMEN ONLY: Other than your first year of menstruation,
have your menstrual periods ever been irregular?

WOMEN ONLY: Have you ever had excessive bleeding with your
menstrual periods?

WOMEN ONLY: Other than your first year of menstruation,
have you ever missed two periods in a row?

Have you ever had to give up work, going to school or
other regular activities for at least several weeks
because you did not feel well enough to carry on
(other than when you were in the hospital)?

Have you ever had a sudden gain or loss of weight,
say 15 pounds in two weeks or less?

Have you ever lost feeling in an arm or a leg other
than when it had just fallen asleep from being in one
position too long?

‡A. Have you lost feeling anywhere else?

Have you ever had a lot of trouble with constipation?

Have you ever been troubled by a period of lots of
crying spells or crying very easily since you've been
an adult?

Has there ever been a period of time when you felt
that life was hopeless?

‡I'm going to mention some of the problems you've told
me about. Then I'll want to know how old you were
when you first had any one of these problems. For instance you've had a problem with (LIST ALL ITEMS POSITIVES)
What's the earliest age you first had one of these problems?

‡How recently have you had any of these problems?

PANIC DISORDER
Have you ever considered yourself a nervous person?

‡At what age did this nervousness begin?

Have you ever had a spell or attack when all of a
sudden you felt frightened, anxious or very uneasy in
situations when most people would not be afraid?

‡During one of your worst spells of suddenly feeling frightened or anxious or uneasy, did you ever notice that you had any of the following problems? During this spell:

A.   Were you short of breath--having trouble catching your breath?

B.   Did your heart pound?

C.   Were you dizzy or light-headed?

D.   Did your fingers or feet tingle?

E.   Did you have tightness or pain in your chest?

F.   Did you feel like you were choking or smothering?

G.   Did you feel faint?

H.   Did you sweat?

I.   Did you tremble or shake?

J.   Did you feel hot or cold flashes?

K.   Did things around you seem unreal?

L.   Were you afraid either that you might die or that you might act in a crazy way?

‡How old were you the first time you had one of these sudden spells of feeling frightened or anxious?

‡Have you ever had 3 spells like this close together--say within a 3-week period?

‡Have spells like this occurred during at least 6 different weeks of your life?

‡How recently have you had a spell like this?

PHOBIAS
Some people have phobias, that is, such a strong fear of something or some situation that they try to avoid it, even though they know there is no real danger. Have you ever had such an unreasonable fear of (INSERT EXAMPLES BELOW) that you tried to avoid (it/them)?

a.   Heights

b.   Tunnels or bridges

c.   Being in a crowd

d. Being on any kind of public transportation like airplanes, buses, or elevators.

e. Going out of the house alone

f. Being in a closed place

g. Being alone

h. Eating in front of other people you know or in public).

i. Speaking in front of a small group of people you know.

j. Speaking to strangers or meeting new people.

k. Storms.

l. Being in water, for instance, in a swimming pool or lake.

m. Spiders, bugs, mice, snakes or bats

n. Being near any (other) harmless animal or a dangerous animal that couldn't get to you.

o. Is there anything else you were unreasonably terrified to do or be near?

‡How old were you the first time you were bothered by any of these fears?

‡How recently (has this fear/have any of these fears) been so strong that you tried to avoid the situation?

‡You mentioned spells of feeling frightened or anxious when you (LIST UP TO 3 SYMPTOMS CODED "YES"). Did those spells occur only when you were (LIST ALL PHOBIAS) or did they occur at other times too?

DEPRESSIVE EPISODE AND DYSTHYMIA
In your lifetime, have you ever had two weeks or more during which you felt sad, blue, depressed, or when you lost all interest and pleasure in things that you usually cared about or enjoyed?

Have you had two years or more in your life when you felt depressed or sad almost all the time, even if you felt OK sometimes?

a) Has there ever been a period of two weeks or longer when you lost your appetite?

b) Have you ever lost weight without trying to--as much as two pounds a week for several weeks [or as much as 10 pounds altogether]?

c) Have you ever had a period when your eating increased so much [Did your eating increase so much] that you gained as much as two pounds a week for several weeks [or 10 pounds altogether]?

d) Have you ever had a period of two weeks or more when you had [Did you have] trouble falling asleep, staying asleep, or with waking up too early?

e) Have you ever had a period of two weeks or longer when you were [Were you] sleeping too much?

f) Has there ever been a period lasting two weeks or more when you felt [Did you feel] tired out all the time?

g) Has there ever been a period of two weeks or more when you talked or moved [Did you talk or move] more slowly than is normal for you?

h) Has there ever been a period of two weeks or more when you had [Did you have] to be moving all the time--that is, you couldn't sit still and paced up and down?

i) Was there ever a period of several weeks when your interest in sex was [Was your interest in sex] a lot less than usual?

j) Has there ever been a period of two weeks or more when you felt [Did you feel] worthless, sinful, or guilty?

k) Has there ever a period of two weeks or more when you had [Did you have] a lot more trouble concentrating than is normal for you?

l) Have you ever had a period of two weeks or more when your thoughts came [Did your thoughts come] slower than usual or seemed mixed up?

m) Has there ever been a period of two weeks or more when you thought [Did you think] a lot about death-- either your own, someone else's, or death in general?

n) Has there ever been a period of two weeks or more when you felt [Did you feel] like you wanted to die?

o) Have you ever felt [Did you feel] so low you thought of committing suicide?

p) Have you ever attempted [Did you attempt] suicide?

‡You said you've had a period of feeling (depressed or
blue/OWN EQUIVALENT) and also said you've had some
other problems like (LIST ALL POSITIVES). Has
there ever been a time when the feelings of depression
and some of these other problems occurred
together--that is, within the same month?
                         OR
You said you have had periods when (LIST ALL POSITIVES)
Was there ever a time when several of these problems
occurred together--that is, within the same month?

‡When you were having some of these problems at
about the same time were you feeling okay, or were
you feeling low, gloomy, blue, or uninterested in
everything?

‡What's the longest spell you've ever had when you felt
blue and had several of these other problems at the
same time?

‡Now I'd like to ask about spells when you felt both
(depressed/OWN EQUIVALENT) and had some of these other
problems like (LIST 2 or 3 POSITIVE ITEMS). In your
lifetime, how many spells like that have you had that
lasted two weeks or more?

‡Did you tell a doctor about (that spell/any of those
spells)?

  ‡A. Did you tell any other professional about (it/any
       of them)?

  ‡B. Did you take medicine more than once because of
       (that spell/any of those spells)?

  ‡C. Did (that spell/those spells) interfere with your
       life or activities a lot?

‡How old were you the first time you had a spell for
two weeks or more where you felt sad and had some of
these other problems?

‡Did (this spell/any of those spells) occur just after
someone close to you died?

  ‡A. Have you had any spell of (depression/OWN EQUILVALENT)
       along with these other problems at times when it wasn't
       due to a death?

‡Are you in one of these spells of feeling low or dis-
interested and having some of these other problems
now?

  ‡A. IF NO. When did your last spell like that end?

‡Now I'd like to know about the time when you were
feeling (depressed/OWN EQUIVALENT) for at least 2
weeks and had the largest number of these other problems at the same time. (IF CAN'T CHOOSE: Then pick
up one bad spell.) How old were you at that time?

During (this/that) spell of (depression/OWN EQUIVA-
LENT) which of these other problems did you have? For
instance, during that spell (when you were _____ years
old) did you -- ASK FOR EACH POSITIVE IN a-p ABOVE, BEGINNING
WITH PHRASE IN BRACKETS.

MANIC EPISODE

Has there ever been a period of one week or more when
you were so happy or excited or high that you got into
trouble, or your family or friends worried about it,
or a doctor said you were manic?

a) Has there ever been a period of a week or more when
   you were [Were you] so much more active than usual
   that you or your family or friends were concerned
   about it?

b) Has there ever been a period of a week or more when
   you went [Did you go] on a spending sprees--spending
   so much money that it caused you or your family some
   financial trouble?

c) Have you ever had a period of a week or more when
   your interest in sex was [At that time was your
   interest in sex] so much stronger than is typical
   for you that you wanted to have sex a lot more
   frequently than is normal for you or with people you
   normally wouldn't be interested in?

d) Has there ever been a period of a week or more when
   you talked [Did you talk] so fast that people said
   they couldn't understand you?

e) Have you ever had a period of a week or more when
   thoughts raced [Did thoughts race] through your head
   so fast that you couldn't keep track of them?

f) Have you ever had a period of a week or more when
   you felt [Did you feel] that you had a special
   gift or special powers to do things others couldn't
   do or that you were a specially important person?

g) Has there ever been a period of a week or more
   when you hardly slept [Did you hardly sleep] at
   all but still didn't feel tired or sleepy?

h) Was there ever a period of a week or more when you
   were [Were you] easily distracted so that any
   little interruption could get you off the track?

‡You said you've had a period of feeling very happy
or excited or manic and also said you've had some
problems like (LIST POSITIVES). Has there ever
been a time when the feelings of being excited or
manic and some of these problems occurred together--
that is, within the same month?
                        OR
You said you had times when (LIST ALL POSITIVES).
Was there ever a time when some of these problems
occurred together--that is, within the same month?

   ‡A. When you were feeling that way, were you unusually
       irritable or likely to fight or argue?

‡What's the longest spell you've had when you felt
(high, manic, or very excited/irritable) for at
least a week and had several of these other problems
like (LIST POSITIVES)?

‡In your lifetime, how many spells like that have
you had that lasted one week or more?

‡Did you tell a doctor about (that spell/any of
those spells)?

   ‡A. Did you tell any other professional about
       (it/any of them)?

   ‡B. Did you take medicine more than once because of
       (that spell/any of those spells)?

   ‡C. Did (that spell/any of those spells) interfere
       with your life or activities a lot?

‡How old were you the first time you had a spell
for one week or more where you felt (high or
excited/irritable) and had some of these problems
(such as)?

‡Are you in one of these spells of feeling (high or
excited/irritable) and having some of these
problems now?

   ‡A. How long ago did your last period like that
       end?

‡Now I'd like to know about the time you were
feeling (high or excited/irritable) and had the
largest number of these other problems at the
same time. (IF CAN'T CHOOSE: Then pick one bad
spell.) How old were you at that time?

‡During (this/that) spell of being (high/irritable),
which of these problems did you do? For instance,
during that spell (when you were ____ years old) (ASK FOR
EACH POSITIVE IN a-h, BEGINNING WITH PHRASE IN BRACKETS)

SCHIZOPHRENIA

Now I want to ask about some ideas you might have had about other people. Have you ever believed people were watching you or spying on you?

Have you ever believed that someone was reading your mind?

    ‡A. Did they actually know what you thought or were they just guessing from the look on your face or from knowing you for a long time?

Have you ever believed you could actually hear what another person was thinking, even though he was not speaking or believed that others could hear your thoughts?

Have you ever believed that others were controlling how you moved or what you thought against your will?

Have you ever felt that someone or something could put strange thoughts directly into your mind or could take or steal your thoughts out of your mind?

Have you ever believed that you were being sent special messages through television or the radio?

Have you ever had the experience of seeing something or someone that others who were present could not see - that is, had a vision when you were completely awake?

    ‡A. What did you see?

Have you more than once had the experience of hearing things other people couldn't hear, such as a voice?

    ‡A. What did you hear?

    ‡B. Did you hear voices commenting on what you were doing or thinking?

Have you ever been bothered by strange smells around you that nobody else seemed to be able to smell perhaps even odors coming from your own body?

    ‡A. What did you smell?

Have you ever had unusual feelings inside or on your body--like being touched when nothing was there or feeling something moving inside your body?

    ‡A. What did you feel?

‡How old were you when you first experienced (READ EXAMPLES CODED POSITIVES)?

‡When was the last time you (saw/heard/smelled) something others thought was not there/felt those sensations]?

‡We've talked about certain beliefs and experiences you had (LIST POSITIVES). Did as much as 6 months go by from the time you first (thought/experienced) any of these to the last time you did?

ANOREXIA NERVOSA

Now I'd like to ask you about problems you might have had with your weight. Have you ever thought that you were too fat or in danger of getting too fat?

Have you ever lost 15 pounds or more, either by dieting or without meaning to (not by having a baby)?

‡A. What is the lowest weight that you ever reached after losing 15 pounds or more?

‡B. How tall were you then?

‡C. How old were you the first time you lost 15 pounds or more?

‡Did you ever think you were overweight when other people such as your parents or friends said you had gotten too thin?

‡Have you ever seen or talked to a doctor because of having lost too much weight?

‡FOR WOMEN ONLY: Did your periods stop shortly before or during any time you were losing weight?

ALCOHOL ABUSE AND DEPENDENCE

Now I am going to ask you some questions about using alcohol. How old were you the first time you ever drank enough to get drunk?

‡Did you get drunk more than once before you were 15?

Has your family ever objected because you were drinking too much?

Did you ever think that you were an excessive drinker?

Have you ever drunk as much as a fifth of liquor in one day, that would be about 20 drinks, or 3 bottles of wine or as much as 3 six-packs of beer in one day?

Has there ever been a period of two weeks when every day you were drinking 7 or more beers, 7 or more drinks or 7·or more glasses of wine?

‡Has there ever been a couple of months or more when at least one evening a week, you drank 7 drinks, or 7 bottles of beer or 7 glasses of wine?

‡A. How long has it been since you drank 7 or more drinks at least once a week, or do you still?

Have you ever told a doctor about a problem you had with drinking?

Have friends, your doctor, your clergyman, or any other professional ever said you were drinking too much for your own good?

Have you ever wanted to stop drinking but couldn't?

Some people promise themselves not to drink before 5 o'clock or never to drink alone, in order to control their drinking. Have you ever done anything like that?

Did you ever need a drink just after you had gotten up (that is, before breakfast)?

Have you ever had job (or school) troubles because of drinking--like missing too much work or drinking on the job (or at school)?

Did you ever lose a job (or get kicked out of school) on account of drinking?

Have you ever gotten into trouble driving because of drinking--like having an accident or being arrested for drunk driving?

Have you ever been arrested or held at the police station because of drinking or for disturbing the peace while drinking?

Have you ever gotten into physical fights while drinking?

Have you ever gone on binges or benders, where you keep drinking for a couple of days or more without sobering up?

Did you neglect some of your usual responsibilities then?

How many times have you gone on benders that lasted at least a couple of days?

Have you ever had blackouts while drinking, that is, where you drank enough so that you couldn't remember the next day what you had said or done?

Have you ever had "the shakes" after stopping or cutting down on drinking (for example, your hands shake so that your coffee cup rattles in the saucer or you have trouble lighting a cigarette)?

‡Have you ever had fits or seizures after stopping or cutting down on drinking?

‡Have you ever had the DT's (Hallucinations and fever) when you quit drinking?

‡Have you ever seen or heard things that weren't really there after cutting down on drinking?

There are several health problems that can result from long stretches of pretty heavy drinking. Did drinking ever cause you to have:

a) liver disease or yellow jaundice?

‡b) vomiting blood or other stomach troubles?

‡c) trouble with tingling or numbness in your feet?

‡d) Memory trouble when you haven't been drinking (not blackouts)?

‡e) inflamation of your pancreas, or pancreatitis?

Have you ever continued to drink when you knew you had a serious physical illness that might be made worse by drinking?

Has there ever been a period in your life when you could not do your ordinary daily work well unless you had had something to drink?

‡I'm going to mention some things you told me about drinking. I'll be asking how old you were the first time any one of these things happened. You mentioned (LIST ALL CODED POSTIVIES). What's the earliest age any of these things happened?

    A. When was the last time any of these (5*) things happened?

OBSESSIVE COMPULSIVE DISORDER

I want to ask you next whether you have ever been bothered by having certain unpleasant thoughts all the time. An example would be the persistent idea that you might harm or kill someone you loved, even though you really didn't want to. Have you ever been bothered by that or by any other unpleasant and persistent thought?

    ‡A. Was this only for a short time or was it over a period of several weeks?

‡B. Did these thoughts keep coming into your mind no matter how hard you tried to get rid of them?

‡Other unpleasant thoughts that keep bothering some people, even when they know they are silly, are that their hands are dirty or have germs on them, no matter how much they wash them, or that relatives who are away have been hurt or killed. Have you ever had any kind of unreasonable thought like that?

‡REPEAT A AND B

‡How old were you when you first had a problem with this kind of thought or worry?

‡How recently have you been bothered by thoughts like this that kept coming back no matter how ridiculous you thought they were?

Some people have problems with feeling that they have to do something over and over again even though they know it is really foolish--but they can't resist doing it--things like washing their hands again and again or going back several times to be sure they've locked a door or turned off the stove. Have you ever had to do something like that over and over?

Was there a time when you always had to do something--like getting dressed perhaps--in a certain order, and had to start all over again if you got the order wrong?

‡Did you have to do this only for a short time, or did you feel you had to do this over a period of several weeks?

Has there ever been a period of several weeks when you felt you had to count something, like the squares in a tile floor, and couldn't resist doing it even when you tried to?

‡How old were you when you first had to (do something over and over/check on things/count/or do things in a special order)?

‡How recently have you been bothered by having to do things like this (do something over and over/check on things/count/or do things in a special order)?

DRUG ABUSE AND DEPENDENCE

Now I'd like to ask about your experience with drugs. (HAND CARD A) Have you ever used any drugs on this list to get high or without a prescription, or more than was prescribed--that is, on your own?

CARD A
AMPHETAMINES, STIMULANTS, UPPERS, SPEED
BARBITURATES, SEDATIVES, DOWNERS, SLEEPING PILLS,
SECONAL, QUAALUDES.
TRANQUILIZERS, VALIUM LIBRIUM.
COCAINE, COKE
HEROIN.
OPIATES OTHER THAN HEROIN (CODEINE, DEMEROL, MORPHIN
METHADONE, DARVON, OPIUM).
PSYCHEDELICS (LSD, MESCALINE, PEYOTE, PSILOCYBIN, DM
PCP).

‡A. Have you taken any other drugs on your own either
     to get high or for other mental effects?

‡Have you ever used (this drug/one of these drugs) on
your own more than 5 times in your life?

A. Which ones?

‡Have you ever used any one of these drugs or any other
illicit drug every day for two weeks or more?
IF YES, ASK FOR SPECIFIC DRUG

‡Have you ever used any of these drugs or any other
illicit drug enough so that you felt like you needed
it or were dependent on it?
IF YES, ASK FOR SPECIFIC DRUG

‡Have you ever tried to cut down on any drugs but found
you couldn't do it?
IF YES, ASK FOR SPECIFIC DRUGS

‡Did you find you need larger amounts of these drugs to
get an effect--or that you could no longer get high on
the amount you used to use?
IF YES, ASK FOR SPECIFIC DRUGS

‡Have you had withdrawal symptoms--that is, have you
felt sick because you stopped or cut down on any of
these drugs?
IF YES, ASK FOR SPECIFIC DRUGS

‡Did you have any health problems like fits, an
accidental overdose, a persistent cough or an
infection as a result of using any of these drugs?
IF YES, ASK FOR SPECIFIC DRUGS

‡Did any drugs cause you considerable problems with your
family, friends, on the job, at school, or with the police?
IF YES, ASK FOR SPECIFIC DRUGS

‡Did you have any emotional or psychological problems
from using drugs--such as feeling crazy or paranoid or
depressed or uninterested in things?
IF YES, ASK FOR SPECIFIC DRUGS

‡Let's go over the problems you told me you had with
drugs. Did you ever tell a doctor about any of these
problems with drugs?

> ‡A. Did you talk to any other professional about any
> problems with drugs?

> ‡B. Did you use medication more than once for any of
> these problems with drugs?

> ‡C. Did any of these problems with drugs interfere with
> your life or activities a lot)?

‡How old were you when you first had any of these
problems with drugs?

‡When was the last time?

‡Which drugs have you had any of these problems with in
the last year?

ANTISOCIAL PERSONALITY

> Now I'd like to ask about your life as a child. Let's
> begin with some questions about school. Did you ever
> repeat a grade?

> > ‡A. Did you get held back more than once?

> How were your grades in school--better than average,
> average, or not so good?

> > ‡A. Did your teachers think you did about as well as
> > you could or did they think you had the ability
> > to do much better?

> > ‡B. How old were you when your teachers first felt that way?

> Did you frequently get into trouble with the teacher
> or principal for misbehaving in school? (ELEMENTARY,
> JUNIOR HIGH, OR HIGH SCHOOL)

> > ‡A. How old were you when you first got into trouble
> > for misbehaving in school?

> Were you ever expelled or suspended from school?
> (ELEMENTARY, JUNIOR HIGH, OR HIGH SCHOOL)

> > ‡A. How old were you when you were first expelled or
> > suspended?

Did you ever play hooky from school at least twice in one year?

    ‡A. Was that only in your last year in school or before that?

    ‡B. Did you play hooky as much as 5 days a year in at least two school years, not counting your last year in school? (Note: Yale question does not include the phrase: "not counting your last year in school.")

    ‡C. How old were you when you first played hooky?

Did you ever get into trouble at school for fighting?

    ‡A. Did that happen more than once?

    ‡B. Were you sometimes the one who started the fight?

    ‡C. How old were you when you first got into trouble for fighting at school?

Before age 18, did you ever get into trouble with the police, your parents or neighbors because of fighting (other than for fighting at school)?

    ‡A. Did that happen more than once?

    ‡B. Were you sometimes the one who started the fight?

    ‡C. How old were you when you first got into trouble for fighting away from school?

    ‡D. Even though you didn't get into trouble for fighting, did you start fights more than once before you were 15?

When you were a kid, did you ever run away from home overnight?

    ‡A. Did you run away more than once?

    ‡B. How old were you when you first ran away from home overnight?

Of course, no one tells the truth all the time, but did you tell a lot of lies when you were a child or teenager?

    ‡A. How old were you when you first told a lot of lies?

When you were a child, did you more than once swipe things from stores or from other children or steal from your parents or from anyone else?

    ‡A. How old were you when you first stole things?

When you were a kid, did you ever intentionally damage
someone's car or do anything else to destroy or
severely damage someone else's property?

‡A. How old were you when you first did that?

Were you ever arrested as a juvenile or sent to
juvenile court?

‡A. How old were you the first time?

Have you ever been arrested since 18 for anything
other than traffice violations?

‡A. Have you been arrested more than once?

‡B. Have you ever been convicted of a felony?

Have you had at least four traffic tickets in your
life for speeding or running a light or causing an
accident?

SOMATIZATION INSERT
Now I'm going to ask you about your sexual experience.
In general, has your sex life been important to you,
or could you have gotten along as well without it?

Has having sexual relations ever been physically
painful for you?

Has there been a period of several months in your life
when having sex was not pleasurable for you (even when
it wasn't painful)?

Have you had any (other) kind of sexual difficulties
(FOR MEN, such as a period of two months or more when
you had trouble having an erection)?

RETURN TO ANTISOCIAL PERSONALITY
Did you ever walk out on your (husband/wife/partner
with whom you were living as married) either
permanently or for at least several weeks?

Did you ever hit or throw things at your
(wife/husband/partner)?

‡A. Were you ever the one who hit or threw things
first, regardless of who started the argument?

‡B. Did you hit or throw things first on more than one
occasion?

Have you ever spanked or hit a child hard enough so
that he or she had bruises or had to stay in bed or
see a doctor?

Since age 18, have you been in more than one fight that came to swapping blows?

Have you ever used a weapon, like a stick, knife, or gun, in a fight since you were 18?

Since you were 18, did you ever hold three or more different jobs within a five-year period?

Have you been fired from more than one job?

Since you were 18, have you quit a job three times or more before you already had another job lined up?

On any job you have had since you were 18, were you late or absent an average of 3 days a month or more?

How many months out of the last five years have you been without a job?

‡For how much of that time did you want to work but were not able to find a job?

‡For how much of that time were you not looking for work because of emotional or mental problems or because of problems with drugs or alcohol?

‡How much time (besides that) were you just not interested in working but not in school, or physically ill (or retired or a housewife)?

Have you ever used an alias or an assumed name?

Have you thought that you lied pretty often since you have been an adult?

Have you ever traveled around for a month or more without having any arrangements ahead of time and not knowing how long you were going to stay or where you were going to work?

Has there ever been a period when you had no regular place to live, for at least a month or so?

Have you sometimes left young children under 6 years old home alone while you were shopping or out doing anything else?

Have there been times when a neighbor fed a child (of yours/you were caring for) because you didn't get around to shopping for food or cooking, or kept your child overnight because no one was taking care of him at home?

Has a nurse, or social worker or teacher ever said that any child (of yours/you were caring for) wasn't being given enough to eat or wasn't being kept clean enough or wasn't getting medical care when it was needed?

Have you more than once run out of money for food for your family because you had spent the food money on yourself or on going out?

‡Did you ever talk to a doctor about any of these things you did like (LIST POSITIVE ANTISOCIAL SYMPTOMS)?

‡Did you do any of these things between the ages of 18 and 25?

‡When is the last time you did any one of these things like (MENTION POSITIVES)?

COGNITIVE IMPAIRMENT

Have you ever had occasion to talk to a doctor about problems with your memory?

Let me ask you a few questions to check your concentration and your memory. Most of them will be easy.

What season of the year is it?

What is the date?

What is the day of the week?

What is the month?

Can you tell me where we are right now? For instance, what state are we in?

What county are we in?

What (city/town) are we in?

    A. What floor of the building are we on?

    B. What is this address (IF INSTITUTIONALIZED: or name of this place)?

I am going to name 3 objects. After I have said them, I want you to repeat them. Remember what they are because I am going to ask you to name them again in a few minutes.

"Apple" "Table" "Penny"

Could you repeat the 3 items for me?

Can you subtract 7 from 100, and then subtract 7 from
the answer you get and keep subtracting 7 until I tell
you to stop?

Now I am going to spell a word forwards and I want you
to spell it backwards. The word is WORLD, W-O-R-L-D.
Spell "WORLD" backwards.

Now what were the 3 objects I asked you to remember?

What is this called? [Watch:]

What is this called? [Pencil:]

I'd like you to repeat a phrase after me: "No if's, and's,
or but's."

Read the words on this page and then do what it says.
(WORDS ARE "CLOSE YOUR EYES")

I am going to give you a piece of paper. When I do,
take the paper in your right hand, fold the paper in
half with both hands, and put the paper down on your
lap.

Write any complete sentence on that piece of paper
for me.

Here's a drawing. Please copy the drawing on the
same paper.

Index of Cited Authors

427

Index of Subjects

NOTE: For specific information on prevalence rates of disorders and on demographic correlates, refer to the following main entries: Age; Race/ethnicity; Rural–urban residence; Sex; Site(s)